AI-driven Healthcare Innovations

AI-driven Healthcare Innovations

Applications in Neurology and Medicine

Edited by

Abhishek Kumar
Priya Batta
J.P. Ananth

iSTE

WILEY

First published 2026 in Great Britain and the United States by ISTE Ltd and John Wiley & Sons, Inc.

ISTE Ltd
27-37 St George's Road
London SW19 4EU
UK

www.iste.co.uk

John Wiley & Sons, Inc.
111 River Street
Hoboken, NJ 07030
USA

www.wiley.com

Library of Congress Control Number: 2026933820

British Library Cataloguing-in-Publication Data
A CIP record for this book is available from the British Library
ISBN 978-1-83669-096-2

The manufacturer's authorized representative according to the EU General Product Safety Regulation is Wiley-VCH GmbH, Boschstr. 12, 69469 Weinheim, Germany, e-mail: Product_Safety@wiley.com.

Contents

Preface

AI-driven Healthcare Innovations: Applications in Neurology and Medicine is conceived to provide a comprehensive and structured understanding of how intelligent computational techniques are reshaping neurological and medical practice. This book integrates fundamental artificial intelligence (AI) concepts with advanced methods such as machine learning (ML), deep learning (DL) and data-driven optimization, highlighting their practical relevance in real clinical settings. Special emphasis is placed on neurological disorders, medical imaging, predictive modeling and personalized care.

In addition, the book discusses data quality, model interpretability, ethical considerations and regulatory challenges essential for responsible adoption. Designed for researchers, clinicians, graduate students and industry professionals, this book aims to bridge the gap between theory and practice and to support the development of robust, trustworthy and patient-centric AI-enabled healthcare solutions.

February 2026

Preface written by Abhishek KUMAR, Priya BATTA and J.P. ANANTH.

1

Artificial Intelligence in Healthcare: Principles, Paradigms and Emerging Trends

Artificial Intelligence (AI) is an emergent revolution in the sphere of contemporary healthcare, and it is producing unique ways to enhance clinical decision-making, diagnostics, treatment planning and patient outcomes. The field of AI is based on computational intelligence and comprises machine learning (ML), deep learning (DL), natural language processing (NLP) and computer vision; these technologies have transformed the way medical data is being processed and interpreted. The introduction of AI into healthcare ecosystems has triggered heightened achievements in the field of predictive analytics, precision medicine, drug discovery, imaging analysis and patient tracking. Digital health products and services using AI have increased the accessibility and efficiency of healthcare, such as cloud-based assistants, wearable devices and telemedicine applications. However, there are issues with the rapid adoption of AI in healthcare: data privacy, the bias of algorithms, interpretability of the model, regulation policies and the necessity of clinical validation. Addressing these obstacles requires interdisciplinary collaboration, ethical governance and the apparent integration of AI into clinical processes. Future trends such as explainable AI, federated learning, multimodal data integration, and blockchain-based healthcare systems are driving the development of more reliable, secure, and scalable AI applications.

This chapter will explore the general principles of AI, paradigms of its application in healthcare and the recent developments that define the profession. This chapter is also a synthesis of the existing literature and innovations and a valuable resource in providing an overview of the way AI is transforming healthcare practices, as well as valuable (and not so valuable) insights into its opportunities and shortcomings. Lastly, this chapter investigates future perspectives that may make AI one of the foundations of the next generation of healthcare systems.

Chapter written by Shilpa C. PATIL and Salim Allauddin CHAVAN.

1.1. Introduction

The use of Artificial Intelligence (AI) is now one of the most prominent 21st-century technologies, particularly in healthcare. This industry generates huge volumes of various data, including medical imaging, electronic health records (EHRs), genomic data, clinical trial outcomes and patient-reported outcomes. The management of this data has posed significant challenges for clinicians due to its vast volume, diversity, and complexity. Now, AI, which can study large datasets and identify the obscure patterns that a person might overlook, can create novel opportunities regarding better clinical decision-making, simplifying the work process and personalizing care to a specific patient (Topol 2019).

1.1.1. *History of AI in healthcare*

We can trace AI, in the domain of healthcare, to the rule-based expert systems of the 1970s and 1980s, including MYCIN and INTERNIST-I. Such rudimentary tools assisted physicians in diagnosing ailments but they were hindered by being inflexible and unscalable. The development of machine learning (ML) and deep learning (DL) made AI a model of dynamic learning that receives complex medical data instead of a set of statistic rules. This development has resulted in the application of AI in numerous fields, including the analysis of medical images or the identification of drugs and real-time patient monitoring (Yu et al. 2018).

Healthcare is becoming progressively more data-oriented, and AI is introducing precision medicine, predictive analytics and care in real time to the stage. AI models can accurately identify malignant masses in medical images, predict the progression of chronic conditions, and discover new treatment targets with remarkable precision. Meanwhile, telemedicine assisted by AI, chatbots and wearables makes care more accessible, particularly to underserved communities. These developments indicate that AI helps clinicians in making critical decisions and also enables patients to take the initiative in managing their health (Rajpurkar et al. 2022).

Still, the introduction of AI in healthcare does introduce issues. Algorithms may be biased and challenging to interpret as well as pose privacy and regulative issues. Also, the implementation of AI in the clinical workflow necessitates the alignment of technology, ethics and policy. However, it must be noted that although AI has enormous potential, we should pay close attention to its boundaries.

This chapter discusses the basics of AI, the ways in which it can be implemented in healthcare and the new tendencies that are predetermining its future. It presents the ways AI is transforming medical practice by entwining its diagnostic, therapeutic and preventive innovations. It also looks at both the ethical and practical dilemmas associated with AI integration, providing recommendations on how it can be used responsibly in medicine.

1.2. Principles of AI in healthcare

1.2.1. *Foundational concepts*

Healthcare organizations can use AI to analyze and interpret medical records to assist in clinical decision-making and prioritize tasks through algorithms that replicate human intelligence. The further subfields of AI are machine learning (ML), deep learning (DL), natural language processing (NLP) and computer vision. These methods enable systems to process large, multipolar health information: structured numeric, unstructured clinical and multidimensional images (Fan et al. 2023).

Modern medical AI is based on ML. Algorithms can gain knowledge and creatively identify trends based on previous data to make predictions. One type of ML is DL; this learns the complex nonlinear relationship using neural networks consisting of multiple layers. This renders DL particularly appropriate with medical imaging and genomics. NLP allows computers to make sense of unstructured text, which is vital in the analysis of physician notes, radiology record and EHR (Electronic Health Records). Computer vision allows automatic insight of pictures in the form of X-rays, MRIs and CT scans.

Such AI concepts have facilitated the transformational health applications. As an example, radiologists can be beaten by DL algorithms regarding the detection of lung nodules on the CT of a chest scanner (Esteva et al. 2019). Long EHRs can be condensed into useful information using NLP systems. With the increase in the volume of healthcare data, AI is able to convert raw data into clinically sound knowledge.

1.2.2. *Core AI methodologies*

Healthcare AI has numerous ways of processing and interpreting data. The most commonly used type is supervised learning, which is trained on labeled data to predict an outcome such as disease classification or a therapeutic effect. Unsupervised learning identifies latent structures in unlabeled data, which can be used in grouping a patient or biomarker discovery. Existence reinforcement learning (RL) is less widespread but thankfully, in selecting the treatment strategy, there is potential to optimize choices by using a sequence of decisions and feedback (Chen and Asch 2017).

Advanced medical AI is based on DL architectures. CNNs are effective in image diagnostics, radiology, dermatology and pathology. Transformers and recurrent neural networks (RNNs) are sequential data models, or networks that process a sequence of data (e.g. a clinical time series). AI systems can be scaled using cloud computing and infrastructure based on big data to handle terabytes of imaging data and huge EHR datasets (Kaul et al. 2020).

These technologies could potentially lead to innovations: specialized AI-based tools in early cancer detection, cardiovascular outcome prediction and custom therapy with the use of genomics. Integrative solutions, such as CNNs with NLP, are becoming more popular as a way of trying to conduct diverse evaluation of a patient.

AI technique	Core function	Healthcare application	Example use case
Machine learning (ML)	Learns patterns from data to make predictions or classifications	Predictive analytics, disease diagnosis, patient risk scoring	Predicting hospital readmission rates using EHR data
Deep learning (DL)	Processes complex data through neural networks with multiple layers	Medical imaging, genomics and signal analysis	Identifying lung nodules in chest CT scans
Natural language processing (NLP)	Extracts meaning from unstructured text	Clinical documentation, EHR analysis and patient feedback	Detecting adverse drug reactions from physician notes
Computer vision	Analyzes and interprets medical images	Radiology, pathology, dermatology	Detecting melanoma or breast cancer lesions
Reinforcement learning (RL)	Learns optimal actions based on feedback loops	Treatment optimization, robotic surgery	Adjusting chemotherapy dosage in oncology care
Federated learning (FL)	Trains models collaboratively without data sharing	Multi-institutional research, privacy-preserving model building	Cross-hospital prediction of chronic disease outcomes
Generative AI (GANs/LLMs)	Synthesizes new data or content	Synthetic data creation, drug discovery, clinical note generation	Creating virtual MRIs for model training

Table 1.1. *Overview of key AI techniques and their applications in healthcare*

1.2.3. *Ethical and philosophical principles*

In addition to technology, AI in healthcare is informed by principles of responsible use that are regulated by ethics and philosophy. They need transparency and interpretability; the AI recommendations should be trusted by the clinicians and the patients. Non-explainable black box models are likely to undermine confidence, particularly when making high-stakes decisions such as cancer diagnosis or surgical planning.

Equity is important and fairness is essential. Bias arising from unrepresentative training data can further marginalize minority groups and exacerbate existing disparities. Ethical AI models promote the use of non-discriminatory datasets and support fair and equitable model development (Amann et al. 2020).

The concept of accountability proves that human practitioners will be accountable for the clinical outcomes, even in cases of AI assistance. AI should not be seen as the replacement. This is based on data privacy and consent as medical data is highly sensitive. Regulations such as GDPR and HIPAA assist in safeguarding the information of patients without hindering AI innovation.

1.3. Paradigms of AI in healthcare

1.3.1. *Diagnostic paradigms*

The most detectable area of AI use is the field of diagnostics, which assists physicians in their interpretation of complicated medical results. The majority of AI applications are motivated by medical imaging. The state-of-the-art deep-learning-based models, such as convolutional neural networks, have compared or surpassed expert radiologists in identifying pneumonia in chest X-rays, cancerous tumors in mammograms and brain lesions in MRIs (McKinney et al. 2020). Such systems increase precision, eliminate variations in readers and reduce the report speed.

Other than imaging, AI also finds application in pathology. Digital pathology systems use computer vision on tissue slides and help in the grading of cancer, the classification of the tissue and the measurement of biomarkers. AI skin-lesion classifiers are also useful in dermatology to assist in the early diagnosis of melanoma, especially in primary care or telemedicine where a dermatologist might not be readily available (Tschandl et al. 2020).

NLP goes beyond diagnostics by extracting meaningful information, even when no predefined structure exists, enabling effective analysis of unstructured data such as EHRs, discharge summaries, and handwritten clinical notes. NLP, powered with AI, identifies comorbidities, notifies about adverse drug reactions and automatic coding of billing. Indicatively, NLP is capable of identifying a high risk of sepsis patients by searching through notes, lab results and vital signs (Rumshisky et al. 2016).

Usually, these diagnostic strategies demonstrate that AI is a decision-support tool and not a replacement of human judgment. However, the wide clinical use requires rigorous validation, high transparency of the model and lack of integration complexity into the existing workflow.

1.3.2. *Therapeutic paradigms*

Treatment, in particular, personalized medicine, drug discovery and robotic surgery can also be affected by AI. Personalized medicine is based on AI that works to customize the plans to the user based on their genes, habits and history. ML algorithms are used to forecast the way cancer patients will react to the treatment, assisting oncologists in selecting the most efficient chemotherapy. In the field of cardiology, AI optimizes the amount of anticoagulant used, reducing the number of adverse events (Krittanawong et al. 2019).

AI has altered drug discovery. The conventional development is time consuming and expensive. AI accelerates this by identifying new targets, drug compounds with interactions and repurposing. In the case of Covid-19, AI has screened vast libraries of chemicals to discover anti-viral hits. Drug manufacturers today incorporate AI at all levels, including molecule structure to initial testing to save money and time (Vamathevan et al. 2019).

Robot surgery is also useful. The AI technology in modern robots focuses on the sharpening of precision, dexterity and safety. AI gives guidance and controllability on the fly, allowing the surgeons to conduct a minimally invasive surgery with fewer complications.

AI, together with augmented reality and the use of computer vision, provides more anatomical views to surgeons, which enhances patient outcomes (Shademan et al. 2016).

These treatment cases demonstrate that AI does not just improve decision-making, but actually defines the type of intervention, which is safer, more efficient and different from each patient.

1.3.3. *Preventive and predictive paradigms*

Preventive care deals with early detection and proactive management of diseases, and AI is instrumental in this. Predictive analytics are able to predict the possibility of developing a disease based on long-term data, lifestyle and genetic information. The likelihood of type 2 diabetes, heart disease or some types of cancer is evaluated using the models, and clinicians can act early using lifestyle change or preventive medications.

On the other hand, wearable and remote monitoring introduce preventive care for day-to-day life. Smartwatches with AI can detect arrhythmias, oxygen and sleep. These devices enable patients to be in control of their health as well as providing physicians with real-time and continuous data, which would be used to act in time (Beam and Kohane 2018). AI-based mobile applications analyze patient information by proposing lifestyle modifications, drug usage and evaluations.

In greater magnitude, AI enhances the health of people and tracks outbreaks. The AI-enhanced models consider mobility, climate and social media to predict the spread of the disease. During the Covid-19 pandemic, AI was being used to track the spread, direct resources and policy-making, and its importance in preparedness cannot be underestimated.

1.4. Emerging trends in AI-driven healthcare

1.4.1. *Explainable AI (XAI) and interpretability*

One of the main problems with healthcare AI is the comprehension of complicated models. DL systems, despite their high power, are black box and do not give clinicians any clue regarding the manner in which the predictions are made. Such a cloud of uncertainty has the potential to destroy credibility and inhibit uptake in such life-or-death areas as oncology and the heart. The explainable AI (XAI) addresses this by developing procedures that reveal the decision-making process, and this renders it more transparent, interpretable and responsible (Holzinger et al. 2020).

Detection of features steering the predictions is aided by such methods as saliency maps, attention layers and SHAP (Shapley Additive Explanations). This can be applied in radiology, such as with a saliency map that reveals to the physician which areas of a CT scan of the chest would lead to an AI prediction of lung cancer. The interpretability is also emphasized as XAI argues that the role of AI must be embedded into everyday clinical work, and AI is not the threat to physicians.

XAI could become the focus of clinical AI due to the increased demand of transparency by regulators. The integration of XAI is ethical and increases the inclination between clinicians and patients.

1.4.2. *Federated and privacy-preserving learning*

The first challenge to AI in healthcare is privacy, since information on patients is delicate and regulated by a strict policy. Training orthodox AI models is required to use centrally assembled data. Federated learning (FL) alters this by enabling institutions to create a common model in a decentralized manner by merely sharing updates to the model and not raw data (Rieke et al. 2020).

In FL, hospitals and research centers collaborate with each other by sharing the model parameters and maintaining their own data locally. This ensures data safety and the ability to create powerful AI models, which are trained using a variety of multi-institutional data. Examples of their application as a form of cross-hospital training are rare-disease training, prediction of chronic conditions and privacy-friendly genomic research.

Privacy-preserving mechanisms such as diffusion privacy and homomorphic cryptography are frequently used with FL to greatly ensure the privacy of sensitive information. Such approaches are becoming more popular because healthcare facilities have discovered the necessity of secure and yet collaborative AI.

1.4.3. *Multimodal and hybrid AI models*

Various sources, such as imaging, genomics, labs, clinical notes and wearables, are used as sources of healthcare data. Classic AI usually runs on a single type, which may be an incorrect representation. Multimodal AI models are new models that combine these sources to create a more complex patient portrait and better predictions (Xu et al. 2021).

As an example, hybrid imaging and EHR models are more accurate in predicting heart attacks and cancer than single-modal systems. Integrating genomics and histopathology extends precision oncology further with the identification of tumor subtypes and the directing of personalized therapy. There is a growing use of hybrid designs which combine CNNs (images), transformers (text) and graph neural networks (molecular data) in order to enhance the advantages of each modality.

The multimodal approach is a significant step toward precision health, allowing clinicians to provide care to an individual patient with greater precision.

1.4.4. *Blockchain and AI synergies*

Integration of blockchain and AI to offer safe and decentralized healthcare is an emerging trend. Blockchain provides retrieval of records that are not mutable or manipulable; it is open and transparent, which is necessary in securing sensitive records. Combined with AI, it helps to share data safely, provides audit trails and provides more confidence regarding medical decisions (Agbo et al. 2019).

Blockchain systems provide patients with the ability to choose who accesses their files, and AI can use the aggregated information to make predictions. Sklearn deals with insurance claim handling, managing trials and consent tracking, all by automatically using smart contracts on the network. Blockchain also ensures the integrity and origin of the data pumped into AI and reduces the risk of manipulation and bias.

Combined, AI and blockchain can address the major issues, namely, interoperability, trust and governance, which makes it a prospective area of healthcare innovation in the future.

1.4.5. *Generative AI in healthcare*

This area of generative AI (also known as GANs and large language models (LLMs)) is attracting rapid interest in health. One important application is the generation of artificial medical data to solve the limited labeled datasets. GANs can produce training images, such as chest X-rays or MRIs, that are similar to real ones (Frid-Adar et al. 2018). This enhances the quality of models and reduces the concerns of privacy as fewer real patients are used.

In other applications, there are virtual patient simulations, in which generative models are created to simulate synthetic scenarios to train and research. Generative AI is another area that designs custom drugs, with the creation of molecules that possess target characteristics (Zhavoronkov et al. 2019). In the meantime, LLC is finding applications in clinical note tuning, medical question answering and patient interaction.

Nevertheless, there are issues to overcome, such as chances of generating incorrect or inaccurate artificial data. The application of generative AI in healthcare requires ethical guidelines and powerful validation measures in order to be incorporated safely (Hayat and Aramvith 2024).

1.5. Challenges and limitations

AI has the potential to be of transformational advantage in the healthcare sector; however, the problems impeding its extensive implementation include technical barriers, ethical challenges and systemic barriers. These should be addressed in order to make use of them responsibly and fairly.

1.5.1. *Bearing data quality and interoperability*

AI models are dependent on the quality, quantity and representativeness of training. Healthcare data takes up a decent portion of space in various systems, is not in a standard algorithm and often lacks completeness or accuracy. This heterogeneity complicates integration and also lowers the reliability of the models (Liu 2018). To take an example, information regarding a single hospital trained into an AI model will not be generalizable to all other populations due to the demographic, method of diagnosis or even equipment differences.

Another barrier is interoperability of the EHR systems. Numerous hospitals use proprietary formats, and it is therefore difficult to generate unified datasets. The presence of AI insights within clinical settings will not increase clinical utility without solid interoperability frameworks.

1.5.2. *Algorithmic bias and fairness*

There is a risk that AI systems may unintentionally strengthen and enlarge the already existing healthcare disparities. In most cases, biases are as a result of non-representative records, where the minority groups are not represented well. As a result, predictive models could provide less precise results on marginalized groups, which results in unfair care (Seyyed-Kalantari et al. 2021).

As an example, algorithms created based mostly on the data made in high-income nations will not be able to measure the risks of the diseases properly in low-resource conditions. Similarly, dermatological models that are trained on the light skin might not work well with the dark skin. The ways of addressing the problem of algorithmic bias include differentiating data, equity-driven training and continuous auditing of deployed systems.

1.5.3. *Regulatory/legal challenges*

AI regulation in the medical field is still developing. In contrast to non-evolutionary medical equipment, AI systems evolve as a result of continuous learning, which increases supervision. The safety approval frameworks applied by agencies such as the U.S. Food and Drug Administration (FDA) and European Medicines Agency (EMA) are progressing and the international harmonization of these approval frameworks is minimal (Benjamens et al. 2020).

Another issue is legal accountability. It is not clear who is liable with regard to the developer, provider or institution, where an AI system provides a wrong recommendation that leads to harm. This ambiguity causes delay in adoption of AI solutions by the stakeholders.

1.5.4. *Clinical validation and barriers to adoption*

Most AI models work in a regulated environment and fail to achieve their objectives in the field. The development and deployment disparity in most of the instances invariably lies in the disparity of data dispensation, combination of workflows and broad acceptance by users (Nagendran et al. 2020).

Clinicians might not be willing to use AI when they cannot comprehend its logic or when its recommendations are inconsistent with their experience.

There are also workflow integration issues which become obstacles to adoption. When an AI system causes clinicians to alter established practice or it introduces administrative responsibilities, its perceived value declines. Successful implementation must be closely aligned with clinical workflows, supported by properly trained clinicians, healthcare staff and AI system operators, and accompanied by continuous monitoring of system performance.

1.5.5. *Cost, scalability and infrastructure*

The creation and implementation of AI systems require a significant amount of computer resources and infrastructure and expertise. HPC processing, storage of data and cybersecurity may prove to be expensive, particularly to health systems that have limited resources. Connecting AI to different environments (including tertiary hospitals and rural clinics) has a high probability of failure due to infrastructure disconnects.

These problems will need sustained effort by policymakers, providers, technologists and patients to solve them. The barriers can only be surmounted through effective implementation of AI in healthcare, which offers fair, efficient and reliable results.

1.6. Future directions

The future of AI in the healthcare sector relies on addressing current restrictions and progressing to combined, ethical, human-oriented applications. There are a number of current opportunities that will transform the integration of AI into health systems.

Precision public health is one of the major trends. In genomic, environmental and behavioral data, AI prediction models are used to determine the risk of diseases in individuals and populations. This allows us to carry out targeted interventions, more effective resource distribution and provide a higher degree of equity through the targeting of strategies according to the vulnerable populations (Khoury et al. 2015).

The next option is the combination of AI with quantum computing. AIs based on quantum computing could help in quickening the drug discovery process, enhancing complicated treatment regimens and handling high-dimensional data that are challenging to compute today (Khoury et al. 2015). Such synergy can reduce pipelines in drug development and enable real-time predictive modeling in critical care.

Future practice will be influenced by the human–AI interaction. Rather than supplanting the clinicians, AI will enhance knowledge. Explainable AI-based decision-support systems allow individuals to verify, interpret and trust recommendations and form a symbiotic relationship between people and machines.

Governments and regulators need to develop complex policy and governance frameworks. The international AI health standards will deal with data regulation, safety and liability (Floridi et al. 2021). Moral standards such as fairness, accountability and transparency will be used to ensure that the advantages of AI will be within the best interest of the patients and therefore reduce the risks.

1.7. Conclusion

AI has rapidly become a theoretical concept and a potent force in healthcare. AI is providing game changers in diagnosis, treatment and prevention through ML, DL, NLP and computer vision technologies. It assists in advanced image analysis, targeted drug research, precog analytics and customized treatment, which demonstrates the potential of transforming healthcare. The latest advances explaining AI, FL, multimodal models and blockchain indicate the rapid rate of change and should therefore lead to safer and more transparent and inclusive systems. Nevertheless, even with such developments, it is not simple to implement

AI into daily clinical practice. The problem of data quality, the absence of interoperability, algorithmic bias, inadequate interpretability and the changing regulations also complicate the process of implementing AI in health systems. Unless such problems are tackled, AI cannot be trusted or used extensively. The gaps in infrastructure and unwillingness of clinicians to use new tools are equally important. It is necessary to find a way to make AI solutions compatible with the current workflows and provide all patient groups with fair access to the technology in order to make it really useful. The future of AI in healthcare will depend on whether it is possible to achieve the correct balance. It will also integrate technical innovations with ethical protection in a balanced set of rules and proactive cooperation between clinicians, engineers and policymakers. Under responsible management and continuous development, AI will become a more comprehensive aspect of healthcare delivery, rather than being merely an assistive resource.

1.8. References

Agbo, C.C., Mahmoud, Q.H., Eklund, J.M. (2019). Blockchain technology in healthcare: A systematic review. *Healthcare*, 7(2), 56.

Amann, J., Blasimme, A., Vayena, E., Frey, D., Madai, V.I., Precise4Q Consortium (2020). Explainability for artificial intelligence in healthcare: A multidisciplinary perspective. *BMC Medical Informatics and Decision Making*, 20(1), 310.

Beam, A.L. and Kohane, I.S. (2018). Big data and machine learning in healthcare. *JAMA*, 319(13), 1317–1318.

Benjamens, S., Dhunnoo, P., Meskó, B. (2020). The state of artificial intelligence-based FDA-approved medical devices and algorithms: An online database. *NPJ Digital Medicine*, 3(1), 118.

Biamonte, J., Wittek, P., Pancotti, N., Rebentrost, P., Wiebe, N., Lloyd, S. (2017). Quantum machine learning. *Nature*, 549(7671), 195–202.

Chen, J.H. and Asch, S.M. (2017). Machine learning and prediction in medicine: Beyond the peak of inflated expectations. *The New England Journal of Medicine*, 376(26), 2507.

Davenport, T. and Kalakota, R. (2019). The potential for artificial intelligence in healthcare. *Future Healthcare Journal*, 6(2), 94–98.

Esteva, A., Robicquet, A., Ramsundar, B., Kuleshov, V., DePristo, M., Chou, K., Cui, C., Corrado, G., Thrun, S., Dean, J. (2019). A guide to deep learning in healthcare. *Nature Medicine*, 25(1), 24–29.

Fan, Y., Song, Z., Zhang, M. (2023). Emerging frontiers of artificial intelligence and machine learning in ischemic stroke: A comprehensive investigation of state-of-the-art methodologies, clinical applications, and unraveling challenges. *EPMA Journal*, 14(4), 645–661.

Floridi, L., Cowls, J., King, T.C., Taddeo, M. (2021). How to design AI for social good: Seven essential factors. In *Ethics, Governance, and Policies in Artificial Intelligence*, Floridi, L. (ed.). Springer, Cham, 125–151.

Frid-Adar, M., Klang, E., Amitai, M., Goldberger, J., Greenspan, H. (2018). Synthetic data augmentation using GAN for improved liver lesion classification. In *2018 IEEE 15th International Symposium on Biomedical Imaging (ISBI 2018)*, 289–293.

Hayat, M. and Aramvith, S. (2024). Transformer's role in brain MRI: A scoping review. *IEEE Access*, 12, 108876–108896.

Holzinger, A., Carrington, A., Müller, H. (2020). Measuring the quality of explanations: The system causability scale (SCS) comparing human and machine explanations. *KI-Künstliche Intelligenz*, 34(2), 193–198.

Kaul, V., Enslin, S., Gross, S.A. (2020). History of artificial intelligence in medicine. *Gastrointestinal Endoscopy*, 92(4), 807–812.

Khoury, M.J., Iademarco, M.F., Riley, W.T. (2015). Precision public health for the era of precision medicine. *American Journal of Preventive Medicine*, 50(3), 398.

Krittanawong, C., Johnson, K.W., Rosenson, R.S., Wang, Z., Aydar, M., Baber, U., Min, J.K., Tang, W.W., Halperin, J.L., Narayan, S.M. (2019). Deep learning for cardiovascular medicine: A practical primer. *European Heart Journal*, 40(25), 2058–2073.

Liu, H.Y. (2018). The power structure of artificial intelligence. *Law, Innovation and Technology*, 10(2), 197–229.

McKinney, S.M., Sieniek, M., Godbole, V., Godwin, J., Antropova, N., Ashrafian, H., Back, T., Chesus, M., Corrado, G.S., Darzi, A. et al. (2020). International evaluation of an AI system for breast cancer screening. *Nature*, 577(7788), 89–94.

Nagendran, M., Chen, Y., Lovejoy, C.A., Gordon, A.C., Komorowski, M., Harvey, H., Topol, E.J., Ioannidis, J.P., Collins, G.S., Maruthappu, M. (2020). Artificial intelligence versus clinicians: Systematic review of design, reporting standards, and claims of deep learning studies. *BMJ*, 368, m689.

Rajpurkar, P., Chen, E., Banerjee, O., Topol, E.J. (2022). AI in health and medicine. *Nature Medicine*, 28(1), 31–38.

Rieke, N., Hancox, J., Li, W., Milletari, F., Roth, H.R., Albarqouni, S., Bakas, S., Galtier, M.N., Landman, B.A., Maier-Hein, K. et al. (2020). The future of digital health with federated learning. *NPJ Digital Medicine*, 3(1), 119.

Rumshisky, A., Ghassemi, M., Naumann, T., Szolovits, P., Castro, V.M., McCoy, T.H., Perlis, R.H. (2016). Predicting early psychiatric readmission with natural language processing of narrative discharge summaries. *Translational Psychiatry*, 6(10), e921.

Seyyed-Kalantari, L., Liu, G., McDermott, M., Chen, I.Y., Ghassemi, M. (2021). CheXclusion: Fairness gaps in deep chest X-ray classifiers. *Pac. Symp. Biocomput.*, 26, 232–243.

Shademan, A., Decker, R.S., Opfermann, J.D., Leonard, S., Krieger, A., Kim, P.C. (2016). Supervised autonomous robotic soft tissue surgery. *Science Translational Medicine*, 8(337), 337ra64.

Topol, E.J. (2019). High-performance medicine: The convergence of human and artificial intelligence. *Nature Medicine*, 25(1), 44–56.

Tschandl, P., Rinner, C., Apalla, Z., Argenziano, G., Codella, N., Halpern, A., Janda, M., Lallas, A., Longo, C., Malvehy, J. et al. (2020). Human–computer collaboration for skin cancer recognition. *Nature Medicine*, 26(8), 1229–1234.

Vamathevan, J., Clark, D., Czodrowski, P., Dunham, I., Ferran, E., Lee, G., Li, B., Madabhushi, A., Shah, P., Spitzer, M. et al. (2019). Applications of machine learning in drug discovery and development. *Nature Reviews Drug Discovery*, 18(6), 463–477.

Xu, J., Glicksberg, B.S., Su, C., Walker, P., Bian, J., Wang, F. (2021). Federated learning for healthcare informatics. *Journal of Healthcare Informatics Research*, 5(1), 1–9.

Yu, K.H., Beam, A.L., Kohane, I.S. (2018). Artificial intelligence in healthcare. *Nature Biomedical Engineering*, 2(10), 719–731.

Zhavoronkov, A., Ivanenkov, Y.A., Aliper, A., Veselov, M.S., Aladinskiy, V.A., Aladinskaya, A.V., Terentiev, V.A., Polykovskiy, D.A., Kuznetsov, M.D., Asadulaev, A. et al. (2019). Deep learning enables rapid identification of potent DDR1 kinase inhibitors. *Nature Biotechnology*, 37(9), 1038–1040.

2

Machine Learning Models for Diagnostic Decision-Making in Neurology

Neurology is a complicated diagnostic task. When making judgments, clinicians make use of their interpretation of symptoms, imaging, electrophysiology and laboratory biomarkers. In recent years, the field of machine learning (ML) has transformed medical diagnostics, increasing the accuracy of the generally performed tasks, speeding them up and contributing to patient-centered care. ML uses large and distinct datasets to identify finer patterns, which could be overlooked by a more traditional approach. This neurology application is where initial and accurate diagnoses are essential in conditions such as Alzheimer disease, Parkinson disease, epilepsy, multiple sclerosis and strokes. Support vector machines and decision trees, as well as ensemble methods, are supervised learning methods, which have demonstrated success with structured clinical data. Convolutional neural networks (CNNs) and recurrent neural networks (RNNs) are deep-learning (DL) architectures that are very useful in interpreting neuroimaging and time-series data on EEG and MEG. Recent developments also incorporate multimodal data, comprising imaging, genetic and clinical data with the view to making holistic decisions. Explainable AI (XAI) approaches are ways to mitigate the interpretation issues to achieve clinician trust in ML-based systems. In spite of this encouraging progress, there exist challenges such as data heterogeneity, algorithm bias, privacy issues and the requirement of achieving large annotated datasets. It takes a joint system, standardized characteristics and regulatory supervision to get over these challenges in order to provide safe and fair clinical implementation.

2.1. Introduction

Neurology is a very broad field that deals with both peripheral and central nervous system disorders. Most of these are characterized by overlapping clinical conditions, which complicates the process of making a diagnosis and in a timely manner. Among the health burdens of the world affecting society are Alzheimer's and Parkinson's diseases, multiple sclerosis, epilepsy and strokes, which not only

Chapter written by Sunil Ramrao YADAV and Kalpana MALPE.

have a great prevalence in the world but also, due to the delayed or wrong diagnosis of the diseases, can have serious social and economic impact on society (Valliani et al. 2019). There are conventional diagnostic tools based on clinical examination, neuroimaging (MRI and CT), electrophysiological (EEG and EMG) and lab biomarkers. Although these tools offer some valuable information, the understanding of the information relies on the professional judgment of the clinicians and interpreters may act differently when confronted with it. This subjectivity may become an obstacle to early diagnosis and formulated treatment plans.

Machine learning (ML) is an artificial intelligence (AI) branch, which provides a novel method of diagnosing decisions in neurology. ML models have the power to find intricate and nonlinear trends on a large body of data, making diagnostic predictions more time-efficient and reliable compared to conventional solutions (Shah and Heiss 2024). They can be trained on a wide range of data sources which include image scans, genetic profiles, clinical notes and electrophysiological signals so that they are able to identify small signs of diseases that would otherwise be invisible to the human eye. Through the use of multimodal data, ML turns out to be a revolutionary tool to use and improve the accuracy of diagnoses and aid clinicians.

The supervised learning algorithms, including the support vector machines (SVMs), decision trees and logistic regression, were used during early applications of ML in neurology. The models proved useful in categorizing patients in terms of diagnostic groups based on organized data, which comprised of demographic and clinical factors (Ramteke and Raut 2025). Even more recent developments in deep learning (DL) have remodeled the world, such that models can directly learn using unstructured data such as MRI images or EEG recordings. Convolutional neural networks (CNNs) are the best at neuroimaging analysis, whereas recurrent neural networks (RNNs) and transformers are used to process sequential signals, including EEG.

Nonetheless, there are still problems with the implementation of ML in clinical practice. In general, diagnostic models frequently have a problem of overfitting to external data as test characteristics, image protocols and imaging settings vary. The black-box nature of most ML models is also a source of concern with interpretability and trust, particularly in a high-stakes area such as neurology (Evangelou et al. 2025). Large-scale adoption has further constraints in the form of ethical concerns, such as favoritism, data privacy and regulatory compliance.

However, studies are underway to develop explainable, generalizable and clinically validated ML systems in neurology. Multimodal integration of imaging, genetic, electrophysiological and clinical data has the potential to construct diagnostic structures in their entirety. Simultaneously, explainable AI (XAI)-related methods are being integrated in order to make the model outputs visible and understandable to a physician, thus increasing trust and acceptance among neurologists.

2.2. Overview of ML in healthcare

The use of ML in the healthcare sector has risen in recent years, largely due to the extensive digital health record, increased computing power and advanced algorithms, which provide an opportunity to process sophisticated, multimodal information. ML automatically identifies genetic patterns in high-dimensional data as opposed to conventional statistical techniques, where we must predetermine certain hypotheses and linear associations. It is also applicable particularly in the field of medicine, where information related to the patient could involve images of the patient, reports, laboratory results, wearable sensor results and even genetic material (Singh et al. 2025).

In its fundamental classification, ML can be distinguished into four categories, namely supervised, unsupervised, semi-supervised and reinforcement learning. The most frequent order of healthcare is supervised learning: labeled data train algorithms to predict or classify results. In one instance, it has been demonstrated that models are capable of handling normal and pathological MRI scans apart or prostitute estimates of disease-progression risk based on patient characteristics. Hidden patterns in original data are discovered through unsupervised learning, which helps in clustering patient subpopulations and identifying novel disease phenotypes. Semi-supervised learning is an amalgamation of the two methods, which uses big, unstructured samples along with smaller labeled samples. Reinforcement learning has been used in the treatment optimization and adaptive clinical decision-making (Usman et al. 2017).

ML is also good at managing large volumes of data generated by the contemporary health systems in diagnostic medicine. Imaging modalities (MRI, fMRI, PET and CT) produce huge data (high-resolution data) which cannot be easily interpreted by human operators. EEG and MEG are examples of electrophysiological signals that generate continuous temporal data, which need complex approaches to identify clinically significant patterns. ML models eliminate non-useful features, find useful features and also discover correlations that are not obvious.

Precision medicine is a field where ML has changed healthcare by providing a transformative effect. Conventional diagnosis and treatment can be based on a one-size-fits-all approach, which may not be optimal due to the heterogeneity of the diseases and differences in response to treatment. ML combines patient unique data, such as genomic, imagining and behavioral data to produce diagnostic and treatment suggestions. In neurology, timely diagnosis of diseases, including Alzheimer's or

Parkinsons, may significantly affect the results, and the accuracy of decisions made with the help of AI may be highly relevant (Deik 2025).

2.3. Supervised learning models in neurological diagnosis

Supervised learning has become the most broadly used field of ML in medical diagnostics. It is based on labeled data and can be interpreted, which can be useful in a clinical practice. In supervised learning, we can assume algorithms are being trained on a set of data in which the values of both the input and the actual result (output) are known. The model is then able to categorize new patient data after training into diagnostic categories or forecast disease outcomes. This method, in particular, has proven to be convenient in the neurological field where, in many instances, the complexity of the disorder and the variability of presentation demand structured deductions and diagnostic assistance (Keerthika and Lal 2023).

2.3.1. *SVMs*

SVMs are knowledge discovery tools such as other ML technologies, which use the information provided by the user to predict and prevent cyberattacks.

SVMs are widely applied in the classification of neurology. Their advantage is that they can deal with high-dimensional data and optimum hyperplanes between diagnostic categories. An example is when SVMs are used to distinguish between patients with Alzheimer's disease, mild cognitive impairment and healthy controls using structural MRI and PET data. These models identify slight morphological variations which may not be evident to the human eye. Thus, early identification is attained. Similarly, SVMs trained on EEG data have performed well at detecting seizures and non-seizures in epilepsy research and thus aid in the real-time monitoring task (Guido et al. 2024).

2.3.2. *Decision trees and random forests*

Decision trees provide more interpretable methods of approach. They are hierarchical in their structure, which is similar to the stepwise decision-making process well known to clinicians. They can be applied in the field of neurology with diagnostic triaging. Basic factors such as age, duration of symptoms and marking of the images may be correlated to raise probable diagnoses. Single decision trees can, however, overfit. Ensemble approaches such as random forests have been used to overcome this drawback. The random forests are a combination of different decision trees, making them robust and generalized. Parkinson's disease has used these models in diagnosing the disease. There is a combination of clinical variables, gait metrics and imaging features, which bring a high level of diagnostic accuracy (Abalde-Cela 2022).

2.3.3. *Logistic regression and linear models*

Logistic regression has commonly been described as a statistical approach but it is actually a supervised learning approach in the field of neurology. It is highly interpretable and does not need a lot of data; hence, it is suitable for small datasets. The model has already been found to be helpful in forecasting the risk of having a stroke based on the vascular risk factors and laboratory outcome. Logistic regression that combines lesion load and demographic variables in multiple sclerosis can be used with a view to predicting the disease's progression probability, in order to assist in prognosis. Logistic regression is not as complex as other ML methods, but it provides helpful baselines to compare with more advanced ones.

2.3.4. *Neural network-based supervised models*

Neurology neural networks with a single or two hidden layers were used as supervised models before the domination of DL. They come in particular handy when it comes to categorizing structured clinical data, such as genetic variants that result in rare neurological conditions. They have also been used to monitor signal classification, including EEG sleep-state determination. Even though DL networks are now superior to them, shallow networks are valuable since they use less computation and are simpler to interpret (Wang 2025).

2.4. Unsupervised and semi-supervised approaches

Although supervised learning characterized early ML usage in neurology, researchers have been motivated by the unavailability of high-quality labeled data to unsupervised and semi-supervised methods. Neurological datasets, especially neuroimaging and electrophysiological data, are vast in scale and highly complex. However, in order to obtain an accurate diagnostic label, we need specific expertise, thus restricting the number of labeled cohorts.

This gap is filled in unsupervised and semi-supervised learning. These datasets allow unlabeled or even partially labeled data to be learnt by algorithms, which means a lot of potential in neurology studies and clinical practice (Wang et al. 2020).

2.4.1. *Unsupervised learning in neurological diagnostics*

The unsupervised models involve the discovery of concealed patterns or unlabeled patterns in data. They particularly possess strong capabilities of clustering, dimensionality reductions and detection of anomalies. In the field of neurology, such techniques are used to find out disease subtypes and characterize various patients:

– *Clustering techniques*: k-means, hierarchical clustering and Gaussian mixture model algorithms can be used to cluster patients with Alzheimer's disease into groups characterized by clear progression patterns. This stratification allows us to conduct specific therapies and gain insight on heterogeneity of disease. The clustering of Parkinson's disease presents subtypes of the disease in relation to motor and nonmotor symptoms, which advocates precision medicine.

– *Dimensionality reduction*: neural imaging or EEG data in high dimensions are reduced, such as PCA, t-SNE and autoencoders, but without losing clinical-relevant features. Indicatively, dimensional reduction of resting-state fMRI data has been used to discover connectivity biomarkers of schizophrenia and epilepsy.

– *Detection of anomalies*: under infrequent neurological conditions, unsupervised algorithms identify abnormal patterns of imaging or signals that do not produce the normative data and which help to identify unusual presentations at an early stage.

2.4.2. *Semi-supervised learning in neurology*

Semi-supervised learning will be between supervised and unsupervised, which involves both block and unblocked databases. In particular, this is essential in neurology, where a large volume of uncoded imaging or EEG data is available but very little annotated.

Through exploitation of the form of unlabeled data, semi-supervised models enhance the classification and reduce expensive manual labeling.

Recent works have used semi-supervised learning to detect epilepsy, in which labeled seizure events are few in number. Models that had been trained on small annotated EEG sections and unlabeled data also achieved the same performance as fully supervised models but with much lower numbers of expert-labeled samples. Similarly, semi-supervised models forecast lesion segmentation on MRI scans, in multiple sclerosis, with a reduction of annotation requirements by a dramatic factor.

2.4.3. *Advantages in neurology*

The major advantages of unsupervised and semi-supervised methods lie in their ability to handle data scarcity, heterogeneity and hidden disease variability. They can:

– *Discover subtypes*: clustering helps identify patient subgroups that may respond differently to treatments.

– *Reduce labeling burden*: semi-supervised learning minimizes reliance on expert annotation, making large-scale applications feasible.

– *Improve generalizability*: by leveraging both labeled and unlabeled data, these models adapt better to new patient cohorts and external datasets.

– *Support biomarker discovery*: dimensionality reduction reveals latent features that may serve as novel diagnostic biomarkers.

2.4.4. *Limitations and challenges*

Also, although they promise a lot, unsupervised and semi-supervised models have a number of weaknesses. Often, clustering depends on the algorithm and parameters that are used and may lead to groupings that are clinically invalid. Stepwise dimensionality reduction may as well be eliminated of its important features unless it is carefully set. Although semi-supervised models do not need a large number of annotations, they nevertheless need a certain number of labeled data to produce clinically meaningful results. Also, interpretation of clusters or latent features is not easy, as their biological sense is not evident without proper validation (Hu et al. 2023).

2.4.5. *Emerging trends*

The latest development incorporates unsupervised and semi-supervised approaches with DL. Variational autoencoders (VAEs) and generative adversarial networks (GANs) provide brain imaging data with a model that is used to generate synthetic samples to scale small datasets. The GANs are used to produce synthetic seizure events in epilepsy research, enhancing the power of classifiers. Self-supervised learning is a strategy that has also proved to be promising, and this strategy bears close relation with the semi-supervised techniques. Through pretext training, where predicting MRI slices which are not needed or repairing damaged EEG signals are used, the model learns practical representations with no explicit labels. Diagnostic tasks may then be performed with only slightly annotated data on the fine-tuning of the representations (Asan and Ercan 2012).

2.5. DL for neuroimaging and signal analysis

Neurology has witnessed the availability of DL as one of the most revolutionizing branches of ML. The reason why it is useful is its unmatched capacity to analyze high-dimensional, complex data, including neuroimaging scans and electrophysiological measures. In contrast to the traditional supervised learning that uses hand-crafted features, the learning process of DL models depends on the raw data directly producing the hierarchical representations. The automatic feature extraction is particularly effective in diagnosing subtle structural/temporal changes that clinicians would fail to detect (Khan et al. 2024).

2.5.1. *CNNs on neuroimaging*

CNNs are the most frequent neuroimaging DL models. They are built with convolutional filters and pooling layers to learn spatial levels in images. CNNs have been effective in diagnosing multiple sclerosis and MRI and PET scans for Alzheimer's and Parkinson's diseases.

Indicatively, CNNs that have been trained on structural MRI are capable of sensing hippocampal atrophy in patients with Alzheimer's disease with high sensitivity, and are hence able to detect early onset. Patients living with Parkinson's disease can also be classified using CNN-based pipelines that indicate the microstructural alteration in the substantia nigra.

Functional MRI (fMRI) is another structural imaging type that can be analyzed using CNNs to map patterns of brain connectivity. They are able to identify disrupted functional suitability of rest without causing disturbances in the rest-state functional connectivity, which are indicators of epilepsy and schizophrenia. CNNs have been used to label lesions in multiple sclerosis automatically and reduce the workload, yet provide reliable and reproducible outcomes (Kim et al. 2022).

2.5.2. *RNNs and time-varying data*

Sequential data, for example, EEG or MEG signals, are frequently used in neurological diagnostics. RNNs, with a particular focus on long short-term memory (LSTM) networks and also gated recurrent units (GRUs), are particularly useful in capturing the temporal dynamics of these signals.

In epilepsy research, RNNs trained in EEG recordings have been used to detect seizure onset with high temporal precision, enabling real-time monitoring systems for patients. Similarly, in sleep medicine, LSTMs classify sleep stages from EEG data, aiding the diagnosis of sleep-related neurological disorders.

2.5.3. *Transformer architectures in neurology*

Transformer models, which were created to work with natural language processing (NLP), have recently been used in studies of the brain. Their attention systems assist them to establish long-range associations of both spatial and temporal information. Vision transformers (ViTs) are effective with MRI classification applications, whereas time-series transformers are used to analyze EEG and MEG data. For example, transformers that are trained on EEG data outperform the traditional RNNs in identifying seizures, which is an indication that they are able to identify global patterns in time (Singh and Malhotra 2023).

2.5.4. *Multimodal DL*

One of the strongest points of DL is the possibility to unite the information of several sources. Neurological diseases can hardly be characterized by a single biomarker, but rather a combination of imaging, electrophysiology, clinical history and genetic information. Multimodal DL models are based on CNNs to work with images and RNNs or transformers to work with time bases, which provide a complete diagnostic view. In the example of Alzheimer's disease, MRI, PET and cognitive test networks outperform single amounts of modal in giving more accurate predictions of the disease's progress.

2.5.5. *Explainability in DL models*

Although they are successful, DL models are still struggling with interpretability. Neurologists require clear charts underlining the rationale that creates the recommendation of a specific diagnosis. Saliency maps, Grad-CAM and layer-wise relevance propagation are examples of techniques that have been introduced to CNN-based neuroimaging pipelines. These methods help to bring out the brain areas that tend to affect the decisions made most in the course of diagnosis. Similarly, weights of the attention in transformer models reflect the EEG segments that are essential in the classification of the seizures. Although these tools enhance trust, using explainable DL in clinical workflows continues to be a priority in research undertakings (Gombolay et al. 2024). Table 2.1 shows a summary of ML techniques and their applications in neurological diagnostics.

ML technique	Learning type	Primary data used	Neurological application	Example outcome/ use case
SVMs	Supervised	MRI, PET, EEG	Classification of Alzheimer's disease, seizure detection in epilepsy	Distinguishes Alzheimer's disease, mild cognitive impairment and healthy controls
Decision trees/random forests	Supervised (ensemble)	Clinical, gait, imaging	Parkinson's disease, stroke prediction	Combines clinical and imaging features to improve diagnostic accuracy
Logistic regression	Supervised	Demographic and lab data	Stroke and multiple sclerosis risk modeling	Estimates probability of disease progression
RNNs/LSTMs	Deep supervised	EEG, MEG, gait data	Epilepsy and sleep disorder detection	Identifies seizure onset and classifies sleep stages
CNNs	Deep supervised	MRI, PET, CT	Alzheimer's disease, Parkinson's disease, multiple sclerosis	Detects hippocampal atrophy and lesion load
Unsupervised learning (k-means, PCA, autoencoders)	Unsupervised	MRI, fMRI, EEG	Subtype discovery, biomarker identification	Reveals hidden disease subgroups in Alzheimer's and Parkinson's diseases
Semi-supervised learning	Hybrid	Partially labeled EEG/MRI	Epilepsy and multiple sclerosis	Reduces labeling effort while maintaining diagnostic accuracy
Transformer models	Deep supervised	EEG, MRI, clinical sequences	Seizure detection, neuroimaging classification	Captures long-range dependencies for accurate pattern recognition
Multimodal DL	Integrative	Imaging + clinical + genetic	Alzheimer's disease, strokes, Parkinson's disease	Combines multiple data types for holistic diagnosis
XAI	Interpretability layer	Any of the above	Transparency and clinician trust	Highlights important imaging regions or biomarkers using SHAP or Grad-CAM

Table 2.1. *Summary of ML techniques and their applications in neurological diagnostics*

2.6. Multimodal and integrative diagnostic models

Neurological disorders are multifactorial and complex in nature as they consist of behavioral, structural, functional and genetic alterations. Using only one diagnostic modality such as MRI or EEG provides useful information, but may fail to capture a larger picture of heterogeneity of the disease. To cover these gaps, multimodal and integrative diagnostic models incorporate different types of data, providing a more detailed perspective on the neurological disorders. Recent developments of ML, in particular, DL, have allowed incorporating multimodal data into single frameworks, and the result is more accurate diagnostic decisions (Yan et al. 2023).

2.6.1. *Rationale for multimodal integration*

The human brain is very complicated, and neurological diseases can hardly manifest themselves in one dimension. Take the example of Alzheimer's disease, where structural atrophy, connectivity, amyloid accumulation and cognitive impairment are all present. Epilepsy, on the other hand, has electrophysiological alterations, which do appear on an EEG, and structural alterations, which are observed or present in an MRI. Through the combination of such signals, ML models will be able to detect complementary information, enhancing the accuracy of the diagnosis and its robustness (Dwivedi et al. 2022).

The multimodal integration works best in situations where one modality presents weak or noisy cues. As an example, microstructural alterations in early-on Alzheimer's disease can be detected with relatively covert changes in MRI that are difficult to observe with MRI alone but become more evident with PET imaging and assessment tests. Using a combination of data streams, the ML systems bring into focus the inefficiencies of each modality and provide more credible clinical information.

2.6.2. *Fusion strategies in multimodal ML*

Multimodal ML models typically use one of three fusion strategies:

– *Early fusion*: different modalities, whether raw or preprocessed, are amalgamated and entered into one model. MRI voxel intensities, along with EEG features, can be paired together to classify epilepsy subtypes.

– *Intermediate fusion*: each modality has its features extracted using specialized networks – imaging and CNNs, EEG and RNNs – and then fused at a latent space.

This helps the models to understand the modality features and the advantages of integration.

– *Late fusion*: independent models are trained on each modality, and their outputs are combined (e.g. via weighted averaging or ensemble methods). This strategy is especially useful when modalities vary in availability, ensuring that missing data from one modality does not prevent diagnostic predictions (Stripelis et al. 2024).

2.6.3. *Applications in neurology*

Multimodal ML models have demonstrated strong performance across a range of neurological conditions:

– *Alzheimer's disease and dementia*: models integrating structural MRI, PET and neuropsychological test scores have significantly improved early detection and prediction of disease progression. In some studies, multimodal integration achieved up to 10–15% higher accuracy than unimodal approaches.

– *Epilepsy*: combining EEG with MRI enhances seizure localization by linking electrophysiological abnormalities with structural lesions. Semi-supervised multimodal frameworks also improve generalization in datasets with limited labels.

– *Parkinson's disease*: multimodal models integrating gait metrics, speech recordings and imaging data provide comprehensive diagnostic profiles, enabling differentiation from other movement disorders.

– *Stroke*: combining clinical data (e.g. vascular risk factors, laboratory results) with imaging features improves risk stratification and prediction of recurrent events.

– *Multiple sclerosis*: multimodal ML incorporating MRI lesion load, cerebrospinal fluid biomarkers and patient-reported outcomes supports personalized prognosis and treatment decisions.

2.7. XAI and clinical interpretability

ML has the potential to bring major improvements to neurological diagnostics, but the major challenge to clinical applications is that many models are black box in nature. Predictions produced by DL are commonly not comprehensibly based, which creates distrust in clinicians and constrains confidence in automated decision support systems. The XAI has become the issue of critical research to resolve this issue. It aims to improve the interpretability without compromising the predictive accuracy (Gulum et al. 2021).

2.7.1. *Importance of explainability in neurology*

Neurology has a high level of stakes in decision-making (e.g. identifying a stroke, seizure foci or neurodegenerative conditions). In such situations, clinicians need more accurate predictions, but they also need an explanation of how a model arrived at its decision. As an example, when an ML model identifies an MRI as early Alzheimer's disease, it should show the brain areas that contributed to the result. A lack of interpretability will make the system reluctant to be relied upon by the physicians, particularly when making decisions on treatment or counseling the patients.

2.7.2. *Approaches to XAI*

Several methods have been developed to enhance the interpretability of ML models in neurology:

1. *Feature attribution methods*: techniques such as SHAP (SHapley Additive exPlanations) and LIME (Local Interpretable Model-agnostic Explanations) provide case-specific explanations by assigning importance scores to features. For instance, in EEG-based seizure prediction, SHAP can highlight which temporal or frequency bands were most influential in the model's output (Fellous et al. 2019).

2. *Saliency maps and heatmaps*: in neuroimaging, saliency maps generated from CNNs indicate which voxels or regions most strongly contributed to a classification. For Alzheimer's disease diagnosis, heatmaps may reveal that the hippocampus and posterior cingulate cortex played a key role in distinguishing patients from controls.

3. *Prototype-based learning*: instead of abstract latent features, some models classify new cases based on similarity to prototypical examples in the training data. This provides clinicians with intuitive comparisons that align more closely with diagnostic reasoning.

4. *Rule-based and hybrid systems*: by combining symbolic reasoning with ML predictions, hybrid models generate human-readable decision rules. For example, a hybrid system may output: "the classification is Parkinson's disease because gait variability and substantia nigra hypo intensity exceeded thresholds".

2.7.3. *Clinical applications of XAI in neurology*

Explainable ML has been applied to a variety of neurological diagnostic tasks:

– *Stroke triage*: heatmaps highlighting vascular occlusion regions in CT angiography improve radiologist confidence in automated stroke detection systems.

– *Epilepsy surgery planning*: XAI applied to EEG analysis enables identification of seizure onset zones, with interpretable features supporting surgical decision-making.

– *Dementia diagnostics*: SHAP-based analysis of multimodal models has clarified the relative contribution of cognitive test scores versus imaging biomarkers, guiding personalized treatment recommendations (Alam et al. 2023; Rudroff et al. 2024).

2.8. Future directions in ML for neurological diagnostics

ML is already very promising in neurological diagnoses, yet the sphere continues to be very dynamic. Further progress will solve the current constraints and provide more opportunities to clinical decision-making with accuracy, efficiency and accessibility. There are several overall trends and innovations in the coming generation of applications in the field of neurology (Gerke et al. 2020).

2.8.1. *Federating and cooperative learning*

The issue of data privacy and scarcity can still be considered a threat in neurology. One of the solutions is federated learning, a distributed method in which the models are trained on many institutions without sharing the raw patient data. Federated learning can be used to privately train on a multitude of diverse data by aggregating updates to the model, which maintains privacy. This mode of approach is particularly optimistic in rare neurological diseases where a single institution may not have sufficient cases to learn powerful models (Shang et al. 2024). Joint consortia are also developing, as are standard repositories of neuroimaging, electrophysiology and clinical data. These efforts enable better generalizability of models and increase the reproducibility of the models as well as ease comparisons of new algorithms with people across diverse backgrounds. The book will also use genomic and molecular data to study lymphocytic leukemia (Sandhu et al. 2023).

2.8.2. *Genomic and molecular data*

Genomic and molecular data will also be used in the book to examine lymphocytic leukemia. Disorders of the nervous system tend to have a complicated genetic and molecular cause. The forthcoming ML paradigm will integrate multi-omic data, genomics, transcriptomics, proteomics and metabolomics with imaging and clinical characteristics. As an example, genetic risk scores in combination with MRI-based biomarkers can add to early Alzheimer's disease diagnosis or to prioritize patients to customized treatment in multiple sclerosis. This holistic methodology goes together with precision medicine since it provides customized diagnostic and prognostic data (Li et al. 2025).

2.8.3. *Self-supervised learning and few-shot learning*

The lack of annotated datasets is an issue that has plagued the field of neurology. Self-standardized learning information models are trained on pretext tasks and few-shot learning, in which models can transfer to new class type on minuscule examples. The strategies minimize the need for expert annotations in preventing diagnostic loss of accuracy. They can, among other things, be used in automated EEG classification, MRI lesion detection and identification of rare disorders, which means that ML is more scalable and reachable in the clinical environment (Finzel 2025).

2.9. Conclusion

ML has recently emerged as a revolutionary technology in the field of neurological diagnostics, providing incomparable opportunities to increase accuracy, speed and an individual approach. Supervised, unsupervised, DL and multimodal models demonstrate that ML can identify subtle patterns in imaging, electrophysiological and clinical data, which humans may overlook. More brain disorders including Alzheimer's, Parkinson's, epilepsy, multiple sclerosis and strokes are diagnosed early, stratified and planned using these models to treat. The inclusion of multimodal information and XAI has transformed the reconstructed ML into a more convenient and accurate tool. The saliency maps and SHAP values and prototype-based models allow the physicians to interpret the findings and align the gap between the raw numbers and clinical judgment. In the meantime, new technologies are addressing the issue of scarce-labeled data and privacy through self-supervised and few-shot learning and federated learning, which makes this technology stronger and more scalable. Despite these advantages, there are still several barriers: data standardization, generalizability, workflow fit and regulatory allowance still prove to be challenging, and ethical problems such as patient privacy, bias and accountability should be managed with considerable attention to provide safe and fair usage. In the future, researchers would be able to refine clinically proven, interpretable, adaptable and alignment of ML systems consistent with daily routine medical practice.

2.10. References

Abalde-Cela, S. (2022). Techniques in biomedical applications. In *SERS for Point-of-care and Clinical Applications,* Fales, A. (ed.). Elsevier, Amsterdam.

Alam, M.N., Kaur, M., Kabir, M.S. (2023). Explainable AI in healthcare: Enhancing transparency and trust upon legal and ethical consideration. *International Research Journal of Engineering and Technology*, 10(6), 1–9.

Asan, U. and Ercan, S. (2012). An introduction to self-organizing maps. In *Computational Intelligence Systems in Industrial Engineering: With Recent Theory and Applications,* Kahraman, C. (ed.). Atlantis Press, Paris, 295–315.

Deik, A. (2025). The role of AI in the management of movement disorders. *Seminars in Neurology*.

Dwivedi, S., Goel, T., Tanveer, M., Murugan, R., Sharma, R. (2022). Multimodal fusion-based deep learning network for effective diagnosis of Alzheimer's disease. *IEEE MultiMedia*, 29(2), 45–55.

Evangelou, K., Kotsantis, I., Kalyvas, A., Kyriazoglou, A., Economopoulou, P., Velonakis, G., Gavra, M., Psyrri, A., Boviatsis, E.J., Stavrinou, L.C. (2025). Artificial intelligence in the diagnosis and treatment of brain gliomas. *Biomedicines*, 13(9), 2285.

Fellous, J.M., Sapiro, G., Rossi, A., Mayberg, H., Ferrante, M. (2019). Explainable artificial intelligence for neuroscience: Behavioral neurostimulation. *Frontiers in Neuroscience*, 13, 1346.

Finzel, B. (2025). Current methods in explainable artificial intelligence and future prospects for integrative physiology. *Pflügers Archiv-European Journal of Physiology*, 477, 513–529.

Gerke, S., Minssen, T., Cohen, G. (2020). Ethical and legal challenges of artificial intelligence-driven healthcare. In *Artificial Intelligence in Healthcare,* Bohr, A. and Memarzadeh, K. (eds). Academic Press, San Diego, 295–336.

Gombolay, G.Y., Silva, A., Schrum, M., Gopalan, N., Hallman-Cooper, J., Dutt, M., Gombolay, M. (2024). Effects of explainable artificial intelligence in neurology decision support. *Annals of Clinical and Translational Neurology*, 11(5), 1224–1235.

Guido, R., Ferrisi, S., Lofaro, D., Conforti, D. (2024). An overview on the advancements of support vector machine models in healthcare applications: A review. *Information*, 15(4), 235.

Gulum, M.A., Trombley, C.M., Kantardzic, M. (2021). A review of explainable deep learning cancer detection models in medical imaging. *Applied Sciences*, 11(10), 4573.

Hu, Y., Huang, Z.A., Liu, R., Xue, X., Sun, X., Song, L., Tan, K.C. (2023). Source free semi-supervised transfer learning for diagnosis of mental disorders on fMRI scans. *IEEE Transactions on Pattern Analysis and Machine Intelligence*, 45(11), 13778–13795.

Keerthika, C. and Lal, A.M. (2023). A methodical and performance-based investigation of Alzheimer disease detection on magnetic resonance and multimodal images. *Current Medical Imaging*, 19(6), 546–563.

Khan, A.A., Mahendran, R.K., Perumal, K., Faheem, M. (2024). Dual-3DM 3 AD: Mixed transformer based semantic segmentation and triplet pre-processing for early multi-class Alzheimer's diagnosis. *IEEE Transactions on Neural Systems and Rehabilitation Engineering*, 32, 696–707.

Kim, I., Kang, K., Song, Y., Kim, T.J. (2022). Application of artificial intelligence in pathology: Trends and challenges. *Diagnostics*, 12(11), 2794.

Li, Y., Yang, Y., Chen, Y., Ye, C., Ma, T. (2025). Self-supervised learning to unveil brain dysfunctional signatures in brain disorders: Methods and applications. *Health Data Science*, 5, 0282.

Ramteke, M. and Raut, S. (2025). Enhancing disease diagnosis: Leveraging machine learning algorithms for healthcare data analysis. *IETE Journal of Research*, 71(2), 688–709.

Rudroff, T., Rainio, O., Klén, R. (2024). Leveraging artificial intelligence to optimize transcranial direct current stimulation for long COVID management: A forward-looking perspective. *Brain Sciences*, 14(8), 831.

Sandhu, S.S., Gorji, H.T., Tavakolian, P., Tavakolian, K., Akhbardeh, A. (2023). Medical imaging applications of federated learning. *Diagnostics*, 13(19), 3140.

Shah, S.P. and Heiss, J.D. (2024). Artificial intelligence as a complementary tool for clincal decision-making in stroke and epilepsy. *Brain Sciences*, 14(3), 228.

Shang, Z., Chauhan, V., Devi, K., Patil, S. (2024). Artificial intelligence, the digital surgeon: Unravelling its emerging footprint in healthcare: The narrative review. *Journal of Multidisciplinary Healthcare*, 17, 4011–4022.

Singh, K. and Malhotra, D. (2023). Meta-health: Learning-to-learn (meta-learning) as a next generation of deep learning exploring healthcare challenges and solutions for rare disorders: A systematic analysis. *Archives of Computational Methods in Engineering*, 30(7), 4081–4112.

Singh, M.S., Thongam, K., Choudhary, P., Bhagat, P.K. (2025). Stroke risk prediction and prevention: Traditional versus machine learning approaches. *Archives of Computational Methods in Engineering*, 1–52.

Stripelis, D., Gupta, U., Saleem, H., Dhinagar, N., Ghai, T., Anastasiou, C., Sánchez, R., Ver Steeg, G., Ravi, S., Naveed, M. et al. (2024). A federated learning architecture for secure and private neuroimaging analysis. *Patterns*, 5(8), 101031.

Usman, S.M., Usman, M., Fong, S. (2017). Epileptic seizures prediction using machine learning methods. *Computational and Mathematical Methods in Medicine*, 2017(1), 9074759.

Valliani, A.A., Ranti, D., Oermann, E.K. (2019). Deep learning and neurology: A systematic review. *Neurology and Therapy*, 8(2), 351–365.

Wang, X.J. (2025). *Theoretical Neuroscience: Understanding Cognition.* CRC Press, Boca Raton.

Wang, Y., Zhao, Y., Therneau, T.M., Atkinson, E.J., Tafti, A.P., Zhang, N., Amin, S., Limper, A.H., Khosla, S., Liu, H. (2020). Unsupervised machine learning for the discovery of latent disease clusters and patient subgroups using electronic health records. *Journal of Biomedical Informatics*, 102, 103364.

Yan, K., Li, T., Marques, J.A., Gao, J., Fong, S.J. (2023). A review on multimodal machine learning in medical diagnostics. *Mathematical Biosciences and Engineering*, 20(5), 8708–8726.

3

Deep Learning Approaches to Neuroimaging and Brain Mapping

Deep learning is a recent method that has achieved strong results in neuroimaging and brain mapping. It has made it possible to extract features, recognize patterns and classify diseases. The conventional methods of analysis were based on manual features and statistical models. Although handy, such techniques could not model the complex nonlinear relations in the brain. Deep learning models, including convolutional neural networks (CNNs), recurrent neural networks (RNNs), autoencoders and transformers can currently be applied to structural and functional imaging due to the increased computing power and large neuroimaging datasets available. The models are superior compared to the traditional approaches in activities, such as image segmentation, tissue classification, functional connectivity analysis and prediction of disease. In addition to classification, deep learning is useful in mapping large neural networks, identifying significant structural deviations and multimodal image data fusion. Such features enable the ease of precision medicine through early detection of neurological diseases such as Alzheimer's disease, Parkinson's disease, epilepsy and brain tumor diseases. Even more sophisticated models of brain organization and functioning are provided by integrating deep learning with graph theory and connectomics. Nonetheless, there are still problems such as interpretability of models, heterogeneity of data, reduced extrapolation to the entire population and the dilemma of privacy. Recent studies have been concerned with explainable AI and federated learning, and integrating multi-omics and imaging to enhance reliability and translational influence. Altogether, deep learning promises a lot to the fields of neuroimaging and brain mapping, and bridges the gap between the advancement of computational and clinical neuroscience.

3.1. Introduction

Neuroimaging has been a staple in neuroscience and clinical neurology, allowing visualization of the brain structure, function and connectivity in a detailed way.

Chapter written by G.V. RAMDAS and G.M. VAIDYA.

Structural magnetic resonance imaging (MRI), computed tomography (CT), functional MRI (fMRI), positron emission tomography (PET) and electroencephalography (EEG) are some of the techniques that have enabled the revolution of how the brain functions and what is wrong in illness. Corpus statists have traditionally analyzed these data using statistical models, handcrafted features and hypothesis-based methods. Although such methods have come a long way, they are not able to reveal the high-dimensional, nonlinear and dynamic behavior of the brain. The advent of AI, and specifically deep learning, has introduced extremely effective tools that circumvent these restrictions and enable the discovery of science and clinical translation to become faster (Avberšek and Repovš 2022).

Deep learning is a subdiscipline of machine learning: it entails the construction of layered neural networks, able to automatically extract features out of raw data, avoiding the manual feature engineering required. Neuroimaging has been successfully used with convolutional neural networks (CNNs), recurrent neural networks (RNNs), autoencoders and transformer models. However, structural image analysis is dominated by CNNs since they are able to extract spatial features, whereas RNNs and transformers are promising in time-dependent data, including fMRI or EEG. These models improve the precision of the classification and segmentation processes and show concealed patterns that are not detected by traditional approaches (Mienye et al. 2025).

In structural neuroimaging, deep learning stimulates the development of brain tissue segmentation, lesion detection, tumor classification and the detection of subtle changes in shapes associated with neurodegenerative diseases. The CNN pipelines have a higher ability to differentiate gray matter, white matter and cerebrospinal fluid compared to the atlas-based or intensity-driven variations. Microstructural alterations of diffusion MRI are also revealed by deep learning, and enhance the sensitivity of the mentioned conditions such as multiple sclerosis and traumatic brain injury (Ahamed et al. 2023). These tools enable clinicians to diagnose more cheaply and successfully in time, which results in timely interventions.

Functional neuroimaging has some other opportunities and challenges. fMRI and PET produce high data which capture spatial and temporal dynamics. As traditional statistical models also include the general linear model, they are not always able to represent complex interdependencies. Spatial and temporal, as well as frequency features can be combined by deep learning frameworks, which leads to improving the detection of a functional network, the prediction of cognitive states and the classification of psychiatric or neurological disorders. Deep learning can also be applied in EEG and magnetoencephalography (MEG) to decode brain signals in brain computer interfaces and when sensing seizures (Xu et al. 2023).

On top of personal modalities, deep learning has transformed brain mapping. Brain mapping aims to map structural and functional organization of individuals and collectives, defining large-scale networks and connectomes. In advanced research applications, the integration of graph-based methods with deep learning is increasingly used to uncover complex connectivity patterns that underlie cognition and neurological diseases. Indicatively, structural and functional connectomes are modeled using graph convolutional networks (GCNs), which allow the forecasting of individual personality and clinical outcomes (Mecheter et al. 2020). Deep learning multimodal imaging data makes comprehensive brain representations that span the structural, functional and molecular spaces.

Deep learning in neuroimaging has huge clinical potential. It has been used in early diagnosis of the Alzheimer's and Parkinson's diseases, as well as in individual therapy design in oncology and epilepsy surgery. Automated pipelines can lower the time and experience requirements to manually analyze images, expand their availability and standardize clinical procedures. Besides, explainable AI advances address the black box problem, which assists clinicians with comprehending and trusting model outputs in decision-making (Lambert et al. 2024).

Although these gains are achieved, there are still challenges. The results of neuroimaging obtained with different scanners, locations and groups differ, meaning that it is difficult to assume that trained models would similarly perform on different populations. A strong performance involves the use of large collections of data, which is exactly what hinders the sharing of data due to privacy issues and regulations.

Federated learning and synthetic data generation are some of the ideas that are being investigated to overcome these challenges. Ethical issues such as training data bias, predictive model abuse and patient privacy need to be approached cautiously, as these technologies transition into the regular use of the clinical procedures (Kaissis et al. 2020).

3.2. Deep learning fundamentals for neuroimaging

Deep learning is a subfield of AI, where hierarchical neural architecture networks are applied to handle complex data with high dimensions. Deep learning models have the ability to learn feature representations as opposed to using traditional, machine-based approaches to machine learning, where features are handcrafted or derived through a separate operation on raw input. It is particularly applicable to neuroimaging, where there are large datasets, which are multidimensional and possess complex patterns, which are difficult to describe using traditional statistical methods (Zhang et al. 2020).

Deep learning is based on artificial neural networks. Such networks are made up of networked nodes, or so-called neurons, which are arranged in layers. There is a weight associated with each connection which can be used to determine the extent to which a particular neuron has an impact on another. It is the adjustment of these weights via the back-propagation process that enables the network to learn by adjusting the weights to minimize the loss metric, based on the difference between predictions and the ground truth. The greater the depth of networks, with numerous layers concealed within them, the greater the ability to model nonlinearity and complexity in the relationships in neuroimaging data (Shulman et al. 2024).

3.2.1. *Convolutional neural networks (CNNs)*

CNNs have been the commonly used deep learning structure in neuroimaging. They are, like the human visual cortex, spatial-data analysis optimized. Local spatial features are represented in convolutional layers; dimension reduction is done on pooling layers; classification or regression is done on fully connected layers. CNNs can be used to segment the brain tissues, detect tumors and use volumes to analyze MRI in neuroimaging. They are also very suitable when we have to perform voxel-based classification alongside strong extraction of structural properties due to their capability to deal with three-dimensional data (Isensee et al. 2021).

3.2.2. *Recurrent neural networks (RNNs) and long short-term memory (LSTM)*

In spite of the fact that CNNs are ideal when it comes to spatial information, the RNNs are capable of detecting dependencies in time. The variants are LSTM and GRU, which are sequential and therefore can be used in fMRI and EEG, which are time-varying. The RNN in the context of fMRI corrects and traces dynamic changes in BOLD signals by brain regions, allowing recognition of the functional connection and prediction of mental states. RNNs have demonstrated this in EEG in detecting seizures, sleep stage classification and bridging the brain computer interface (Cisotto et al. 2024).

3.2.3. *Autoencoders and generative models*

Autoencoders reduce data input to low-dimensional latent representation, which is subsequently used to reconstruct the original input. This method can be deployed to reduce dimensions, and in neuroimaging denoising and feature extraction. Variational autoencoders (VAEs) incorporate probabilistic mechanisms, enabling the generation of synthetic data with the ability to recover the statistical characteristics of data. This type of generative model ensures data scarcity in neuroimaging research is reduced. Other uses of generative adversarial networks (GANs) are data augmentation, MRI super-resolution and across-center scan harmonization (Kebaili et al. 2023).

3.2.4. *Transformer architectures*

Regular models have been developed that take the form of transformer-based models originally designed to process natural language, and adapted to medical imaging, including neuroimaging. Transformers have self-attention capabilities that learn long-distance-dependent features among the data points. This provides them with an edge with CNNs and RNNs on complicated spatial and temporal relationships. Transformers may be used in the imaging of the brain to achieve image classifications, lesion localization and multimodal data analysis. Brain mapping and connectomics are gaining growing popularity due to their scalability and ability to model them in global context (Li et al. 2023).

3.2.5. *Training strategies and optimization*

There are a number of difficulties in training deep learning models to do neuroimaging: imbalance between classes, high-dimensionality and small datasets. Data augmentation, transfer learning and pretraining with large non-medical datasets such as ImageNet are the common ones to enhance generalization. This model is better assisted to converge with the aid of optimization algorithms such as Adam or RMSprop. Regularization techniques, including dropout and batch normalization, help prevent overfitting, which is particularly important in neuroimaging due to small sample sizes relative to model complexity (Raghu et al. 2019).

3.2.6. *Interpretability and explainability*

The primary drawback of deep learning in the medical field is that it is a black box. To be used in clinical practice, interpretable results that are trustable by the clinicians need to be provided. Saliency maps, class activation mapping (CAM), and layer-wise relevance propagation (LRP) techniques are used to visualize the data that provides the highest contribution to model predictions of neuroimaging data. Such explainable ways of AI do not only boost transparency, but also provide insights into the underlying neurobiological processes, which may be useful in generating hypotheses in neuroscience studies (Montavon et al. 2018). Table 3.1 shows an overview of deep learning architectures and their neuroimaging applications.

Deep learning model	Core mechanism	Primary neuroimaging modality	Key application area	Example outcome
Convolutional neural networks (CNNs)	Extract spatial features through convolution and pooling layers	MRI, CT	Brain tissue segmentation, tumor detection, morphometric analysis	Improved gray/white matter delineation and early Alzheimer's detection
Recurrent neural networks (RNNs)/LSTMs	Capture temporal dependencies in sequential data	fMRI, EEG	Cognitive state decoding, seizure prediction, dynamic connectivity analysis	Accurate seizure onset prediction using EEG signals
Autoencoders/ variational autoencoders (VAEs)	Encode input data into low-dimensional latent space and reconstruct	MRI, DTI	Denoising, feature extraction, data compression	Enhanced image reconstruction and noise reduction in MRI
Generative adversarial networks (GANs)	Learn generative distribution via generator–discriminator framework	MRI, PET	Image synthesis, super-resolution, modality translation	PET image synthesis from MRI with improved realism
Transformer models	Use self-attention mechanisms for global dependencies	MRI, fMRI, multimodal	Lesion localization, multimodal fusion, functional mapping	Accurate cross-modality representation learning
Graph convolutional networks (GCNs)	Operate on brain graphs and connectivity matrices	DTI, fMRI, Connectomics	Brain network analysis, connectome classification	Classification of mild cognitive impairment using structural connectomes
Multistream/ multimodal CNNs	Integrate multiple imaging modalities simultaneously	MRI + PET + EEG	Multimodal fusion, disease progression prediction	Enhanced accuracy in Alzheimer's progression prediction
Explainable AI (XAI) frameworks	Visualize decision mechanisms via saliency and relevance maps	Any modality	Interpretability and model validation	Highlighting disease-relevant regions for clinician trust

Table 3.1. *Overview of deep learning architectures and their neuroimaging applications*

3.3. Applications in structural neuroimaging (MRI, CT)

Structural neuroimaging provides finer anatomical images of the brain that assist in evaluating the composition of tissues, shapes and changes of diseases. Two of the most common techniques include MRI and CT. Deep learning has delivered a significant contribution in terms of automating the segmentation, classification and detection of anomalies, improving speed, consistency and accuracy due to the outdated approaches (Al-Rahbi et al. 2025).

3.3.1. *Brain tissue segmentation and morphometric analysis*

Automatic tissue segmentation became the first significant structural neuroimaging AI breakthrough of deep learning. Previous techniques were based on the atlases or intensity clustering, and they frequently failed due to individual anatomy or motion, or due to scanners. Current CNNs, and in particular, 3D U-Net architectures, can now segment gray matter, white matter and cerebral fluid with a lot of accuracy. These models also excel over traditional algorithms, as they are more accurate and robust, which allows them to conduct credible morphometric analysis to study neurodevelopment and neurodegeneration (Rasool and Bhat 2025). The cortical thickness, subcortical volumes and white-matter lesions in multiple sclerosis, schizophrenia, Alzheimer's and other diseases are sensitive biomarkers of the automated pipelines.

3.3.2. *Cancer detection and classification*

Neuro-oncology imaging has also been transformed by deep learning. CNNs can be used to locate and classify brain tumors, and differentiate between gliomas, meningomas and metastases when trained on large annotated sets of MRI images. They do not only predict tumor grade and growth patterns, but also molecular subtypes, which makes them useful in supporting precision oncology. Radiomics and deep learning representations outperform each other in providing better predictive accuracy when combined in a hybrid form. Such tools are also useful in surgical planning to outline the limits of tumors to be resected safely, which is essential (Gullo et al. 2024).

3.3.3. *Lesion detection and abnormality detection*

Clinical care requires the detection of non-tumor abnormalities, such as ischemic lesions, hemorrhages and malformations. A CNN and GAN have the capacity to identify small ischemic infarcts or microbleeds that may be missed by radiologists.

Deep learning stroke imaging assists in the long-term outcome forecasts and the acute treatment decision support in stroke imaging. Developmental disorders of subtle malformations are also better detected by use of algorithms that identify atypical morphometric patterns (Zhang et al. 2022).

3.3.4. *Diffusion MRI and microstructural analysis*

Diffusion-weighted (DWI) and diffusion tensor (DTI) imaging provide information on the microstructural integrity of the white matter. Traditional diffusion analysis, however, involves a large amount of prior processing and is noisy. Diffusion data processing can be simplified with deep learning, fiber tracts can be assessed and the prediction of microstructural parameters can be carried out without using complex mathematical models. CNN-based super-resolution methods are used to improve spatial resolution in the process of diffusion imaging, and deep generative models are able to refine or harmonize diffusion data with scanners. The advances allow the improvement of the characterization of conditions such as traumatic brain injury and demyelinating disorders (Liu et al. 2024a).

3.3.5. *CT imaging applications*

The gold standard of neuroimaging is MRI, and CT is still a necessity in cases of emergency, since it is rapid and very common. The recent developments in the field of deep learning have significantly contributed to CT neuroimaging, particularly the detection of acute conditions. A number of algorithms have been developed and are currently able to identify intracranial bleeding, skull fracture and hydrocephalus. CNNs that have been trained using big datasets of CT images can be used to triage urgent patients, guaranteeing that the stroke or trauma patients receive timely services. Besides, transfer learning allows models that are trained on MRI to transfer to CT and enhance cross-imaging generalizability (Dayarathna et al. 2024).

3.3.6. *Multimodal structural integration*

Multimodal integration, or deep learning models using MRI, CT and other imaging measures to enhance the accuracy of the diagnosis, is a growing trend in structural neuroimaging. Multi-stream CNN backbones can process this multimodal information at the same time and extract more features that are complementary and encode topography and pathology alike. As an illustration, CT provides a benefit of providing hemorrhagic transformation after a stroke and T1- and T2-weighted MRI sequences allow a better characterization of the tumor. Such strategies introduce the concept of imaging-based biomarkers that can be clinically used (Raza et al. 2025).

3.4. Applications in functional neuroimaging (fMRI, PET, EEG/MEG)

Functional neuroimaging is aimed at mapping brain functional and connectivity by monitoring dynamic physiology and metabolism. Functional MRI (fMRI), positron emission tomography (PET), electroencephalography (EEG) and magnetoencephalography (MEG) represent different modalities which provide complementary, real-time operation of the neural activity. Compared to structural imaging, the data of functional imaging is always high-dimensional, and there are time courses at thousands of voxels or electrodes. Traditional methods of analysis, such as the general linear models and independent component analysis, find it hard to deal with this complexity. The application of deep learning, which integrates both spatial and time factors, is becoming a highly effective tool in conducting research in the field of functional neuroimaging (Cheng et al. 2021).

3.4.1. *Functional MRI (fMRI)*

fMRI captures blood oxygen level-dependent (BOLD) signals as anatomical proxies of brain activity. Deep learning has significantly advanced the analysis of the BOLD data, including the automation of features, the discovery of dynamic patterns of connections and the modeling of the behavioral or clinical results. The default mode network is among the resting-state networks that have been recognized by CNNs more precisely than the traditional methods. This is done with the RNNs and LSTM-based models that are sensitive to changes in cognitive state in BOLD data and have the ability to capture temporal dependencies.

FMRI with deep learning can be used in clinical practice to detect psychiatric and neurological diseases at the earliest stage. Depression, schizophrenia or autism spectrum disorder patients can be distinguished among functional connectivity signatures with patients with a different condition, such as a healthy control on the basis of models trained on large datasets. In addition, multimodal architectures, which integrate structural MRI and FM MRI, make predictions of treatment response in disorders such as major depressive disorder. These achievements highlight how deep learning can bring positive change in individualized psychiatry and neurology (Kaur and Kaur 2023).

3.4.2. *Positron emission tomography (PET)*

PET imaging provides metabolic and molecular information that complements anatomical and fMRI. Deep learning models have been applied for denoising, reconstruction and interpretation of PET images. Traditionally, PET suffers from low spatial resolution and high noise; however, CNN-based super-resolution techniques significantly improve image quality without increasing radiation dose.

Deep learning of PET data on neurodegenerative diseases has the potential to identify amyloid and tau pathology at its initial stages, even prior to any symptoms. Multimodal deep learning pipelines composed of PET and MRI enhance disease progression and cognitive decline prediction accuracy. Besides, GANs are capable of generating PET images out of MRI data, which is a noninvasive and inexpensive alternative to radiation-based imaging (Fujita et al. 2024).

3.4.3. *Electroencephalography (EEG)*

EEG measures the electrical activity in milliseconds, which is critical in the analysis of quick neural activity. However, unfortunately, EEG signals are often polluted with noise and artifacts, and cannot be easily interpreted. EEG can be significantly enhanced by deep learning because useful temporal and frequency-domain features are automatically acquired and can greatly enhance analysis. CNNs have been used to identify sleep, decode motor images and detect epileptic seizures with good sensitivity.

Seizure prediction is one of the prominent uses of deep learning in the field of EEG. The EEG LSTM-based models learn the temporal patterns of different EEG sequences and are capable of predicting seizure occurrence long before they take place. This allows real-time tracking and prompt intervention, which can greatly enhance the quality of life of an epileptic. Deep learning on EEG can also be applied in brain–computer interfaces (BCIs). It can be said that these systems directly encode neural signals into control signals for assistive machines, for example, prosthetic limbs or communication devices disabled with paralysis (Roy et al. 2019).

3.4.4. *Magnetoencephalography (MEG)*

MEG provides complementary information to EEG by measuring magnetic fields generated by neural currents. It offers high temporal resolution and better spatial localization than EEG, although its availability is more limited due to cost and technical requirements. Deep learning has been applied to MEG data for cognitive decoding, language mapping and identification of pathological activity in epilepsy. CNN-based models trained on MEG time-series data have demonstrated high accuracy in distinguishing patients with neurological disorders from healthy controls. Additionally, deep learning methods enable source localization by modeling the inverse problem more effectively than traditional algorithms, thus enhancing clinical utility in pre-surgical planning (Pan et al. 2023).

3.4.5. *Multimodal functional integration*

The concept of multimodal imaging is one of the new frontiers in functional neuroimaging, which functions to solve the complementary angle of brain activity. The multi-stream CNNs and transformer deep learning models make it possible to examine fMRI, PET and EEG/MEG data simultaneously. Indicatively, fMRI and PET are more sensitive to hemodynamic and metabolic abnormalities when used together, which is essential in sensitive detection of neurodegenerative disorders. Similarly, a combination of EEG and fMRI offers an effective compromise in both time and space resolution, and a greater understanding of the mechanisms in a brain network.

Multimodal fusion is increasingly being carried out via transformer-based architectures, which have the benefit of modeling global dependencies. These models enhance the accuracy of classification and generate cross-modal knowledge transfer, such as when predicting EEG connectivity with fMRI connectivity signals. This integration preconditions accurate brain mapping and all-inclusive models of neurological disease (Ahmad et al. 2017).

3.5. Brain mapping and connectomics with deep learning

Brain mapping seeks to map the structural and functional organization of the brain, focusing on microscopic brain circuits to large-scale networks. One subfield of brain mapping is known as connectomics, and it aims to describe the network architecture of the brain. It is usually graphically described as a graph, with nodes being brain regions and edges structural or functional connections. Deep learning is now an effective platform to make progress in brain mapping and connectomics, and to deal with the enormous dimensionality, non-homogeneous and complex data of imaging (Brown and Hamarneh 2016).

3.5.1. *Structural connectomics*

Structural connectomes tend to be as a diffusion MRI tractography, a map of the white matter fiber pathways. Graph-theoretical metrics such as degree centrality, modularity and efficiency are used in traditional methods of analysis. Although informative, these methods may be missing a higher-order pattern in the form of connectivity matrices. Structural connectomes represent the comprehensive maps of physical neural connections in the brain, typically derived from diffusion-based neuroimaging data, and are used to analyze brain architecture, connectivity patterns, and their relationship to cognition and neurological disorders. As an example, GCNs that are trained on structural connectomes have demonstrated better fidelity to the separation of patients with mild cognitive impairment and healthy controls than graph measures.

3.5.2. *Functional connectomics*

Functional connectomics takes correlations or causal dependencies between brain regions based upon dynamic activity maps that have been measured with fMRI, PET or EEG/MEG. Deep learning is efficient in learning these complicated interactions. Transformers and RNNs have already been used on time-series data to estimate time-based dependencies on functional connectivity. This allows a better understanding of the cognitive states and also forecasting clinical progressions.

3.5.3. *Multiscale brain mapping*

Deep learning has the application of multiscale brain mapping that focuses on the combination of information on cellular, regional and network scales, which is uniquely prepared. Multimodal imaging datasets are a type of MRI which are trained to combine structural MRI, diffusion MRI and fMRI to compose single brain architecture maps. Through hierarchical representations of features, CNNs, as well as transformers, are able to recognize local anatomical information, as well as global network topology. This helps us to better understand how a change in microstructure can be converted into a change on a large-scale network and clinical symptoms.

3.5.4. *The research has a clinical/translational relevance*

The clinical effects of brain mapping and connectomics based on deep learning are significant. Biomarkers based on connectivity are becoming more frequently applied in the early detection of neurological and psychiatric conditions, risk-sharing and in tracking the disease progression. As an example, deep learning can have functional connectivity alterations, which are suggested as biomarkers to predict mild cognitive impairment to the Alzheimer's disease conversion. In the same way, structural connectome alteration identified using deep learning is predictive of prognosis in traumatic brain injury and multiple sclerosis.

3.6. Clinical applications and translational potential

3.6.1. *Neurodegenerative disorders*

Early prediction and diagnosis of neurodegenerative diseases, including Alzheimer's and Parkinson's diseases, are among the most potentially promising clinical applications of deep learning. Deep learning models which are developed on structural MRI and PET images can detect subtle brain changes in the Alzheimer's disease long before symptoms develop, and thus allow themselves to be diagnosed earlier and potentially be enrolled in preventive trials (Cheng et al. 2021; Zhang et al. 2022; Kaur and Kaur 2023; Gullo et al. 2024; Dayarathna et al. 2024; Fujita et al. 2024; Liu et al. 2024a; Al-Rahbi et al. 2025; Rasool and Bhat 2025; Raza et al. 2025). In a similar manner, the subtypes of the Parkinson's disease can be distinguished by deep learning analysis of the feature of functional connectivity in resting-state fMRI, in order to provide clinically relevant information on the heterogeneity of the disease (Kaur and Kaur 2023).

3.6.2. *Neuro-oncology*

Brain tumor detection and classification are areas where deep learning has already shown tangible clinical benefits. Automated tumor segmentation pipelines reduce the time and variability associated with manual delineation, improving surgical and radiotherapy planning (Gullo et al. 2024). Furthermore, deep learning models are being developed to predict tumor grade and molecular subtype directly from imaging, reducing reliance on invasive biopsies. In the future, integration of imaging-based predictions with genomic and clinical data may enable noninvasive "virtual biopsies", significantly transforming neuro-oncology workflows.

3.6.3. *Cerebrovascular disorders*

Fast and accurate image interpretation is highly essential in acute scenarios, such as ischemic stroke, when making treatment decisions. Models of deep learning, based on CT and MRI images, can detect hemorrhages, the ischemic core and penumbra, and predict the recovery outcome of a patient (Zhang et al. 2022; Dayarathna et al. 2024; Liu et al. 2024a). The automated tools prove particularly helpful during emergency care, as every minute counts and a radiologist may be unavailable. In addition to the acute stroke triage, deep learning tools can track the changes of vascular lesions. These are endowed with customized secondary prevention strategies.

3.6.4. *Epilepsy and seizure prediction*

The neuroimaging built on deep learning has enhanced the management of epilepsy. The analysis of structural MRI assists in the identification of subtle cortical malformations, associated with drug-resistant epilepsy, and the epileptic seizures can be detected and predicted by deep neural networks using EEG and MEG signals

(Roy et al. 2019; Pan et al. 2023). These devices will help in surgical planning processes because they localize the epileptogenic foci, and eventually they are capable of performing real-time monitoring, initiating preventive measures before the onset of a seizure.

3.7. Challenges, limitations and future directions

3.7.1. *Data availability and quality*

One of the most urgent issues is the absence of big and heterogeneous datasets. Deep learning needs large labeled datasets. Neuroimaging patient privacy and high data acquisition costs, as well as inter-scanner and protocol variations, make data sharing challenging. In spite of the open efforts of the Human Connectome Project and the Alzheimer's Disease Neuroimaging Initiative, datasets remain too small to make them useful in creating strong models (Kebaili et al. 2023).

In the institution of learning, a promising way out has been identified in federated learning, which allows the institutions to train the models jointly without needing to share raw data. Nonetheless, it also comes with several new data harmonization challenges and heavy computing infrastructure requirements (Rasool and Bhat 2025).

3.7.2. *Generalizability and reproducibility*

The generalizability of the models that have been trained on particular datasets is also another significant shortcoming. Deep learning models are usually effective based on internal data, but are less effective on external cohorts due to changes in population distributions, disease–diseases or even imaging modalities (Shulman et al. 2024). This brings up the issue of reproducibility, as clinical rollout is the need to reliably provide the same results with varying patient groups. Domain adaptation and transfer learning methods are under development to address this issue, but they have to be validated cautiously prior to their clinical use.

3.7.3. *Interpretability and trust*

Deep learning models are sometimes referred to as black boxes as they do not explain the way they got to making such decisions. In high-stakes situations such as medicine, interpretability is a condition, clinicians must realize why a model sounded an alarm over a certain part of the brain or what reason made it predict a certain outcome (Montavon et al. 2018). Saliency maps and LRP are explainable AI methods that can be used to identify the features behind predictions, but have had little to no clinical applications. Innovation in the future should be sustained around intrinsically explainable architectures that can create confidence in the clinical community and regulatory approval.

3.7.4. *Computational and resource demands*

Deep neural networks require a lot of computing strength to be trained and used. The cloud services and powerful GPUs have enabled an overall acceleration in the research, but still, numerous hospitals, especially those that lack adequate resources in both low- and middle-income countries, are not equipped to run heavy models.

Consequently, scientists are developing leaner architecture and more intelligent optimization so that AI-based neuroimages may be implemented beyond their use in top academia.

3.7.5. *Future directions*

Looking ahead, several research avenues promise to overcome current limitations:

– *Multimodal integration*: combining structural MRI, fMRI, PET, EEG and genomic data within unified deep learning frameworks may yield more comprehensive biomarkers of brain function (Dayarathna et al. 2024). Such approaches will enable precision medicine by capturing disease signatures that are invisible to single-modality analyses.

– *Self-supervised and few-shot learning*: to reduce reliance on large labeled datasets, researchers are increasingly adopting self-supervised learning techniques that leverage unlabeled data to pretrain models, followed by fine-tuning with smaller annotated datasets (Liu et al. 2024b). This direction is particularly promising in rare neurological conditions where data scarcity is inevitable.

– *Real-time applications*: advances in model optimization could enable real-time analysis of neuroimaging data, supporting intraoperative guidance during neurosurgery or rapid triage in acute stroke care.

– *Integration with clinical workflows*: for broad adoption, AI systems must integrate seamlessly into radiological and neurological workflows, providing user-friendly interfaces and decision-support tools rather than standalone systems.

3.8. Conclusion

Deep learning is one of the most potent paradigms of further development of neuroimaging and brain mapping. It provides functionality that is much more than conventional methods of computation. These methods, with the help of massive data flow and intricate neural network architectures, provide higher than ever accuracy. They are outstanding in the detection of disease, tracking brain networks and predicting neurological and psychiatric disorders. Clinical use is already being applied in neurodegenerative diseases and neuro-oncology in the cerebral vascular, epilepsy and psychiatry. Deep learning provides greater diagnostic accuracy in every region, targets medical decision-making and provides a personalized intervention. Nevertheless, despite such progress, there are still obstacles. The most notable ones are data availability, model interpretability, reproducibility and equitable clinical translation. The legal, ethical and infrastructural barriers further emphasize the necessity to be careful and transparent as the technologies transition between research and practice. Still, there is a trend toward the creation of explainable AI, federated learning and multimodal integration. Such attempts indicate that the restrictions are overcome. Significantly, the application of deep learning in neuroscience will be extended in the future by emerging innovations in self-supervised learning and real-time neuroimaging analysis. Finally, deep learning is not supposed to replace clinicians. Rather, it gives them the instruments that advance the cognition regarding the brain structure and functioning. Its capability to discover obscured patterns, assemble multimodal information and sell off personalized prediction places it as a fundamental block of accuracy in neuroscience. With the challenges being solved in the technical domain, and clinical confidence increasing, deep learning will radically change the outlook of neuroimaging and brain mapping. It is going to introduce a new period of data-driven discovery and patient-centered care.

3.9. References

Ahamed, M.F., Hossain, M.M., Nahiduzzaman, M., Islam, M.R., Islam, M.R., Ahsan, M., Haider, J. (2023). A review on brain tumor segmentation based on deep learning methods with federated learning techniques. *Computerized Medical Imaging and Graphics*, 110, 102313.

Ahmad, R.F., Malik, A.S., Kamel, N., Reza, F., Amin, H.U., Hussain, M. (2017). Visual brain activity patterns classification with simultaneous EEG-fMRI: A multimodal approach. *Technology and Health Care*, 25(3), 471–485.

Al-Rahbi, A., Al-Habsi, T., Al-Suli, A., Al-Saadi, T. (2025). Artificial intelligence use in diagnosis, grading, and segmentation of neuro-oncology: A narrative review. *The Egyptian Journal of Neurology, Psychiatry and Neurosurgery*, 61(1), 54.

Avberšek, L.K. and Repovš, G. (2022). Deep learning in neuroimaging data analysis: Applications, challenges, and solutions. *Frontiers in Neuroimaging*, 1, 981642.

Brown, C.J. and Hamarneh, G. (2016). Machine learning on human connectome data from MRI. *arXiv preprint*. doi: 10.48550/arXiv.1611.08699.

Cheng, Z., Wen, J., Huang, G., Yan, J. (2021). Applications of artificial intelligence in nuclear medicine image generation. *Quantitative Imaging in Medicine and Surgery*, 11(6), 2792.

Cisotto, G., Zancanaro, A., Zoppis, I.F., Manzoni, S.L. (2024). hvEEGNet: A novel deep learning model for high-fidelity EEG reconstruction. *Frontiers in Neuroinformatics*, 18, 1459970.

Dayarathna, S., Islam, K.T., Uribe, S., Yang, G., Hayat, M., Chen, Z. (2024). Deep learning based synthesis of MRI, CT and PET: Review and analysis. *Medical Image Analysis*, 92, 103046.

Fujita, S., Hagiwara, A., Kamagata, K., Aoki, S. (2024). Clinical neuroimaging over the last decade: Achievements and what lies ahead. *Investigative Radiology*, 10–97. doi: 10.1097/RLI.0000000000001192.

Gullo, R.L., Marcus, E., Huayanay, J., Eskreis-Winkler, S., Thakur, S., Teuwen, J., Pinker, K. (2024). Artificial intelligence-enhanced breast MRI: Applications in breast cancer primary treatment response assessment and prediction. *Investigative Radiology*, 59(3), 230–242.

Isensee, F., Jaeger, P.F., Kohl, S.A., Petersen, J., Maier-Hein, K.H. (2021). nnU-Net: A self-configuring method for deep learning-based biomedical image segmentation. *Nature Methods*, 18(2), 203–211.

Kaissis, G.A., Makowski, M.R., Rückert, D., Braren, R.F. (2020). Secure, privacy-preserving and federated machine learning in medical imaging. *Nature Machine Intelligence*, 2(6), 305–311.

Kaur, P. and Kaur, A. (2023). Review of progress in diagnostic studies of autism spectrum disorder using neuroimaging. *Interdisciplinary Sciences: Computational Life Sciences*, 15(1), 111–130.

Kebaili, A., Lapuyade-Lahorgue, J., Ruan, S. (2023). Deep learning approaches for data augmentation in medical imaging: A review. *Journal of Imaging*, 9(4), 81.

Lambert, B., Forbes, F., Doyle, S., Dehaene, H., Dojat, M. (2024). Trustworthy clinical AI solutions: A unified review of uncertainty quantification in Deep Learning models for medical image analysis. *Artificial Intelligence in Medicine*, 150, 102830.

Li, J., Chen, J., Tang, Y., Wang, C., Landman, B.A., Zhou, S.K. (2023). Transforming medical imaging with Transformers? A comparative review of key properties, current progresses, and future perspectives. *Medical Image Analysis*, 85, 102762.

Liu, F., Yao, Y., Zhu, B., Yu, Y., Ren, R., Hu, Y. (2024a). The novel imaging methods in diagnosis and assessment of cerebrovascular diseases: An overview. *Frontiers in Medicine*, 11, 1269742.

Liu, Z., Kainth, K., Zhou, A., Deyer, T.W., Fayad, Z.A., Greenspan, H., Mei, X. (2024b). A review of self-supervised, generative, and few-shot deep learning methods for data-limited magnetic resonance imaging segmentation. *NMR in Biomedicine*, 37(8), e5143.

Mecheter, I., Alic, L., Abbod, M., Amira, A., Ji, J. (2020). MR image-based attenuation correction of brain PET imaging: Review of literature on machine learning approaches for segmentation. *Journal of Digital Imaging*, 33(5), 1224–1241.

Mienye, I.D., Swart, T.G., Obaido, G., Jordan, M., Ilono, P. (2025). Deep convolutional neural networks in medical image analysis: A review. *Information*, 16(3), 195.

Montavon, G., Samek, W., Müller, K.R. (2018). Methods for interpreting and understanding deep neural networks. *Digital Signal Processing*, 73, 1–5.

Pan, R., Yang, C., Li, Z., Ren, J., Duan, Y. (2023). Magnetoencephalography-based approaches to epilepsy classification. *Frontiers in Neuroscience*, 17, 1183391.

Raghu, M., Zhang, C., Kleinberg, J., Bengio, S. (2019). Transfusion: Understanding transfer learning for medical imaging. In *33rd Conference on Neural Information Processing Systems (NeurIPS 2019)*, Vancouver.

Rasool, N. and Bhat, J.I. (2025). Brain tumour detection using machine and deep learning: A systematic review. *Multimedia Tools and Applications*, 84(13), 11551–11604.

Raza, M.L., Hassan, S.T., Jamil, S., Hyder, N., Batool, K., Walji, S., Abbas, M.K. (2025). Advancements in deep learning for early diagnosis of Alzheimer's disease using multimodal neuroimaging: Challenges and future directions. *Frontiers in Neuroinformatics*, 19, 1557177.

Roy, S., Kiral-Kornek, I., Harrer, S. (2019). ChronoNet: A deep recurrent neural network for abnormal EEG identification. In *Conference on Artificial Intelligence in Medicine in Europe*. Springer, Cham, 47–56.

Shulman, D., Israeli, A., Botnaro, Y., Margalit, O., Tamir, O., Naschitz, S., Gamrasni, D., Shir, O.M., Dattner, I. (2024). Physics-guided inverse regression for crop quality assessment. *Journal of Agricultural, Biological and Environmental Statistics*, 1–24 [Online]. Available at: https://link.springer.com/article/10.1007/s13253-024-00643-9#citeas.

Xu, M., Ouyang, Y., Yuan, Z. (2023). Deep learning aided neuroimaging and brain regulation. *Sensors*, 23(11), 4993.

Zhang, L., Wang, M., Liu, M., Zhang, D. (2020). A survey on deep learning for neuroimaging-based brain disorder analysis. *Frontiers in Neuroscience*, 14, 779.

Zhang, Y., Liu, S., Li, C., Wang, J. (2022). Application of deep learning method on ischemic stroke lesion segmentation. *Journal of Shanghai Jiaotong University (Science)*, 27(1), 99–111.

4

Predictive Analytics for Early Detection of Neurodegenerative Disorders

Neurodegenerative diseases, such as Alzheimer's, Parkinson's, Huntington's and amyotrophic lateral sclerosis are emerging as a growing health problem in the world, due to the increasing population and the unavailability of treatment. It is important to detect the disease early since early intervention can slow down the progression, enhance the outcome and reduce costs. Conventional diagnostic methods rely on symptoms that are manifested in the end stages, and the preventive or treatment opportunities are overlooked. Machine learning, AI, neuroimaging and biomarker research have been used to create a tool, known as predictive analytics, which is a game changer in terms of early detection. Models are able to reveal hidden trends before they turn into symptoms by integrating various data genomics, proteomics, electronic health records, imaging and wearable sensors. It enables the protocol of risk stratification, early detection of biomarkers and individualized disease tracking. Furthermore, predictive analytics serves precision medicine, tailoring interventions to any risk profile and improving the efficacy of treatments. Nevertheless, even though they hold a lot of promise, model interpretability, data privacy and training set bias remain signifcant issues. Scholars are interested in multimodal data fusion, long-term cohort research and federated learning as a way to enhance accuracy and safeguard privacy. This chapter looks at the present situation of predictive analytics in neurodegenerative studies, new approaches, and translational issues and opportunities. The application of predictive analytics into clinical practice may transform reactive treatment into proactive prevention.

4.1. Introduction

Neurodegenerative disorders (NDDs) are a significant health problem all over the world. These include Alzheimer's disease, Parkinson's disease, Huntington's disease and amyotrophic lateral sclerosis (AD, PD, HD and ALS, respectively). These diseases progressively and irreversibly reduce brain neurons, resulting in

Chapter written by Debabrata SAHANA and K. GAVHALE.

brain damage, leading to a decline in cognitive functions, motor impairments and reduced quality of life (Nies et al. 2021). The rising elderly population is augmenting the incidences of NDDs, and this has piled a lot of strain on healthcare, caregivers and society in general (Nichols et al. 2022).

The conventional approaches to NDD diagnosis are based on clinical evaluation, neurological examination and X-rays. But not all pathological changes are visible in the acute stages of the disease as such tools are not capable of detecting this kind of disease at its initial stages (Jack 2018). This is the case with AD, where amyloid plaques and tau tangles accumulate decades prior to the manifestation of memory loss and cognitive impairment. In PD, when dopamine secreting neurons start degenerating, it takes a long time for tremors or rigidity to occur, and in this phase/stage, there is a silent period where the damage could best be reversed with an early intervention (Poewe et al. 2017).

The fact that these disorders are often not diagnosed in time shows that there is an urgent demand that can be satisfied by means of the tools that can identify individuals who are at risk before the limbic neurons have been lost to a large extent. To fulfill this requirement, predictive analytics, an emerging area that combines artificial intelligence (AI) and machine learning (ML) with health data science, intervenes. It is able to identify patterns in big, varied datasets to reveal diseases, conditions and risk factors in the early stages, even before they develop (Brogi and Calderone 2021).

Predictive analytics of neurodegenerative diseases covers a number of areas. Multimodal imaging is sensitive to minor changes in the brain; genetic indicators and protein markers are indicators of the risk of disease; and electronic health records (EHRs) can be used to follow the progress of the illness. Mobility apps and wearables engage in real-world data collection (movement, speech and other signals of physiology) 24/7. The models are all connected by weaving these streams of data together to form individualized risk profiles that are used to guide precision medicine on an individual basis.

In its own right, predictive analytics is transforming healthcare at a broader, systemic level. Early identification could prevent the process of the disease, reduce incurring hospitalization and long-term care costs, and facilitate the shortening of clinical trials by optimizing the recruiters to identify high-risk subjects, making the clinical trials more effective and accelerating drug discovery. On a social scale, these tools allow policymakers to predict the future cost of neurodegenerative diseases, use resources in the wisest way and implement preventive programs.

Adoption is challenged even though it is a promising area. The adaptive lack of transparency of algorithms and possible bias are some of the primary concerns. The tools should also integrate easily into normal clinical operations and be accepted by clinicians, as well as by the regulations. To break these hurdles, a cross-disciplinary team of clinicians, data scientists, ethicists and policymakers is needed.

In this chapter, the authors provide a review of the present state of predictive analytics when detecting neurodegenerative diseases at their early stages. It includes the basic modeling methods, the progress in the multimodal data integration, the practical constraints and the prospects of the future. In the end, predictive analytics can change the treatment of neurodegenerative conditions and provide better results to both patients and the rest of the population as it will stop being symptom-focused and so reactive, and become data-centered and thus proactive.

4.2. Predictive analytics framework for neurodegenerative disorders

To minimize NDDs with the help of predictive analytics, an adequate framework is necessary that would transform various biomedical data into practical clinical conclusions. This model usually entails four major steps, which include (1) data acquisition, (2) data preprocessing, (3) model development and (4) clinical integration. With these steps, predictive analytics can be useful in identifying and tracking organs with the onset of such diseases as Alzheimer's disease (AD), Parkinson's disease (PD), Huntington's disease (HD) and amyotrophic lateral sclerosis (ALS) (Obermeyer and Emanuel 2016).

4.2.1. *Data acquisition*

The foundation of predictive analytics lies in robust and diverse data sources. In the context of NDDs, data acquisition involves collecting multimodal information from patients, including:

– *Neuroimaging data*: techniques such as magnetic resonance imaging (MRI), positron emission tomography (PET) and functional MRI (fMRI) provide insights into structural and functional changes in the brain long before clinical symptoms emerge (Rajkomar et al. 2019).

– *Omics data*: genomics, transcriptomics and proteomics aid us in recognizing molecular biomarkers that are associated with neurodegeneration. For example, Alzheimer's related diseases can be worsened by the presence of the APOE ε4 allele, whereas the SNCA gene mutations are related to PD. Transcriptomic and proteomic signatures are better predictors when combined with genetic risk factors.

– *Clinical and demographic data*: EHRs are long-term stores of information regarding the medical history of a patient, co-morbidities, medications and lifestyle.

This information is examined in predictive models in order to detect minor shifts that can indicate the development of a disease.

– *Digital and wearable data*: recent advancements in wearable sensors and smartphone-based monitoring allow the real-time tracking of motor activity, gait, voice patterns and sleep cycles.

Collectively, these datasets create a comprehensive picture of patient health and disease progression, forming the input for predictive models (Beam and Kohane 2018).

4.2.2. *Data preprocessing and feature engineering*

Raw biomedical data can usually be noisy, incomplete and heterogeneous. Hence, analysis can only be reliable when preprocessed. This stage involves the normalization of imaging data, setting missing values in healthcare data and artifact detection in wearable sensor records.

Feature engineering transforms raw data into variables that make sense to clinically enhance the performance of the model. Indicatively, cortical thickness can be measured by an MRI scan. The data of wearable devices may be converted to gait variability measures. The selection of the best features applied to the inputs further narrows the task to select the most predictive variables, dimensionality reduction and overfitting (Rashidi et al. 2019).

Multimodal data fusion is a prospective strategy in which the imaging, genetic, clinical and behavioral characteristics of the patient are used to create a comprehensive profile of the patient. Bringing all of this together enhances the prediction through the combination of complementary information from various types of data.

4.2.3. *Model development*

Machine learning (ML) and artificial intelligence (AI) are the leading techniques that are used to construct predictive models of neurodevelopmental disorders (NDDs). Such models range from basic statistical techniques to sophisticated deep learning models:

– *Statistical models*: Cox proportional hazards models and logistic regression are often applied for risk prediction and survival analysis, particularly in longitudinal cohorts.

– *ML models*: random forests, support vector machines and gradient boosting machines are extremely helpful in the interpretation of complicated and nonlinear biomedical data.

– *Deep learning models*: specifically, convolutional and recurrent neural networks are gaining more and more popularity regarding the assessment of sequential and imaging data. Spatial convolutional neural networks (CNN) incorporate important patterns in an MRI or PET scan, whereas recurrent neural networks incorporate time-varying data such as EHRs and speech files.

– *Hybrid models*: recent research has registered the extent to which the interruption of diverse algorithms can result in the strengthening of systems. As an example, ensemble learning combines the outputs of multiple models, which aids in balancing bias and variance (Lundberg and Lee 2017).

4.2.4. *Clinical integration and decision support*

The main purpose of predictive analytics is to convert computational results into actionable insights for clinicians. Predictive systems should meet the following criteria for successful predictive clinical integration:

– *Interpretability*: for clinicians to trust predictive models and adopt them into their practice, models must articulate the reasoning behind each prediction. Outcomes must demonstrate how various risk factors influence results and calculations.

– *Workflow compatibility*: predictive tools must fit seamlessly into the existing clinical information systems and diagnostic workflows without interrupting the routine practice.

– *Regulatory approval*: for predictive systems to be adopted, they must comply with regulatory standards for safety, accuracy and reproducibility.

– *Ethical considerations*: safeguards are required to ensure patient privacy, address algorithmic bias and promote equitable access to predictive technologies.

Decision-support systems based on predictive analytics are already being piloted in some clinical contexts. For instance, early-warning systems for cognitive decline can notify clinicians of high-risk individuals, prompting additional testing or lifestyle interventions. The development of user-friendly interfaces and visualization dashboards further enhances clinical usability (Tonekaboni et al. 2019). Table 4.1 shows a predictive analytics framework for NDDs.

Stage	Key components	Example techniques/tools	Clinical significance
1. Data acquisition	Neuroimaging, omics, clinical, wearable and digital health data	MRI, PET, EEG, genomic sequencing, wearable sensors	Enables early identification of biomarkers such as cortical thinning, tau buildup and altered gait patterns
2. Data preprocessing and feature engineering	Cleaning, normalization and feature extraction	Dimensionality reduction, feature selection, signal denoising	Improves model interpretability and minimizes bias by standardizing heterogeneous data
3. Model development	Statistical, machine learning, deep learning and hybrid models	Logistic regression, random forest, CNNs, RNNs, ensemble learning	Predicts disease onset, progression and prognosis for AD, PD, ALS and HD
4. Clinical integration and decision support	Model interpretability, regulatory compliance, workflow embedding	Explainable AI (SHAP, LIME), clinical dashboards, EHR integration	Facilitates clinician trust, real-time decision-making and risk stratification
5. Ethical and regulatory oversight	Data privacy, fairness and accountability	Federated learning, GDPR, HIPAA compliance tools	Ensures ethical data use, equity in prediction and patient privacy

Table 4.1. *Predictive analytics framework for neurodegenerative disorders*

4.2.5. *Challenges and future directions*

Although the predictive analytics framework of NDDs is an established concept, there are still problems. The heterogeneity of sets, the absence of standardized biomarkers and the black box characteristics of deep learning models are impeding its translation into regular practice. The problem of scalability, in particular, in low-resource environments, needs to be resolved as it can guarantee equal access to positive outcomes among populations.

Future prospects include federated learning (FL) where collaborative model training is conducted without the need to share data, explainable AI where the predictive models of the future are verified by first-mover studies, and longitudinal cohort designed to determine the predictive value of the model and its validity in the future. The advances in these aspects will play a crucial role in achieving the promise of predictive analytics regarding the early detection of NDDs.

4.3. Applications of predictive analytics in specific neurodegenerative disorders

NDDs are becoming common in the application of predictive analytics, in which disease trends and progression can be predicted and detected early. With multimodal datasets, computational models provide helpful information on the risk and development of diseases, and therapy responses. In the following, we discuss the implementation of these approaches to four significant NDDs: Alzheimer's disease (AD), Parkinson's disease (PD), amyotrophic lateral sclerosis (ALS) and Huntington's disease (HD).

4.3.1. *Alzheimer's disease*

AD is the most prevalent type of neurodegeneration and cause of dementia across the globe. It is progressive (coming with a gradual reduction in cognition) and is characterized by amyloid-b plaques, tau tangles and neuroinflammation. Traditional diagnostic methods diagnose AD when the patient exhibits cognitive impairment to a noticeable degree, which will minimize the opportunity to intervene at an earlier stage. Consequently, predictive analytics will be important in identifying people at preclinical or prodromal stages (Livingston et al. 2020).

– *Neuroimaging-based prediction:* ML on structural MRI and PET scans can identify any subtle change in the brain well before the disease develops. Hippocampal atrophy, cortical thinning and amyloid load can be predicted many years before. Deep learning and, in particular, CNNs are significantly accurate in the process of differentiating between mild cognitive impairment (MCI) and AD, and provide insight into what patients with MCI will transition into (Petersen et al. 2018).

– *Biomarker integration:* proteomic and genomic indicators are important in the prediction of AD. The APOE allele ε4 is the most robust genetic risk factor which is enhanced by plasma biomarkers, including phosphorylated tau and neurofilament light chain (NfL). Hybrid imaging-genetic-fluid biomarker models are more effective than single-modality models (Warren and Moustafa 2023).

– *EHR and cognitive data:* EHRs and longitudinal data from digital cognitive assessments can be used to predict clinical outcomes and disease progression and, in turn, may themselves be predicted or enriched through advanced computational modeling and analytics. Natural language processing (NLP) of clinical notes identifies early language indicators of bad health (Vieira et al. 2017). Longitudinal EHR data can be analyzed using predictive models to identify people at high risk, and trigger proactive diagnostic preparations and preventive measures sooner.

4.3.2. *Parkinson's disease*

The second NDD is known as Parkinson's disease (PD). It has both motor and non-motor symptoms, including rigidity, motor tremors, bradykinesia, sleep disturbance, depression and cognitive impairment. Notably, there is a prodromal stage of PD where non-motor symptoms manifest decades prior to motor impairment, thereby offering a significant predictive analytics window (Woo et al. 2017).

– *Gait and motor analytics*: as a demonstration of wearable and mobile sensor technologies, it is possible to mention continuous gait, tremors and fine motor activity detection. Accelerometer and gyroscope-based predictive models are able to identify abnormal motor behavior, which indicates prodromal PD. Machine learning programs which study the dynamics of handwriting and typing have also been useful in identifying the signs of early motor impairments.

– *Neuroimaging approaches*: neuroimaging, not to mention dopamine transporter (DAT) SPECT imaging, is a source of valuable biomarkers to predict PD. Deep learning models that use imaging data deliver high performance when detecting people at risk of PD before they develop clinical motor symptoms. Sensitivity and specificity in prediction arc better when imaging is coupled with clinical features.

– *Non-motor symptom data*: predictive analytics also include non-motor symptoms such as sleeping behavior disorders, constipation and loss of sense of smell. The analysis of these features along with imaging and genetic information can be very helpful in predicting the onset of PD. Multimodal predictive methods can categorize people in high- and low-risk groups, and direct efforts towards monitoring and assisting in the recruitment of participants in clinical trials (Hampel et al. 2019).

4.3.3. *Amyotrophic lateral sclerosis*

Amyotrophic lateral sclerosis (ALS) is a terminal NDD, which degenerates motor neurons. This damage causes muscle weakness, respiratory failure and death, normally three to five years after the development of symptoms. The early diagnosis of ALS is not very easy as its symptoms are diverse and can be confused with other motor disorders. Predictive analytics can provide an opportunity to diagnose the disease earlier and model the outcome of patients more precisely (Rizzo et al. 2016):

– *Clinical and genetic predictors*: ALS may be episodic or familial. Genetic mutations play a major role as they include C9orf72 repeat expansions. Genetic information and clinical data such as age of onset, age at symptom onset and modulation rate of the disease can now give a patient a more reliable estimate of their survival.

– *Neuroimaging and electrophysiology*: making an ML of structural and diffusion MRI, researchers are able to identify white-matter alterations, which aid in the differentiation between ALS and other related conditions. When used as inputs in predictive models, electromyography (EMG) and motor-unit recordings are able to reveal very subtle neuromuscular issues that could be undetected by routine tests, which also contributes to the promptness of diagnosis.

– *Prognostic prediction*: in addition to ALS diagnosis, predictive analytics are also broadly used to predict patient outcomes. Ensemble learning has been used to construct survival models that enable clinicians to categorize patients to obtain trials and develop customized treatment strategies. The tools are in particular useful in making decisions about ventilation and nutrition plans, which are instrumental in enhancing patient survival (Pagano et al. 2016).

4.3.4. *Huntington's disease*

Huntington's disease (HD) is an NDD that is inherited due to extended repeats of CAG in the huntingtin (HTT) gene. However, as opposed to other genetic disorders, testing is able to help easily identify the likely suspects, but the age of onset and the rate at which the condition advances vary highly among carriers. Predictive analytics can be used to predict the possibility of phenotypic conversion and map the disease process (Parnetti et al. 2019):

– *Genetic and imaging integration*: although it is possible to determine with absolute certainty the carriers of genetic mutations, predictive analytics determine when clinical symptoms may appear. Imaging biomarkers, including striatal atrophy, white-matter alterations, among others, can be used together with genetic information to predict the onset of the disease more effectively.

– *Motor and cognitive monitoring*: predictive models analyzing motor performance (e.g. finger tapping, gait analysis) and cognitive testing data have been effective in forecasting disease conversion in premanifest carriers.

– *Longitudinal modeling*: HD research has benefited from large longitudinal datasets, such as the TRACK-HD study, which provided rich multimodal data for predictive modeling. ML applied to these datasets can estimate both the onset and rate of progression, enabling more precise patient monitoring and earlier intervention.

4.4. Emerging trends and methodological advances

4.4.1. *Multimodal data fusion*

Conventional predictive models typically make use of a single source of information, for example, neuroimaging or genetics. However, neurodevelopmental disorders are complex, and the integration of multiple sources of data results in much stronger predictions.

Multimodal data fusion involves combining imaging biomarkers, genetic risk factors, fluid-based data (such as plasma tau or neurofilament light chain) and clinical data together into concerted predictive models. With respect to Alzheimer's, it was revealed that the structural MRI, PET imaging and plasma biomarker models do better in predicting the onset of dementia compared to single-modality predictors at MCI (Miotto et al. 2018).

4.4.2. *Longitudinal modeling*

Another key trend is the shift from cross-sectional to longitudinal predictive modeling. Neurodegeneration is a dynamic process, and single-time-point measurements often fail to capture the full trajectory of disease progression.

Longitudinal models analyze repeated observations over time, allowing predictions of not only disease onset, but also progression speed and future clinical outcomes. In PD, for instance, longitudinal gait and motor activity data collected from wearables have been used to predict motor decline trajectories years in advance (Topol 2019). Similarly, in ALS, survival prediction models based on longitudinal clinical and electrophysiological data provide more accurate prognostic estimates than baseline-only models.

4.4.3. *Deep learning and advanced AI techniques*

Deep learning continues to transform predictive analytics in healthcare. Its ability to process high-dimensional data, such as neuroimaging scans and genetic profiles, makes it particularly relevant for NDDs. CNNs have been used extensively in brain imaging studies, while recurrent and transformer-based architectures are applied to sequential data such as clinical notes or speech recordings.

Graph neural networks (GNNs) are used to model the data of brain connectivity, which is one of the emerging trends. GNNs have the ability to learn advanced topological properties which are connected with early neurodegeneration because they represent the brain as a graph of interconnected nodes (Holzinger et al. 2019). Such methods have been successful in forecasting the course of AD and also in distinguishing subtypes of PD.

4.4.4. *Explainable artificial intelligence (XAI)*

The main issue with predictive analytics is that many ML models are black box plots, which is a critical impediment to the clinical adoption of predictive analytics. Clinicians do not want to make decisions they do not understand when it may end up being a life-altering decision, such as deciding when to start treatment or place patients in a clinical trial.

XAI addresses this problem by providing clinicians with clear understandable results. Tools such as SHapley Additive exPlanations (SHAP) and local interpretable model-agnostic explanations represent how individual features contribute to prediction and allow doctors to determine why a patient may be considered high risk (Kaissis et al. 2020).

4.4.5. *Federated learning and data privacy*

One of the biggest issues in predictive models is data privacy, as in most cases sensitive patient data needs to be exchanged across institutions in order to create a strong model. The conventional centralized solutions pose a threat of undermining privacy and security. FL can deliver an answer to this problem, as it allows model training to be collaborative using distributed datasets without sharing raw data (Warin et al. 2022).

In the federated standards, the sites develop their model on their own and send only the updated parameters to a central aggregator. This technique has been tested in AD and PD experiments, and federated models have been found to be as equally accurate as centralized models and maintain privacy. FL plays a major role, particularly in unusual neurodegenerative diseases such as HD, where the inter-center pooling of information is critical in order to come up with predictive instruments.

4.4.6. *Real-world digital health integration*

The emergence of digital health technologies, such as wearables, smartphones and home-based monitoring technology, has opened up new possibilities for predictive analytics. Ecologically valuable neurodegenerative markers are obtained through continuous streams of data (including gait dynamics, sleep patterns, speech features and fine motor activity).

A case in point is that wearable-based predictive models can forecast early gait variability in PD or small changes in speech in ALS, which are otherwise undiagnosed through clinical means. Remote monitoring can also be done with these tools, which creates better accessibility to care, used in addition to the necessity to visit the hospital regularly (Van der Schaar et al. 2021). Notably, the integration of real-world data enables predictive analytics to go beyond clinical controlled processes to offer population-wide scalable solutions to early detection.

4.5. Challenges, ethical considerations and future directions

The potential of predictive analytics to detect NDDs in their early stages is immense, yet a number of factors do not allow predictive analytics to become a widespread practice. These barriers include legal barriers, technical barriers, ethical barriers and social barriers. To achieve accuracy, fairness, trust in prediction tools and protect the rights of patients, it is important to overcome them. The following section summarizes the key challenges, discusses the ethical considerations and identifies a way forward for predictive analytics within NDD research and practice.

4.5.1. *Data-related challenges*

The complexity and heterogeneity of biomedical data is a significant obstacle on the way to predictive modeling. The data on NDDs are usually small, decentralized between institutions and of differing quality. Small samples are a problem as they prevent the training of generalizable machine learning models, particularly with rare conditions, such as HD. The skewed model performance is also due to the data imbalance of a smaller number of cases of disease positivity compared to the controls (McMackin et al. 2023).

The aspect of multimodal integration increases the challenge. Digital health data are in different formats and resolutions, which include neuroimaging, omics, clinical records and neuroimaging. To match these sources, extensive harmonization and preprocessing pipelines are needed, which are not yet standardized between laboratories. Devoid of common frameworks, the models can be too specific to one dataset and cannot be generalized.

Analytics are complicated by the limiting of information sharing. Privacy, ownership issues and regulation, including GDPR and HIPAA, may restrict access to being able to mix datasets between centers. The frameworks must be validated with caution and development, as the solutions may be offered by FL, yet these ideas are still in their infancy stage of deployment.

4.5.2. *Model-related challenges*

Interpretability, reproducibility and robustness influence the predictive model performance. Most deep learning algorithms are black boxes, making it difficult to determine why a prediction was taken. To clinicians, such transparency diminishes the levels of trust and hinders its integration into diagnostic processes.

The problem of reproducibility is different. The models are known to work on controlled experiments, but fail on outside data. This gap is caused by overfitting, a lack of standard protocols and disproportionate validation. A high level of robustness in population, imaging and health systems is essential to clinical translation (Roberts et al. 2021).

Another significant aspect of concern is prejudice. When there is an imbalance in feeding models with data not representative of women, ethnic minorities or low-resource societies, they may not work well with such populations. This kind of bias will hamper equity and deteriorate current healthcare disparities.

4.5.3. *Social and ethical exposures*

There exist profound ethical concerns in the integration of predictive analytics into neurodegenerative care. The most known problem is that of the psychological effects of early-risk prediction. Notifying a person that they have a high risk of a fatal disease that has no cure, such as AD or ALS, can be stressful, depressing and result in discrimination by employers or insurance companies. There should be clear guidelines on how to convey predictive results and at what time (Winter and Davidson 2019).

Another issue is algorithmic fairness. If models incorrectly categorize certain groups, they can deny the vulnerable community's preventive care. The best way to overcome these threats is to transparently report on model limitations and actively involve different cohorts in the training data.

There are other ethical issues such as privacy and consent. Patients need to know and manage the ways in which their data is collected, shared and used.

4.5.4. *Clinical translation and adoption*

Even in the cases where predictive models are effective in research, they remain hard to transform into clinical instruments. The major challenges include their integration into EHR systems, integrating the corresponding pattern and speed of clinician activity, and regulatory approval. To make the tools useful, they should provide easy-to-understand and interpretable data, such as individual risk scores or graphics that explain visual imaging biomarkers, which can be used by clinicians to make decisions.

Another significant problem is cost-effectiveness. Imposing the use of advanced imaging, multi-omics sequencing and constant wearable monitoring is costly. Achieving access to such technology in low and middle-income countries (LMICs) means scalable and affordable predictive products that will not expand the disparities already present in healthcare (Kelly et al. 2019).

Procedural authorities are starting to make use of cutting-edge AI-driven predictive instruments, but the permissions procedure can be convoluted. Some agencies such as the U.S. Food and Drugs Administration (FDA) and the European Medicines Agency (EMA) are formulating AI-specific guidelines to the use of clinical devices, but still, there is a lack of clear guidelines regarding validation, transparency and continuous monitoring.

4.5.5. *Future directions*

– *Internationalization of data and protocols*: design an international data collection, labeling and preprocessing standard to support inter-center collaboration and reproducible models. Innovations such as the Alzheimer's Disease Neuroimaging Initiative (ADNI) are useful blueprints towards a standardized data infrastructure.

– *Explainable and trustworthy AI*: build explainable AI (XAI) systems in such a way that clinicians are able to make sense of, and validate their predictions. The models that highlight important biomarkers or brain regions are going to develop trust and enhance usability.

– *Combination of multimodal and real-world information*: future models need to go beyond controlled clinical data and include wearable-based and normal health data. This will lead to risk assessments that are an indication of real-life conditions.

– *Federated and collaborative learning*: predictive analytics can only be scaled by using federated and secure frameworks, which allow institutions to keep data private and share it with other institutions. Building strong and varied models will require the use of international consortia and cloud-based platforms.

– *Ethical frameworks and engaging patients*: ethics policies should change to cope with the psychosocial consequences of predictive analytics. Engaging the patients in the process of designing and validating models will ensure that the tools cater to real-life needs and expectations.

– *Policy and regulation*: regulators and policymakers should learn to be in tandem with advancements in AI. There must be clear guidelines on validation, liability and equitable access so that there is responsible deployment.

4.6. Conclusion

NDD research and care is transforming with the help of predictive analytics. It is shifting healthcare from a reactive diagnostic approach toward proactive forecasting and prediction. The tools identifying minor disease signs detect them regularly before their manifestation, through AI advancements, the synthesis of various types of data and real-world digital health monitoring. Early diagnosis may result in early treatment, healthier patients and reduced pressure on society. Different important prediction frameworks have been discussed in this chapter, as well as their application in imaging, omics, clinical records and wearables. We also referred to explainable AI and federated learning. Combined with the advances, the field is tending towards more precise neurology, with customized risk evaluation and treatment design becoming commonplace. Nevertheless, there is limited information, low reproducibility, bias in the algorithm and ethical concerns that should be approached with caution. Addressing these issues is crucial to ensure predictive analytics enhances clinical decisions instead of making them confusing. A step forward requires collaboration between clinicians, data scientists, policymakers and patients. We should implement standardized data facilities, comprehensible and readable algorithms and privacy-preserving technology. We should also have ethical standards that would convey findings in a responsible manner and make access to care equitable. Predictive analytics is the new game-changer as the number of patients with neurodegenerative disease, and their age, increase. With responsible production and the utilization of such tools, healthcare will be able to move towards earlier care, improved quality of life and a more sustainable disease management system.

4.7. References

Beam, A.L. and Kohane, I.S. (2018). Big data and machine learning in health care. *JAMA*, 319(13), 1317–1318.

Brogi, S. and Calderone, V. (2021). Artificial intelligence in translational medicine. *International Journal of Translational Medicine*, 1(3), 223–285.

Hampel, H., Vergallo, A., Perry, G., Lista, S. (2019). Alzheimer precision medicine initiative (APMI). The Alzheimer precision medicine initiative. *Journal of Alzheimer's Disease*, 68(1), 1–24.

Holzinger, A., Langs, G., Denk, H., Zatloukal, K., Müller, H. (2019). Causability and explainability of artificial intelligence in medicine. *Wiley Interdisciplinary Reviews: Data Mining and Knowledge Discovery*, 9(4), e1312.

Jack Jr, C.R., Bennett, D.A., Blennow, K., Carrillo, M.C., Dunn, B., Haeberlein, S.B., Holtzman, D.M., Jagust, W., Jessen, F., Karlawish, J. et al. (2018). NIA-AA research framework: Toward a biological definition of Alzheimer's disease. *Alzheimer's & Dementia*, 14(4), 535–562.

Kaissis, G.A., Makowski, M.R., Rückert, D., Braren, R.F. (2020). Secure, privacy-preserving and federated machine learning in medical imaging. *Nature Machine Intelligence*, 2(6), 305–311.

Kelly, C.J., Karthikesalingam, A., Suleyman, M., Corrado, G., King, D. (2019). Key challenges for delivering clinical impact with artificial intelligence. *BMC Medicine*, 17(1), 195.

Livingston, G., Huntley, J., Sommerlad, A., Ames, D., Ballard, C., Banerjee, S., Brayne, C., Burns, A., Cohen-Mansfield, J., Cooper, C. et al. (2020). Dementia prevention, intervention, and care: 2020 report of the Lancet Commission. *The Lancet*, 396(10248), 413–446.

Lundberg, S.M. and Lee, S.I. (2017). A unified approach to interpreting model predictions. *Advances in Neural Information Processing Systems*, 30.

McMackin, R., Bede, P., Ingre, C., Malaspina, A., Hardiman, O. (2023). Biomarkers in amyotrophic lateral sclerosis: Current status and future prospects. *Nature Reviews Neurology*, 19(12), 754–768.

Miotto, R., Wang, F., Wang, S., Jiang, X., Dudley, J.T. (2018). Deep learning for healthcare: Review, opportunities and challenges. *Briefings in Bioinformatics*, 19(6), 1236–1246.

Nichols, E., Steinmetz, J.D., Vollset, S.E., Fukutaki, K., Chalek, J., Abd-Allah, F., Abdoli, A., Abualhasan, A., Abu-Gharbieh, E., Akram, T.T. et al. (2022). Estimation of the global prevalence of dementia in 2019 and forecasted prevalence in 2050: An analysis for the Global Burden of Disease Study 2019. *The Lancet Public Health*, 7(2), e105–e125.

Nies, Y.H., Mohamad Najib, N.H., Lim, W.L., Kamaruzzaman, M.A., Yahaya, M.F., Teoh, S.L. (2021). MicroRNA dysregulation in Parkinson's disease: A narrative review. *Frontiers in Neuroscience*, 15, 660379.

Obermeyer, Z. and Emanuel, E.J. (2016). Predicting the future – big data, machine learning, and clinical medicine. *The New England Journal of Medicine*, 375(13), 1216.

Pagano, G., Niccolini, F., Politis, M. (2016). Imaging in Parkinson's disease. *Clinical Medicine*, 16(4), 371–375.

Parnetti, L., Gaetani, L., Eusebi, P., Paciotti, S., Hansson, O., El-Agnaf, O., Mollenhauer, B., Blennow, K., Calabresi, P. (2019). CSF and blood biomarkers for Parkinson's disease. *The Lancet Neurology*, 18(6), 573–586.

Petersen, R.C., Lopez, O., Armstrong, M.J., Getchius, T.S., Ganguli, M., Gloss, D., Gronseth, G.S., Marson, D., Pringsheim, T., Day, G.S. et al. (2018). Practice guideline update summary: Mild cognitive impairment: Report of the Guideline Development, Dissemination, and Implementation Subcommittee of the American Academy of Neurology. *Neurology*, 90(3), 126.

Poewe, W., Seppi, K., Tanner, C.M., Halliday, G.M., Brundin, P., Volkmann, J., Schrag, A.E., Lang, A.E. (2017). Parkinson disease. *Nature Reviews Disease Primers*, 3(1), 1–21.

Rajkomar, A., Dean, J., Kohane, I. (2019). Machine learning in medicine. *New England Journal of Medicine*, 380(14), 1347–1358.

Rashidi, H.H., Tran, N.K., Betts, E.V., Howell, L.P., Green, R. (2019). Artificial intelligence and machine learning in pathology: The present landscape of supervised methods. *Academic Pathology*, 6, 2374289519873088.

Rizzo, G., Copetti, M., Arcuti, S., Martino, D., Fontana, A., Logroscino, G. (2016). Accuracy of clinical diagnosis of Parkinson disease: A systematic review and meta-analysis. *Neurology*, 86(6), 566–576.

Roberts, M., Driggs, D., Thorpe, M., Gilbey, J., Yeung, M., Ursprung, S., Aviles-Rivero, A.I., Etmann, C., McCague, C., Beer, L. et al. (2021). Common pitfalls and recommendations for using machine learning to detect and prognosticate for COVID-19 using chest radiographs and CT scans. *Nature Machine Intelligence*, 3(3), 199–217.

Tonekaboni, S., Joshi, S., McCradden, M.D., Goldenberg, A. (2019). What clinicians want: Contextualizing explainable machine learning for clinical end use. In *Machine Learning for Healthcare Conference*, 28 October, 359–380. PMLR.

Topol, E.J. (2019). High-performance medicine: The convergence of human and artificial intelligence. *Nature Medicine*, 25(1), 44–56.

Van der Schaar, M., Alaa, A.M., Floto, A., Gimson, A., Scholtes, S., Wood, A., McKinney, E., Jarrett, D., Lio, P., Ercole, A. (2021). How artificial intelligence and machine learning can help healthcare systems respond to COVID-19. *Machine Learning*, 110(1), 1–4.

Vieira, S., Pinaya, W.H., Mechelli, A. (2017). Using deep learning to investigate the neuroimaging correlates of psychiatric and neurological disorders: Methods and applications. *Neuroscience & Biobehavioral Reviews*, 74, 58–75.

Warin, K., Limprasert, W., Suebnukarn, S., Jinapornthan, S., Jantana, P., Vicharueang, S. (2022). AI-based analysis of oral lesions using novel deep convolutional neural networks for early detection of oral cancer. *Plos One*, 17(8), e0273508.

Warren, S.L. and Moustafa, A.A. (2023). Functional magnetic resonance imaging, deep learning, and Alzheimer's disease: A systematic review. *Journal of Neuroimaging*, 33(1), 5–18.

Winter, J.S. and Davidson, E. (2019). Big data governance of personal health information and challenges to contextual integrity. *The Information Society*, 35(1), 36–51.

Woo, C.W., Chang, L.J., Lindquist, M.A., Wager, T.D. (2017). Building better biomarkers: Brain models in translational neuroimaging. *Nature Neuroscience*, 20(3), 365–377.

5

AI-Enhanced Stroke Diagnosis, Prognosis and Rehabilitation Pathways

Stroke is considered to be the major cause of mortality and sever impairment throughout the world. It places a huge burden on healthcare systems and society. Despite new neuroimaging, medications and rehabilitation, it is hard to diagnose a stroke fast and precisely. Another significant challenge is to predict functional outcomes and design rehabilitation plans. Artificial intelligence (AI), such as machine learning, deep learning and multimodal data analytics, is transforming into a revolution in stroke care. CT and MRI scans are almost as accurately analyzed by AI-based diagnostic models as the most talented radiologists. Clinical, imaging and genomic prognostic models have the ability to forecast the outcome for a patient in terms of recovery, risk of recurrence and treatment response. Moreover, AI-based rehabilitation systems include robotics, wearable and brain–computer interfaces to enhance therapy. They identify real-time progress and enable individualized neurorehabilitation programs. These technologies also enhance the decision-making processes at the clinic and expand access to underserved populations via telemedicine and home-based systems. However, issues of data privacy, model generalizability, lack of interpretability and the obstacles of incorporating AI into clinical operations are still critical issues. This chapter will recall the present developments in AI-assisted stroke diagnosis, prognosis and rehabilitation. It covers new innovations, present limitations and future research directions. Integrating computational intelligence with clinical practice, AI can radically transform the treatment of stroke and a shift to precision-based and patient-centered treatment.

5.1. Introduction

Stroke is perpetually among the foremost fatal and persistent causes of disability across the globe. Millions of people sufferer annually from stroke, and many who survive are left with permanent disabilities, affecting their ability to move, talk, think

Chapter written by Rahul PATIL and Fazil SHEIKH.

and feel. These individual impacts include independence, quality of life and mental health (WHO 2021). At the societal level, stroke leads to high direct costs in emergency and continuous care, and indirect costs due to work loss and necessitating the presence of informal caregivers. Stroke continues to be one of the three leading causes of death in the world; thus, there is a pressing need to find alternative methods of diagnosing, prognosticating and reinstating patients. Despite significant improvements in treatment during the first critical hour, further optimization is still required to enhance patient outcomes. (Millán 2024).

Stroke patient care can be split into three linked processes. First, such diagnosis involves early and precise identification of the kind of stroke – ischemic or hemorrhagic – and the location of the damage, to be able to begin treatments such as clot-breaking drugs or mechanical clearing of the clot at the appropriate time. Wrong categorizing or delays may severely impair the quality of treatment. Second, prognosis entails prediction of the recovery capacity of a patient, probability of the occurrence of another stroke and the likelihood of surviving. The conventional methods such as the NIH Stroke Scale and modified Rankin Scale provide general estimations but do not help in customizing the predictions. Third, rehabilitation attempts to achieve maximum recovery based on physical training, cognitive activities, speech therapy and emotional aid. Depending on individual patients, the results vary widely, and the current programs tend to be inefficient in changing with the progress of every patient (Deo 2015).

AI, such as machine learning, deep learning and advanced analytics, has been perceived to be a revolutionary tool throughout the stroke continuum. Datasets, which are massive and heterogeneous, such as brain scans, electronic health records, genetics and readings by wearable sensors, can be analyzed by AI models in ways that cannot be covered by typical statistics. AI can analyze CT and MRI images in diagnosis automatically, detect small ischemic lesions, delineate lesions and automatically classify the type of stroke with the same level of accuracy as expert radiologists. During prognosis of recovery, predictive models may combine clinical and imaging as well as time-based data, to identify high-risk patients and advise individual care strategies. In rehabilitation, AI provides innovation, such as adaptive robotic assistance, brain–computer interface and tele-rehab, where the intensity and type of therapy are adjusted to actual performance in real-time (van der Weijden et al. 2023).

The inclusion of AI in stroke care fits into the larger trend of precision medicine, where treatment is adjusted to each individual biological, clinical and lifestyle profile. AI has the ability to transform the process of stroke management – both in the emergency room and in home recovery by providing earlier detection, personalized risk prediction and tailored therapy. Nevertheless, there are a number of hurdles. There are concerns regarding data quality and the compatibility of systems, algorithm bias and fairness, answer explanations and clinician trust, and regulatory consensus and payment. In addition, the majority of AI models are developed and tested in small environments, and it is uncertain how effective they will be when applied to different patients and health systems across the globe.

This chapter is a comprehensive overview of the existing and novel applications of AI in stroke care, which is structured based on the main spheres of stroke care, diagnosis, prognosis and rehabilitation. It also brings attention to technological advancements, clinical advantages, current issues and future research directions that will promote large-scale adoption. Associating computational intelligence and medical expertise, AI has the capacity to transform stroke management, enhance patient outcome and alleviate the global burden of this complicated disease.

5.2. AI in stroke diagnosis

5.2.1. *Importance of early and accurate diagnosis*

Stroke is a health crisis. Early diagnosis is critical for isolating the illness, as well as decreasing mortality. Early detection of a stroke enables the physician to administer clot-busting therapy in the case of an ischemic stroke or the rapid planning of surgery in the event of a hemorrhagic stroke. The traditional practices depend on the examination of imaging, patient history and physical examination by a clinician. Nevertheless, human judgment is subject to error, individuals become weary and professional radiologists are frequently unavailable, particularly in low-resource or more remote locations (Bojsen et al. 2024). A late diagnosis implies reduced efficacy of reperfusion therapy, increased stay in the hospital and adverse long-term outcomes. Stroke can be quickly and automatically identified with the help of AI, which can potentially reduce the critical so-called door-to-needle time and save lives.

5.2.2. *AI applications based on neuroimaging*

Stroke diagnosis relies on neuroimaging. The most widespread scans are CT and MRI. AI, and more specifically, the deep learning architectures such as convolutional neural networks (CNN), has demonstrated high accuracy in detecting ischemic lesions on CT scans and at times more accurate than a trained neuroradiologist (Koska and Selver 2023). As an example, CNNs that are trained on large datasets are capable of detecting early low-density areas, distinguishing core infarcts and penumbral tissue, and generating volume segmentation. Other deep-learning-based applications to diffusion-weighted MRI (DWI) are useful to identify small or subtle infarcts, which can be overlooked during regular examination

(Jiang et al. 2025). Hematoma volumes can also be determined with precision with the help of automated segmentation of hemorrhagic strokes, which is essential when it comes to predetermining the outcomes and performing surgery (Adablanu et al. 2025).

5.2.3. *Stroke subtype differentiations*

It is important to know whether an attack is ischemic or hemorrhagic as different treatments are required. AI classifiers using imaging characteristics, clinical and lab data may precisely differentiate between stroke subtypes (Liu et al. 2024). On CT angiography (CTA) and MR angiography (MRA), they can identify the large-vessel occlusions, assisting in making quick decisions regarding mechanical thrombectomy (Bani-Sadr n.d.). Some AI systems can also combine a variety of imaging modalities such as CT perfusion, CTA and MRI sequences to form complex stroke profiles that provide diagnostic and prognostic data. This kind of integration is particularly handy during an emergency, when it is imperative to have speed and precision.

5.2.4. *Incorporating multimodal biomarkers*

In other imaging modes, clinical, lab and physiological biomarkers are becoming increasingly integrated into AI frameworks to enhance diagnosis. Machine learning algorithms have the ability to combine vital signs, laboratory measures (such as glucose or coagulation indicators), EEG monitoring and patient demographics to identify when (and what type of) stroke takes place (Klug et al. 2024). The preliminary experience of using wearable and AI-assisted devices indicates that portable blood pressure monitors can monitor blood pressure, heart rhythm and other parameters in real-time and report possible cerebrovascular events before the patient arrives at a hospital. These methods make AI better suited to in-hospital diagnoses and pre-hospital triage, so the AI can respond more quickly with potentially improved outcomes in underserved areas (Lee et al. 2023).

5.2.5. *The use of AI in rapid triage and workflow optimization*

AI can be used, not only to make a diagnosis, but also in operations. There are triage systems powered by AI that are applied in some emergency departments to identify potential strokes, put imaging first, and notify specialized teams. Research has shown that the system will be able to reduce the time taken to make a diagnosis and even enhance compliance with the recommended treatment windows given by guidelines. The real-time analysis of AI images may assist in giving rapid readouts prior to official radiology analysis when clinicians need to make quicker decisions, which remain safe and accurate (Koska and Selver 2023; Bojsen et al. 2024). Moreover, AI will be able to track patient movement, identify possible bottlenecks and streamline the use of resources in centers with a large volume of stroke patients.

5.2.6. *Challenges and limitations*

AI stroke care presents difficulties regardless of its potential. Most models are conditioned with information from a particular population or large resource institution, restricting their generalization. The accuracy for minority groups may be lower due to algorithmic prejudice, which should encourage the need to include such groups in datasets. Lack of regulatory barriers, standards and liability issues also interfere with mass adoption. The privacy of data and communication within current hospital systems are serious concerns, where large-scale implementation will have to be solved (Adablanu et al. 2025; Jiang et al. 2025). Finally, clear, interpretable AI outputs are required to increase clinicians' faith in automated decisions and integrate them successfully into patient care.

5.3. AI in stroke prognosis

5.3.1. *The need for accurate prognostic models*

The outcomes of stroke are diverse and depend on a lot of different factors such as the size or location of the lesion, the age of a patient, other medical disorders, the initial neurological impairment and the type of treatment applied. Proper prediction of functional recovery, recurrence risk and mortality, is important in order to customize treatment, resource allocation and offer realistic expectations to patients and caregivers. The most commonly used prognostic instruments such as the National Institutes of Health Stroke Scale (NIHSS) and the modified Rankin Scale (mRS) give a cross-sectional view of the initial severity but they do not reflect the multifactorial relationships between clinical, imaging and biological factors that influence recovery (Huang et al. 2024).

The solutions to these limitations are provided by AI, which manifests itself by linking high-dimensional and multimodal data to predictive models. Machine learning and deep learning programs can detect trends in imaging and electronic health records, and data produced by wearable sensors, enhancing the prediction of who can be affected and in what way.

5.3.2. *Predicting functional outcomes*

An important aspect of patient care after a stroke is the ability to predict their post-stroke functioning status. Functional independence is typically determined by the mRS when the doctor is three- or six-months post-stroke. Recent studies indicate that the ensemble learning models, comprised of random forests, gradient ready machines and neural networks, have proven to be more effective in forecasting mRS scores, compared to their regular regression counterparts (Otieno et al. 2024). For example, models integrating CT lesion volume, diffusion-weighted MRI data, clinical variables (age, baseline NIHSS), and laboratory biomarkers have shown improved prediction of motor and cognitive recovery. Deep learning models can also capture nonlinear relationships and complex spatial patterns in imaging data, providing individualized recovery trajectories (Li et al. 2023).

Such predictive insights can guide decisions regarding the intensity and type of rehabilitation, early discharge planning and the likelihood of requiring long-term care or assistive devices. Additionally, identifying patients at risk for poor outcomes enables early initiation of targeted interventions and family counseling.

5.3.3. *Mortality and recurrence risk prediction*

Secondary prevention and risk stratification requires the accurate prediction of mortality and recurrent stroke. Dynamically predicting risks over time is possible using AI models based on longitudinal EHR data and vital signs and imaging biomarkers. RNNs and TCNs are particularly useful when time-based data is involved, such as time-series data, where trends and movements of patient physiology can be analyzed (Wang et al. 2024). Both early and late complications can be predicted using these models so that the clinician can more precisely target the pharmacologic therapies (antiplatelet or anticoagulant medication) and lifestyle interventions.

5.3.4. *Treatment planning*

Customizing the intervention with each individual requires a thorough evaluation of personal factors, needs and preferences, especially considering the age and cognitive development.

An individualized treatment plan may also be guided via AI prognostic models. Radiomic-based predictive algorithms, which incorporate the radiomic features of CT scans and MRI with clinical and genomic data, are being formulated to predict the patient's reaction to thrombolysis, thrombectomy or rehabilitation treatment

(Abujaber et al. 2024). This method is in line with precision medicine, which seeks to select interventions that can achieve the optimal functional recovery with the minimum adverse events.

Moreover, these models are able to simulate the what-if scenarios, which approximate the results based on alternative treatment plans. As an illustration, they will be able to forecast the probability of successful recovery in the case of higher intensity rehabilitation being escalated, and manage to allocate resources effectively while maximizing patient-centered care.

5.3.5. *Explainability and clinical trust*

One of the largest obstacles in the clinical implementation of AI prognostic tools is the non-transparency surrounding model decisions. Most deep learning models are black boxes, and clinicians have problems understanding the mechanisms underlying the generation of a prediction. Explainable AI (XAI) methods, such as feature importance analysis, SHapley Additive exPlanations (SHAP) and saliency mapping, provide insight into the factors driving predictions (Malviya et al. 2025). For example, highlighting which imaging features or clinical variables most strongly influenced an adverse outcome prediction can enhance clinician confidence, support shared decision-making and facilitate validation in local patient populations.

5.3.6. *Integration with clinical workflow*

Effective use of AI prognostic tools requires integration into existing clinical workflows. Models must provide actionable, interpretable outputs that can inform multidisciplinary team decisions without adding undue cognitive or operational burden. Early studies indicate that embedding prognostic dashboards into stroke units improves planning for rehabilitation services, discharge and follow-up, while also allowing ongoing monitoring of model performance and recalibration as patient populations evolve (Ahmed and Husien 2024).

5.4. AI in stroke rehabilitation pathways

5.4.1. *Importance of personalized rehabilitation*

Post-stroke rehabilitation is a cornerstone of recovery, aiming to restore motor function, cognitive abilities, language skills and independence in daily activities. Traditional rehabilitation often follows generalized protocols, which may not account for individual differences in stroke severity, lesion location, age, comorbidities or neuroplastic potential. This one-size-fits-all approach can lead to suboptimal outcomes and inefficient use of therapy resources. AI offers the ability to personalize rehabilitation programs by analyzing patient-specific data, adapting therapy intensity and providing continuous feedback, ultimately optimizing recovery trajectories (Zhang et al. 2024).

5.4.2. *Robotics-assisted rehabilitation*

In robotics-assisted rehabilitation, a robot is designed to work with a patient and a therapist to achieve recovery.

AI-based rehab has now become inclusive of robots. Exoskeleton and end-effector robots provide patients with high-intensity, controlled, and repetitive training, which is essential for promoting brain plasticity. Machine learning algorithms can modify resistance, speed and the difficulty of the task in real-time depending on parameters such as range of motion, strength and smoothness (Elashmawi et al. 2024). As an example, an adaptive system is capable of identifying minute progress or plateaus and adjusting the training program to challenge the patient without overburdening them. Robot therapy has been demonstrated to be more effective in enhancing amputation – arm and leg – recovery compared to conventional treatment.

5.4.3. *Wearable sensors and real-time monitoring*

Wearable sensors, including IMUs, EMG units and pressure sensitive insoles, are used to monitor the quality of movement, gait and muscle motion in real-time. AI analyzes such complicated data to quantify improvements, identify compensations and propose individual modifications (Kim et al. 2025). Real-time interventions, such as constant gait symmetry and joint angle monitoring, can be launched by constant analysis and could make lower-limb rehabilitation more efficient; it could also decrease the risk of falls.

5.4.4. *Neurofeedback and brain–computer interfaces*

BCIs are brain-based interventions that assist patients who are not able to exercise normally. AI can convert brain activity, via decoding EEG or ECoG actions, into signals that can control the robots or virtual avatars passing through the damaged portions of the motor nexus (Raffin and Hummel 2018). Neurofeedback incorporates visual/auditory feedback to the patients regarding their brain activity stimulating cortical rearrangements. Research indicates that BCI-aided therapy improves arm and hand activity, motor imagery and brain connectivity, particularly with conventional rehabilitation.

5.4.5. *Virtual reality and game-based rehabilitation*

VR and gamification enhance interest and favoritism – which is essential to compliance and malleability. VR based on AI generates immersions wherein the intensity is automatically changed in response to the performance of the patient (Kien et al. 2024). AI is capable of modifying the speed, complexity and feedback of virtual reach or grasp tasks based on an assessment of movement accuracy that is being conducted. The gamified VR has been found to enhance arm dexterity, balance, as well as patient independence and satisfaction when compared to traditional therapy.

5.4.6. *The use of tele-rehabilitation and remote monitoring*

AI tele-rehab platforms provide therapy beyond the hospital, which enhances access to remote/underserved patients. They use wearable sensors + cloud analytics, video calls and AI to track the progress and performance, and offer personalized therapy recommendations (Ostrowska et al. 2021). Exercises are effective and challenging due to real-time feedback. Tele-rehab demonstrated the continuity that can be achieved by remote delivery while still not affecting the outcome during Covid-19. AI helps to monitor compliance, exhaustion and risk analysis, and makes customizing programs fast for clinicians.

5.4.7. *Integration of multimodal data*

One of the key advantages of AI in rehabilitation is the integration of multimodal data sources. By combining imaging biomarkers, clinical assessments, wearable sensor outputs and neural activity measures, AI models can predict recovery potential and recommend individualized therapy plans (Burns et al. 2022). Multimodal learning frameworks can forecast functional outcomes, identify patients at risk of delayed recovery and guide intensity modulation in real-time. This holistic approach enhances precision in rehabilitation and supports data-driven clinical decision-making.

5.5. Integration into clinical workflows

5.5.1. *The need for seamless integration*

For AI to meaningfully improve stroke outcomes, algorithms must move beyond research settings and integrate seamlessly into everyday clinical workflows. Standalone AI tools, no matter how accurate, have limited impact if their outputs are not accessible or interpretable by clinicians at the point of care. Integration requires that AI systems provide timely, actionable insights, such as automated detection of large vessel occlusions, lesion segmentation, risk predictions or personalized rehabilitation recommendations, directly within imaging, EHR or decision support platforms (Duncan and Bernhardt 2021).

5.5.2. *Decision support systems in practice*

AI-driven decision support systems (DSS) can improve triage, diagnosis and treatment planning. For example, systems embedded in stroke units can automatically flag suspected stroke cases, prioritize imaging and alert multidisciplinary teams, reducing time-to-treatment. Predictive dashboards can provide risk stratification for functional outcomes, recurrence or mortality, guiding therapy intensity and discharge planning. Real-world implementation studies indicate that AI-assisted workflows can shorten "door-to-needle" times, improve adherence to guideline-recommended interventions and reduce the length of stay in hospitals, demonstrating tangible clinical value (Duncan and Bernhardt 2021).

5.5.3. *Interoperability and data standards*

Data interoperability is a critical requirement for integration. Stroke AI systems must communicate with heterogeneous clinical data sources, including PACS imaging systems, EHRs and wearable sensor platforms. Standardized data formats such as DICOM for imaging and FHIR for clinical records facilitate model deployment and continuous learning. Consistent labeling and harmonization of datasets are essential for model generalization across multiple hospitals and patient populations. Without standardization, AI outputs risk being unreliable or inconsistent, undermining clinician trust (Munce et al. 2023).

5.5.4. *Privacy and regulatory considerations*

Data privacy in healthcare is a priority issue. Privacy-friendly machine learning methods, known as federated learning, are available to progressively train AI models in institutions without necessarily revealing sensitive patient information. These approaches contribute to the observance of data protection rules, access to a variety of datasets, enhanced generalizability and the bias of algorithms. The regulatory systems are also undergoing change to regulate AI in clinical practice. Continuously or constantly updating prediction models poses special problems regarding approval and monitoring; it must have clear instructions and validation criteria to promote safety and efficacy when developing clinician confidence.

5.5.5. *Acceptance and explainability of clinicians*

Acceptance by clinicians is essential to integration. The predictions made with AI need to be understandable, practical and they should integrate seamlessly with the current processes. XAI methods, including feature-importance maps, saliency visualizations and confidence scores, enable clinicians to better understand the logic behind model results, which leads to increased trust and acceptance. To transform AI tools and make them useful in the real-world setting, it is necessary to have training programs and multidisciplinary cooperation and continuous feedback between the clinicians and developers (Duncan and Bernhardt 2021; Munce et al. 2023).

Domain	AI techniques used	Key applications	Clinical benefits
Diagnosis	Deep learning (CNNs), machine learning	Automated detection of ischemic and hemorrhagic lesions on CT/MRI; stroke subtype classification; workflow triage	Early and accurate diagnosis; reduced "door-to-needle" time; improved emergency decision-making
Prognosis	Ensemble learning, random forest, gradient boosting, deep neural networks, RNNs	Prediction of functional outcomes (mRS), mortality, recurrence; treatment response modeling	Individualized care planning; early identification of high-risk patients; enhanced resource allocation
Rehabilitation	AI-driven robotics, brain–computer interfaces (BCI), wearables, virtual reality	Adaptive robotic therapy; real-time monitoring; neurofeedback and tele-rehabilitation	Personalized therapy; enhanced recovery; continuous patient engagement, even at home
Integration and Workflow	Explainable AI (XAI), decision support systems (DSS), federated learning	Clinical workflow integration; privacy-preserving data sharing; interoperability with EHR systems	Improved clinician trust; ethical and secure AI implementation

Table 5.1. *Applications of artificial intelligence in stroke care*

5.6. Future directions

5.6.1. *Understandable and reliable AI*

Increasing AI in the process of stroke care, explainability, transparency and trustworthiness are crucial. Clinicians need to be aware of why a model is making a prediction so that they can be confident in using the model. XAI systems allow clinicians to visualize the parts of an image, clinical phenomenon or physiological measurements that have contributed most to a finding (Uddin et al. 2024). In the future, the field of research should concentrate on models that prevent tradeoffs among accuracy, interpretability, and thus clinicians should be in a position to use AI at crucial moments. Regulatory acceptance and extended clinical practice will also depend on the standardized reporting guidelines of interpretability.

5.6.2. *Equity, bias mitigation and fairness*

The issue of algorithmic bias is still an overwhelming challenge, in particular in heterogeneous patient groups. The future AI needs to be able to tackle age-related, sex, ethnicity and socioeconomic disparities. The possibility of training models, using heterogeneous multicenter datasets to minimize bias, and constant monitoring of real-world performance can make sure that it is applied fairly. The strategies include the bias audits, subgroup performance analysis and fairness–conscious learning algorithms, which are crucial for developing trust in AI and implementing it in stroke care in an ethical manner (Uddin et al. 2024).

5.6.3. *Federated and privacy-preserving learning*

Federated learning, secure multiparty computation and differential privacy are privacy-preserving approaches, which will become the focus of future AI. These methods enable various institutions to prepare models jointly without having access to raw patient data, increasing the diversity of the data and compliancy with privacy regulations (Yadav et al. 2025). As more electronic health records, imaging archives and wearable sensor data are available, federated learning is scalable to apply distributed data, producing robust AI models that are applicable across populations and healthcare systems.

5.6.4. *Multimodal and continuous prognostication*

Future AI systems are likely to leverage multimodal data integration to provide continuous prognostication throughout the acute, subacute and chronic phases of stroke. Combining neuroimaging, clinical records, physiological monitoring and genomic data enables dynamic risk assessment and individualized care planning. AI models capable of continuous learning can update predictions in real-time, supporting adaptive treatment and rehabilitation strategies. Such systems will be particularly valuable for monitoring patients remotely, optimizing therapy intensity and anticipating complications before they manifest clinically (Yadav et al. 2025).

5.6.5. *Scalable tele-rehabilitation and home-based therapy*

Tele-rehabilitation platforms, enhanced by AI, are expected to become increasingly widespread. These platforms combine real-time monitoring via wearable sensors, adaptive therapy algorithms, gamified virtual exercises and remote clinician supervision. AI can personalize exercise programs, detect deviations or plateaus, and provide feedback to both patients and therapists. Scalable, AI-driven home rehabilitation will improve access for patients in rural or resource-limited regions, reduce healthcare costs and maintain therapy adherence over long recovery periods.

5.6.6. *Neurotechnology and advanced brain–computer interfaces*

Emerging neurotechnologies, including non-invasive and minimally invasive BCIs, closed-loop neurostimulation and AI-enhanced neurofeedback, offer unprecedented opportunities for patients with severe motor deficits. Future studies should focus on large-scale, longitudinal trials to evaluate efficacy, safety and long-term neuroplasticity outcomes. Integration of these neurotechnologies with multimodal AI prognostic models could further personalize rehabilitation, optimize therapy schedules and accelerate functional recovery.

5.7. Conclusion

AI is transforming stroke care across the entire continuum – from rapid diagnosis to individualized prognostication and personalized rehabilitation. In diagnosis, AI algorithms, particularly deep learning models, enhance neuroimaging interpretation by detecting ischemic lesions, quantifying hemorrhage volumes and distinguishing stroke subtypes with speed and accuracy comparable to expert clinicians. Early and precise identification enables timely interventions, reduces "door-to-needle" times and improves patient outcomes. In prognosis, AI models integrate multimodal data, including imaging biomarkers, clinical parameters, laboratory results and longitudinal physiological data, to predict functional recovery, recurrence risk and mortality. These models are more accurate and personalized than the traditional scoring systems. They endorse precision medicine and allow clinicians to customize interventions to the recovery process of every patient. Explainable AI facilitates clinician trust through providing actionable insights and being transparent. AI-based rehabilitation is one of the most significant integrations. Therapy through robotics, brain–computer interfaces, virtual reality, wearable sensors and tele-rehabilitation platforms is provided at a level that is responsive to the performance of the person. It results in increased motor recovery, increased cognitive performance and increased treatment adherence, which can be provided outside of a clinical environment and improve access to underserved populations. However, challenges persist. There are data heterogeneity, algorithmic bias, regulatory concerns, workflow integration and privacy concerns. It will be essential to address them with explanatory, fair and privacy-aware AI, as well as maintaining the strict focus on prospective validation, to achieve safe and effective clinical use.

5.8. References

Abujaber, A.A., Albalkhi, I., Imam, Y., Nashwan, A., Akhtar, N., Alkhawaldeh, I.M. (2024). Machine learning-based prognostication of mortality in stroke patients. *Heliyon*, 10(7), e28869.

Adablanu, S., Barman, U., Das, D. (2025). Advancing deep learning for automated stroke detection: A review. *Brain Hemorrhages*, 6(5), 247–260.

Ahmed, M. and Husien, I. (2024). Heart disease prediction using hybrid machine learning: A brief review. *Journal of Robotics and Control (JRC)*, 5(3), 884–892.

Bani-Sadr, A. (n.d.). Impact de l'IRM multimodale dans la prise en charge des AVC ischémiques à la phase aigüe. Doctoral Dissertation, Université Claude Bernard-Lyon I.

Bojsen, J.A., Elhakim, M.T., Graumann, O., Gaist, D., Nielsen, M., Harbo, F.S.G., Krag, C.H., Sagar, M.V., Kruuse, C., Boesen, M.P. et al. (2024). Artificial intelligence for MRI stroke detection: A systematic review and meta-analysis. *Insights Imaging*, 15(1), 160.

Burns, S.P., Fleming, T.K., Webb, S.S., Kam, A.S., Fielder, J.D., Kim, G.J., Hu, X., Hill, M.T., Kringle, E.A. (2022). Stroke recovery during the COVID-19 pandemic: A position paper on recommendations for rehabilitation. *Archives of Physical Medicine and Rehabilitation*, 103(9), 1874–1882.

Deo, R.C. (2015). Machine learning in medicine. *Circulation*, 132(20), 1920–1930.

Duncan, P.W. and Bernhardt, J. (2021). Telerehabilitation: Has its time come? *Stroke*, 52(8), 2694–2696.

Elashmawi, W.H., Ayman, A., Antoun, M., Mohamed, H., Mohamed, S.E., Amr, H., Talaat, Y., Ali, A. (2024). A comprehensive review on brain–computer interface (BCI)-based machine and deep learning algorithms for stroke rehabilitation. *Applied Sciences*, 14(14), 6347.

Huang, Q., Shou, G.L., Shi, B., Li, M.L., Zhang, S., Han, M., Hu, F.Y. (2024). Machine learning is an effective method to predict the 3-month prognosis of patients with acute ischemic stroke. *Frontiers in Neurology*, 15, 1407152.

Jiang, B., Pham, N., van Staalduinen, E.K., Liu, Y., Nazari-Farsani, S., Sanaat, A., van Voorst, H., Fettahoglu, A., Kim, D., Ouyang, J. et al. (2025). Deep learning applications in imaging of acute ischemic stroke: A systematic review and narrative summary. *Radiology*, 315(1), e240775.

Kien, N.M., Long, V.T., Chau, M.T., Anh, N.T. (2024). A VR–BCI system to support rehabilitation for stroke patients. In *International Conference on Brain Informatics*, 12 December, 125–136. Springer, Singapore.

Kim, M.S., Park, H., Kwon, I., An, K.O., Kim, H., Park, G., Hyung, W., Im, C.H., Shin, J.H. (2025). Efficacy of brain-computer interface training with motor imagery-contingent feedback in improving upper limb function and neuroplasticity among persons with chronic stroke: A double-blinded, parallel-group, randomized controlled trial. *Journal of NeuroEngineering and Rehabilitation*, 22(1), 1.

Klug, J., Leclerc, G., Dirren, E., Carrera, E. (2024). Machine learning for early dynamic prediction of functional outcome after stroke. *Communications Medicine*, 4(1), 232.

Koska, I.O. and Selver, A. (2023). Artificial intelligence in stroke imaging: A comprehensive review. *The Eurasian Journal of Medicine*, 55(Suppl 1), S91.

Lee, J., Park, K.M., Park, S. (2023). Interpretable machine learning for prediction of clinical outcomes in acute ischemic stroke. *Frontiers in Neurology*, 14, 1234046.

Li, Q., Chi, L., Zhao, W., Wu, L., Jiao, C., Zheng, X., Zhang, K., Li, X. (2023). Machine learning prediction of motor function in chronic stroke patients: A systematic review and meta-analysis. *Frontiers in Neurology*, 14, 1039794.

Liu, Y., Wen, Z., Wang, Y., Zhong, Y., Wang, J., Hu, Y., Zhou, P., Guo, S. (2024). Artificial intelligence in ischemic stroke images: Current applications and future directions. *Frontiers in Neurology*, 15, 1418060.

Malviya, R., Singh, A.K., Sharma, R. (2025). *Photodynamic Therapy for the Management of Disease: Advances and Perspectives*. Apple Academic Press, Palm Bay, FL.

Millán, J.S. (2024). *Control Strategies for Robotic Exoskeletons to Assist Post-Stroke Hemiparetic Gait: An Assistive Approach Based on Technology Embodiment*. Springer, Cham.

Munce, S., Andreoli, A., Bayley, M., Guo, M., Inness, E.L., Kua, A., McIntyre, M. (2023). Clinicians' experiences of implementing a telerehabilitation toolkit during the COVID-19 pandemic: Qualitative descriptive study. *JMIR Rehabilitation and Assistive Technologies*, 10, e44591.

Ostrowska, P.M., Śliwiński, M., Studnicki, R., Hansdorfer-Korzon, R. (2021). Telerehabilitation of post-stroke patients as a therapeutic solution in the era of the COVID-19 pandemic. *Healthcare*, 9(6), 654.

Otieno, J.A., Häggström, J., Darehed, D., Eriksson, M. (2024). Developing machine learning models to predict multi-class functional outcomes and death three months after stroke in Sweden. *PLoS One*, 19(5), e0303287.

Raffin, E. and Hummel, F.C. (2018). Restoring motor functions after stroke: Multiple approaches and opportunities. *The Neuroscientist*, 24(4), 400–416.

Uddin, M., Ganapathy, K., Syed-Abdul, S. (2024). Digital technology enablers of tele-neurorehabilitation in pre-and post-COVID-19 pandemic era – A scoping review. *International Journal of Telerehabilitation*, 16(1), e6611.

Wang, Z., Yang, W., Li, Z., Rong, Z., Wang, X., Han, J., Ma, L. (2024). A 25-year retrospective of the use of AI for diagnosing acute stroke: Systematic review. *Journal of Medical Internet Research*, 26, e59711.

van der Weijden, C.W., Biondetti, E., Gutmann, I.W., Dijkstra, H., McKerchar, R., de Paula Faria, D., de Vries, E.F., Meilof, J.F., Dierckx, R.A., Prevost, V.H. et al. (2023). Quantitative myelin imaging with MRI and PET: An overview of techniques and their validation status. *Brain*, 146(4), 1243–1266.

World Health Organization (2021). Global Burden of Stroke—Facts and Figures. WHO, Geneva.

Yadav, J., More, A., Ghosh, B., Sinha, D., Chavane, N., Kumari, A., Datta, A., Borah, A., Bhattacharya, P. (2025). Implications of artificial intelligence in stroke intervention and care. *Iradiology*, 3(2), 115–131.

Zhang, M., Zhu, F., Jia, F., Wu, Y., Wang, B., Gao, L., Chu, F., Tang, W. (2024). Efficacy of brain–computer interfaces on upper extremity motor function rehabilitation after stroke: A systematic review and meta-analysis. *NeuroRehabilitation*, 54(2), 199–212.

6

Computational Biomarker Discovery for Neurological and Psychiatric Disorders

Neurology and psychiatry oversee some of the most common causes of disability in the world, but it is challenging to diagnose and treat them due to the lack of homogeneity in the manifestations of the diseases and a shortage of objective methods. Biomarkers have become essential in the initial diagnosis, following up on the disease and monitoring response to treatment. With advanced algorithms – machine learning and deep learning – complex patterns that would be difficult to identify through traditional statistical techniques can be identified, and predictive and prognostic biomarkers be determined more frequently, resulting in the possibility of precision medicine in neurology and psychiatry. This chapter discusses the current state of the computational biomarker discovery which is applied in key neurological disorders such as Alzheimer's disease, Parkinson's disease, epilepsy and multiple sclerosis, and psychiatric disorders such as major depressive disorder, schizophrenia, bipolar disorder and autism spectrum disorder. The role of computational models in managing multimodal data, recognizing disease-specific patterns and giving clinical interpretable results is emphasized. This chapter also identifies challenges that inhibit clinical translation, such as data inconsistency, absence of standards, ethical concerns and regulatory hurdles. Lastly, the perspectives on the future directions are addressed, focusing on integrative frameworks to incorporate artificial intelligence (AI), systems biology and digital phenotyping towards the creation of robust and clinically actionable biomarkers.

6.1. Introduction

Neurological and psychiatric disorders represent some of the most significant public health challenges of the 21st century. Conditions such as Alzheimer's disease (AD), Parkinson's disease (PD), epilepsy, multiple sclerosis, major depressive disorder (MDD), schizophrenia, bipolar disorder and autism spectrum disorder (ASD) collectively affect hundreds of millions of people worldwide and contribute

Chapter written by Chaitnya GODBOLE and Shamla MANTRI.

substantially to disability and reduced quality of life (Glewwe et al. 2025). Beyond the personal toll, these disorders impose a considerable socioeconomic burden due to long-term healthcare needs, loss of productivity and caregiving demands. Despite decades of research, diagnosis and treatment remain suboptimal, largely because current methods rely heavily on clinical observation and self-reported symptoms, which are often subjective and imprecise.

The need to find objective and quantifiable biomarkers has come to the fore in the world of neurology and psychiatry.

6.1.1. *Biomarkers defined*

Biomarkers are quantifiable variables of biological conditions, pathophysiology or treatment effects. They are able to offer important information on disease pathologies, enable early diagnosis and aid in patient stratification and monitoring treatment. Neuroimaging biomarkers, for example, hippocampal atrophy in cases of AD or dopaminergic dysfunction in PD, have been extensively investigated in neurological conditions. Electrophysiological patterns, genetic variation and digital behavioral signatures are becoming the most likely biomarkers used in psychiatric disorders (Asif et al. 2025). However, the range of promising results is shadowed by the fact that not many biomarkers have reached clinical utility due to reproducibility, scalability and mechanistic validation problems.

In the last 10 years, computation has revolutionized the discovery of biomarkers. Machine learning, artificial intelligence (AI) and data-driven modeling can now analyze complex and high-dimensional datasets, which incorporate genomics, transcriptomics, proteomics, metabolomics, neuroimaging, electrophysiology and digital health records. These methods detect nonlinear but subtle trends in nonhomogeneous sources of data, trends that standard statistics would not be likely to detect. To illustrate, a genetic and neuroimaging algorithm can be used to identify a disease risk or evidence of progression, whereas a natural language processing algorithm will retrieve the digital biomarkers of a patient through speech or text. These methods aid the narrowing of research to practice disconnects in clinical research (Chan et al. 2025).

The other aspect of great significance is the combination of multimodal data. There are seldom instances of neurological and psychiatric disorders that are caused by one biological change. They are a product of interaction between genetic disposition, environmental effects, brain connectivity and the expression of behavior. Combined computational models between these layers, for example, the correlations between transcriptomic responses and neuroimaging connections, or combined wearable-based behavioral responses with clinical scale, provide a more comprehensive disease perspective. This system-level approach makes it easier to discover predictive and yet informative biomarkers that can be mechanistic, which can further precision medicine.

These opportunities notwithstanding, there are still barriers to implementation. The manifestations of neurological and psychiatric conditions are highly diverse, varying not only between patients but also over time within the same individual. Data collection procedures differ across the board, which would make computational modeling difficult. Translation ability is also a problem in many machine learning approaches, which may increase concerns about their black-box behavior. Furthermore, computational biomarkers cannot be used fully in clinical workflows because of privacy concerns, biased algorithms and approval by the regulators.

This chapter will endeavor to give a holistic analysis of the computational biomarker discovery in the application of neurological and psychiatric conditions. We will initially explain computation methods, such as omics-based methods, neuroimaging analytics, electrophysiological signal processing and digital phenotyping. After this, we will cover machine learning and AI with a focus on supervised, unsupervised and deep learning, and newly emerging models of multimodal integration, and explainable AI (XAI). Then, we will comment on disorder-specific biomarker applications in the neurological and psychiatric fields, namely, AD, PD, epilepsy, multiple sclerosis, depression, schizophrenia, bipolar disorder and ASD. Lastly, we will discuss data heterogeneities, ethical concerns and the translational gap and suggest the way forward to improve the clinical implementation of computational biomarkers.

This chapter highlights the fact that computational approaches are transforming the process of biomarker discovery through synthesis of existing knowledge. These inventions have an early and more precise diagnosis, and they are the way towards individualized methods of treatment that have the potential to revolutionize the approach to managing neurological and psychiatric diseases.

6.2. Computational approaches for biomarker discovery

The discovery of credible biomarkers of neurological and psychiatric illnesses increasingly depends on the computational methods that are able to manipulate the high-dimensional and heterogeneous data. Conventional statistical procedures are finding it hard to represent the nonlinear interactions and multimodal patterns that are typical of biomedical data. Computational approaches, including omics applications, pipeline neuroimaging and electrophysiological signal processing, and digital phenotyping, are all key to finding compelling, clinically useful biomarkers today (Calhoun et al. 2021).

6.2.1. *Omics-based biomarker discovery*

The sources of biomarker discovery are highly abundant using high-throughput omics technologies such as genomics, transcriptomics, proteomics, metabolomics and epigenomics. Computer software is useful in spotting meaningful trends in these massive datasets, identifying disease-related signatures and prioritizing candidate biomarkers for further validation.

Genome-wide association studies (GWAS) have implicated a large number of genetic variations in nerve and mental illnesses. Nevertheless, the transfer of such findings to a clinical practice presupposes computational solutions that take into account the gene–gene and gene–environment interaction (Dai et al. 2025). Machine learning algorithms, random forests and support vectors may rank variants according to functional annotations and use them with clinical and imaging data.

Transcriptomics and proteomics provide the opportunity of dynamically profiling the expression of genes and proteins. Dysregulated pathways are detected as the possible biomarkers, which are network-based analyses and clustering algorithms, and are carried by a number of dysregulated pathways instead of just one gene (Ricetti et al. 2025). As an example, postmortem brain tissue transcriptomic profiles have been trained in machine learning classifiers to differentiate between schizophrenia and bipolar disorder. Proteomic profiling of cerebrospinal fluid (CSF) through the use of computational modeling has enhanced identifying diagnostic and prognostic biomarkers in AD (Możaryn and Szczegielniak 2025).

6.2.2. *Imaging-based biomarkers*

Neuroimaging is of prime focus in finding a biomarker of neurological and psychiatric disorders. Quantitative indicators of brain morphology, connectivity and function are offered by structural MRI (sMRI), functional MRI (fMRI), positron emission tomography (PET) and diffusion tensor imaging (DTI). Computational pipelines make it possible to process, extract features and model statistical imaging data.

Neuroimaging pipelines such as FreeSurfer, FSL and SPM can be used to analyze the structure and connection of the brain on a large scale. Disease states, and predictive effects of progression, can be classified and predicted using machine learning algorithms on imaging characteristics, such as cortical thickness, volumetric characteristics and functional connectivity. In one example, the classifier of support vector machines (SVM) applied to resting-state fMRI has differentiated between the AD patients and the normal population (Rosca and Stancu 2025).

A combination of imaging data is increasingly being multimodeled with the objective of enhancing the reliability of biomarkers. When sMRI is used along with fMRI, PET and DTI, a researcher can obtain the complementary features of brain pathology. Canonical correlation analysis, multimodal deep learning architectures and tensor decomposition are also some of the methods that have been used to identify convergent biomarkers. As an example, the combination of amyloid 185 PET and sMRI can enhance the early diagnosis of the AD, contrasted with analyses of individual modalities (Calhoun et al. 2021).

FmMRI-based connectivity biomarkers are associated with default mode; salience and executive network activity change in psychiatric disorders. These calculation indices indicate levels of disease and can be used to predict treatment response (Dai et al. 2025).

6.2.3. *Electrophysiological signals and digital phenotyping*

Electroencephalography (EEG) and magnetoencephalography (MEG) offer high temporal resolution for measuring brain activity. Computational signal processing methods, such as wavelet transforms, independent component analysis (ICA) and graph-theoretical approaches, extract features that serve as electrophysiological biomarkers.

For epilepsy, EEG data can be analyzed using a computer to identify and anticipate the seizures early. Machine learning, component-based models that are trained on pre-ictal EEGs have demonstrated that machine learning can pinpoint the most accurate biomarkers to predict seizures. Event-related potentials (ERPs) and oscillatory activity, when considered similarly in computational terms, are able to differentiate between schizophrenia, ADHD or depression and healthy controls in psychiatric disorders (Ricetti et al. 2025).

One of the most recent approaches is known as digital phenotyping, where smartphone and wearable data among other digital devices are used to monitor the pattern of behavior and physiology (Możaryn and Szczegielniak 2025). These continuous data streams are analyzed using machine learning models to detect biomarkers, including speech patterns, which indicate depression relapse or gait measurements, which are associated with PD.

6.2.4. *Multimodal data integration*

Single-modality biomarkers are frequently not robust, since neurological and psychiatric disorders are not homogeneous. Integrating information across a wide range of sources including omics, imaging, electrophysiology and digital health will allow us to find similar signatures that enhance prediction ability.

Multimodal integration algorithms include matrix factorization, multi-kernel learning, graph models and deep learning, such as multimodal autoencoders and graph convolutional networks. For example, integrating transcriptomic data with neuroimaging measures in schizophrenia has revealed multimodal biomarkers that outperform unimodal predictors (García-Gutiérrez et al. 2020). Multimodal integration also supports patient stratification, enabling precision medicine approaches tailored to biologically distinct subgroups.

6.3. Machine learning and AI in biomarker identification

There is currently more data available on neurology and psychiatry than ever before; this gives new opportunities to discover valuable biomarkers. Machine learning and AI are both appropriate in the treatment of large, diverse and multifarious data. They are able to identify some of the smallest trends that would not be detected by simple statistical procedures. Having these techniques, physicians are able to categorize illnesses more precisely, determine the patient's prospects, segment poor-risk and high-risk patients, and design individualized treatment plans (Lam et al. 2022).

6.3.1. *Supervised learning approaches*

Supervised learning accommodates algorithms by using labeled data to predict results such as disease condition, progress or reaction to therapy. SVMs, random forests, gradient boosting machines and logistic regression are common models.

SVMs used on resting-state fMRI or sMRI in neuroimaging can effectively distinguish between patients with either AD or PD, and normal controls (Eslami et al. 2019). Multi-omics-based random forest models have predicted psychiatric diseases including schizophrenia and MDD, based on predictive molecular biomarkers. Such features as LASSO regression and recursive feature elimination (RFE) are of great importance in dealing with high-dimensional omics data and enhancing the legibility of models (Zhang et al. 2020).

6.3.2. *Unsupervised learning approaches*

Unsupervised learning discovers concealed patterns within data which has no labels and can thus prove beneficial in the exploration of novel biomarkers. Some of the commonly used methods are k-means clustering, hierarchical clustering, Gaussian mixture models, principal component analysis (PCA) and t-stochastic neighbor embedding (t-SNE). These procedures provide an insight into the structure of complex data.

An example use is unsupervised clustering of multi-omics and neuroimaging data which has yielded biologically significant patient subsets in MDD and schizophrenia, which are helpful in discovering biomarkers unique to the subtype (Zheng et al. 2024). Unsupervised methods of networks, including weighted gene co-expression network analysis (WGCNA), find dysregulated modules of genes which could be used as potential biomarkers of disease.

6.3.3. *Deep learning in biomarker discovery*

Convolutional neural networks (CNNs), recurrent neural networks (RNNs), autoencoders and transformers are deep learning technologies that have demonstrated themselves to be capable of extracting hierarchical, nonlinear features of complex biomedical data. CNNs can particularly be useful with spatial data such as MRI data, PET images and histopathology images, whereas RNNs and transformers work better with sequential data such as EEGs or speech recordings.

Patterns of hippocampal atrophy, cortical thinning and white mark lesions can be easily detected using CNNs on sMRI, enhancing diagnostic accuracy in the AD (Alves et al. 2022). Deep learning on untreated EEG signals has boosted the ability to predict seizures and classify psychiatric disorders without the extra handcrafted features. Uncovered latent representations of features, small datasets and improved discovery of biomarkers in rare neurological diseases are accomplished through variational autoencoders (VAEs) and generative adversarial networks (GANs) (Lam et al. 2022).

6.3.4. *Multimodal data fusion and integration*

Several biological and behavioral domains exist in neurological and psychiatric disorders including genetics, brain imaging, electrophysiology and digital health. AI can integrate these diverse data types to identify biomarkers, enhancing predictive accuracy through their combined analysis.

Multimodal autoencoders, graph neural networks and multi-kernel learning are research avenues that help researchers to relate sMRI and fMRI, as well as transcriptomic data (Uyanik et al. 2025). The resultant biomarkers represent opposite sides of the disease. These combined methods also assist in isolating the patients into biologically different subsets that can react differently to treatments.

Computational approach	Data modalities used	Target disorders	Example applications/ biomarkers identified	Clinical significance
Omics-based modeling	Genomics, transcriptomics, proteomics, metabolomics	Alzheimer's, schizophrenia, bipolar disorder	Gene expression patterns, CSF protein markers, metabolic signatures	Enables identification of molecular pathways and potential diagnostic biomarkers
Neuroimaging analytics	MRI, fMRI, PET, DTI	Alzheimer's, Parkinson's, depression, ASD	Cortical thinning, hippocampal atrophy, altered connectivity networks	Supports early diagnosis and tracking of neurodegeneration
Electrophysiological signal analysis	EEG, MEG	Epilepsy, schizophrenia, depression	Pre-ictal EEG features, gamma oscillations, ERP components	Provides real-time functional biomarkers and seizure prediction
Digital phenotyping	Smartphone, wearable sensor data	Depression, Parkinson's, anxiety	Speech rhythm, gait changes, activity and sleep patterns	Enables continuous, remote monitoring and relapse prediction
Machine learning (supervised/ unsupervised)	Multimodal datasets	All major neuropsychiat ric disorders	Classification, clustering, subtype identification	Improves diagnostic accuracy and patient stratification
Deep learning (CNNs, RNNs, autoencoders)	Imaging, EEG, genomics	Alzheimer's, epilepsy, ASD	Structural MRI feature extraction, seizure forecasting	Detects nonlinear complex patterns, boosts prediction performance

Multimodal integration	Imaging + omics + digital	Schizophrenia, MS, depression	Combined biomarkers from transcriptomics and MRI	Provides comprehensive disease signatures for precision medicine
Explainable and federated AI	Distributed clinical data	Cross-disorder models	SHAP/attention maps, privacy-preserving modeling	Improves interpretability, clinician trust and multi-site collaboration

Table 6.1. *Computational approaches and applications in biomarker discovery for neurological and psychiatric disorders*

6.3.5. *Explainable AI for biomarker discovery*

While deep learning models achieve high predictive performance, their "black-box" nature limits clinical adoption. XAI provides interpretability by revealing the features driving model predictions. Methods such as SHapley Additive exPlanations (SHAP), layer-wise relevance propagation (LRP) and attention-based saliency maps allow identification of the most influential biomarkers.

For instance, in AD, XAI applied to CNNs has highlighted hippocampal atrophy and posterior cingulate cortex connectivity as key imaging biomarkers (Lam et al. 2022).

6.3.6. *Transfer learning and federated learning*

Data scarcity and privacy concerns are major obstacles in computational biomarker discovery. Transfer learning and federated learning offer solutions.

Transfer learning leverages pretrained models developed on large datasets to improve performance on smaller disease-specific cohorts. For example, CNNs pretrained on large-scale MRI datasets can be fine-tuned for Alzheimer's or PD classification, reducing the need for extensive labeled data (Eslami et al. 2019; Zhang et al. 2020).

Federated learning allows collaborative model training across multiple institutions without sharing raw patient data, preserving privacy while enabling larger sample sizes. This approach has been successfully applied to multicenter neuroimaging studies, facilitating robust biomarker discovery (Alves et al. 2022; Zheng et al. 2024).

6.4. Biomarkers in neurological disorders

Neurological disorders relate to the alteration of the structure, functioning and molecules of the nervous system, resulting in aggravated disability in most cases. Computational approaches have played a vital role in identifying biomarkers which can be used for early diagnosis, to monitor the course of the disease and predict a response to therapy (Uyanik et al. 2025). This section discusses four of the largest disorders, namely, Alzheimer's, Parkinson's, epilepsy and multiple sclerosis, and describes the recent advances in the field of computational biomarker discovery.

6.4.1. *Alzheimer's disease*

The most prevalent type of dementia is Alzheimer's disease (AD). It is characterized by deterioration of cognition, memory impairment and behavioral changes. Conventional biomarkers of AD would entail the accumulation of amyloid-2 and tau proteins, findings of neurodegeneration on sMRI, as well as diverse indicators in cerebral spinal fluid (CSF). The development of the recent computational approaches significantly enhanced the process of detecting the early signs of the disease and the process of its monitoring (Wankhede et al. 2025).

The machine learning tools that have been used to process various types of data, including sMRI, PET scans, CSF proteomic profiles and genomic data, have demonstrated high accuracy difference between AD and mild impaired cognitive (MCI), as well as normal aging. Deep learning algorithms, particularly CNN, identify scars, such as the shrinkage and thinning of the hippocampal and cortex automatically (Wang et al. 2024). Imaging data are combined with the transcriptomic data that prompts researchers to identify molecular signatures as they depict changes in structure resulting in the biomarkers that give mechanistic insight.

Digital biomarkers are also emerging in use. Computer algorithms can identify the slightest behavioral changes that can be early signs of cognitive deterioration by analyzing speech patterns, gait and activity on smartphones. These non-invasive measurements, which are continuous, are used to complement the conventional imaging and molecular tests and to provide clinicians with a chance to determine the disease progression over a period of time (Şerban et al. 2025).

6.4.2. *Parkinson's disease*

Parkinson's disease (PD) is a neurodegenerative condition that primarily affects dopaminergic neurons in the substantia nigra, causing both motor and non-motor symptoms. Neuroimaging, electrophysiology, molecular profiling and digital health metrics are some of the areas that scientists have focused on to find the computational biomarkers of PD.

Machine learning and resting-state fMRI with diffusion-tensor imaging (DTI) have revealed alterations in connectivity networks that monitor the progression of PD (Khaleghi et al. 2022). A PET scan of dopaminergic activity when manipulated by computational pipelines provides extremely sensitive biomarkers of diagnosis and monitoring.

Motor dysfunction is assessed by electrophysiological biomarkers EEG and local field potential recordings which are measured using the advanced signal processing and machine learning techniques. Use of beta band oscillatory activity is a strong indicator that will be used in guiding therapy interventions such as deep brain stimulation (de Oliveira et al. 2025).

Tremor, bradykinesia and gait abnormalities are recorded by wearable devices and smart phone sensors. The machine learning algorithms for these continuous signals can be used to detect patients with diseases in real-time and objectively evaluate the severity of a disease outside of a clinical environment (Cheung et al. 2025).

6.4.3. *Epilepsy*

Epilepsy is a disorder characterized by frequent seizures as a result of hyperirritability of neurons. Researchers have been seeking biomarkers in three principal directions, namely, electrophysiology, imaging and genetics. Recent progress in computing methods allows us to forecast unwanted events as well as locate their sources, with a lot of accuracy.

EEG profiles give out the most valuable biomarkers. Applying scenarios such as wavelet analysis, nonlinear dynamics and deep learning, scientists are able to consider seizures at an early stage and even predict them prior to a seizure taking place (Wankhede et al. 2025). Continuous EEG processing deep neural networks are able to predict an impending seizure several minutes before it happens, such that clinicians are able to gather actionable information, which can be used to trigger real-time treatment.

MRI images display function-related and structural alterations of the brain, which suggest epileptogenic locations. Machine learning pipes are useful in detecting these abnormalities, and can detect them much better than human hand-checking. This enhanced detection facilitates better preparation of the surgery and predictions of the outcomes on the patients (Wang et al. 2024).

The genetic data, along with the EEG and imaging, makes a multimodal biomarker set. For example, genetic variation with specific epilepsy conditions may be correlated with specific EEG patterns. This combination enhances the quality of diagnosis and assists clinicians in developing therapies specific to particular patients (Şerban et al. 2025).

6.5. Biomarkers in psychiatric disorders

Common psychiatric conditions include MDD, schizophrenia, bipolar, anxieties and ASD; these are significant worldwide disabilities. When compared to several neurological illnesses, psychiatric illnesses cannot be indicated in terms of visual, structural or molecular indicators, which is why physicians rely primarily on clinical examination and patient self-reporting. To discover objective biomarkers that might enhance diagnosis, predict outcome and personalize treatment, researchers are turning to computational techniques to identify the objective biomarkers (Boes 2021).

6.5.1. *Major depressive disorder*

MDD includes a low mood that is persistence, loss of pleasure, cognitive and neurovegetative functional changes. Neuroimaging, electrophysiology, genomics and digital phenotyping have been the areas of biomarker research in MDD.

Machine learning of resting-state and task-based fMRI has revealed disrupted functional connectivity, particularly in the default mode network, salience network and prefrontal-limbic circuits. The results facilitate the anticipation of depression and the management of treatment (Boes 2021). Predictive models include sMRI phenotypes such as cortical thinning and decreased volume of the hippocampal and amygdala to diagnose depression and predict treatment response.

Alpha and theta variability, ERPs and frontal asymmetry are EEG-based biomarkers that are processed using advanced signal processing and classification algorithms to reveal the predictive ability on antidepressant efficacy (Meyler et al. 2007).

Digital phenotyping is a powerful instrument to track depressive symptoms. We can forecast the onset of relapse or response using machine learning based on smartphone data, such as activity, sleep, social interaction and speech (Park et al. 2019). These digital-based, continuous markers complement neuroimaging and molecular data, and allow a longitudinal evaluation of the dynamics of the disease.

6.5.2. *Schizophrenia*

Schizophrenia is a chronic mental disorder that is characterized by psychosis, issues in thinking and lack of social skills. Neuroimaging, brain electrical recordings and overall multi-omics investigations are methods used by researchers to find biomarkers.

This is demonstrated by MRI studies, both structural and functional, which reveal that schizophrenia cell connectivity is impaired in the default-mode network, thalamocortical pathways and prefrontal cortex. A combination of various types of imaging, machine learning models can distinguish patients and healthy individuals with high accuracy (Billeri and Naro 2021).

EEG responses (abnormal neutrons of gamma waves, the pattern of ERP, etc.) show the issues with cognition and sensory processing. EEG time-series classification and subgrouping using deep learning algorithms are useful in improving patient classification.

Markers that are identified with machine learning techniques and the network approaches go by the name of genomic and transcriptomic and are indicative of the altered pathways in the functioning of the synaptic systems, inflammation in the brain and neurotransmitter signaling. A combination of these molecular biomarkers and imaging and behavioral data enhances prediction and assists in disclosing the specific biological subgroups of patients (Boes 2021).

6.5.3. *Bipolar disorder*

Bipolar disorder is characterized by frequent incidences of mania and depression that may differ in terms of impact on thinking and normal functioning. Computational biomarkers in bipolar disorder have been sought by the researchers primarily through neuroimaging, electrophysiology and omics.

MRI research has observed variations in limbic-prefrontal networks, the volume of amygdala and connectivity, which vary depending on the mood. Bipolar disorder can be classified by machine learning models made out of these MRI features with predictions of the time a mood outburst may start (Meyler et al. 2007).

EEG biomarkers, particularly changes in oscillatory power and connectivity, are strongly associated with mood states as well as treatment response in patients. Multi-omics techniques are a combination of transcriptomics, proteomics and metabolomics finding derailed pathways that influence neurotransmission, circadian rhythms and energy metabolic processes (Park et al. 2019). A combination of these types of data, which can be done by computation, will provide robust biomarkers that will aid in the diagnosis of bipolar disorder and forecast its progression.

6.5.4. *Anxiety disorders*

High hyperarousal, impaired ability to control cognitive processes, as well as disturbed responses to stress, are associated with anxiety disorders, such as generalized anxiety disorder (GAD) and post-traumatic stress disorder (PTSD). The neuroimaging biomarkers and, in particular, amygdala–prefrontal connection have been revealed using fMRI and machine learning algorithms (Billeri and Naro 2021).

Autonomic biomarkers (heart-rate variability and skin conductance) and EEG are sent through computational models to determine the severity of symptoms and response to treatment. There are additional biomarkers of behavioral phenotyping, which is digital phenotyping passive oversight of activity, sleep and social interactions, and which can assist in early diagnosis and prediction of relapse (Bufano et al. 2023).

6.6. Challenges and future directions

6.6.1. *Data heterogeneity and quality*

The heterogeneity in biomedical data analysis is one of the key issues in the process. Neurological and psychiatric disorders are very complicated systems that are classified by genes, molecules, neurons, behavior and by the environment. The sources and platforms of data are extremely varied and, hence, the data could vary in terms of quality, resolution and format. As an illustration, neuroimaging datasets might vary in terms of the scanner type, scanner acquisition and scanner processing. Omics data are different in terms of sequencing depth, platform and normalization.

This heterogeneity makes it challenging to train models and achieve reliable generalization. Machine learning algorithms can fit to the specific tendencies of a certain group of observations, which results in poorer predictive accuracy for new groups. Thus, it is essential to standardize the data collection procedures, pre-data-processing steps, as well as benchmark sets in order to maintain reproducibility and reliability of computational biomarkers (Das 2025).

6.6.2. *Sample size and data scarcity*

Small, imbalanced datasets are common in the many neurological and psychiatric conditions, particularly in rare diseases or in the early phases of the disease. Whereas high-dimensional datasets, including whole-genome sequencing or voxel world image analysis, contain more features than samples, the potential number of false discoveries and increasing overfitting makes them more vulnerable to risk factors.

Researchers suggest such methods as data augmentation, transfer learning and federated learning to address these issues. Transfer learning applies models which have been ready-trained using large sample companies, to enhance the performance of application to small cohort companies. Federated learning benefits include several institutions cooperating but with no direct sharing of raw patient data, hence preserving privacy as well as effectively increasing the size of the sample (Kokare and Revathy 2024).

6.6.3. *Interpretability and clinical adoption*

The black-box character of deep learning models presents a significant challenge. Biomarkers obtained through computation require interpretability so clinicians can rely on them to make an action plan. The use of XAI tools, including SHAP, LRP and attention-based visualizations, could help to indicate the importance of features and the relevance of a particular mechanistic nature; however, their implementation in the clinical work process is not widespread. It is very important to bridge the gap between the high predictive accuracy and interpretability that would permit regulatory approval and daily usage (Zheng et al. 2024).

6.6.4. *Ethical, legal and privacy concerns*

There are ethical and legal concerns regarding using patient information to identify computational biomarkers. Privacy would be of particular concern when the data, comprising genomic, neuroimaging and digital phenotyping, is combined. When there is no diversity between the training data and the diverse populations, the existence of algorithmic bias can exacerbate healthcare disparities. The clinical use of these biomarkers must be reported ethically, employing machine learning models that are fair and designed to preserve patient privacy (Das 2025).

6.6.5. *Future directions*

The future of computational biomarker discovery lies in several key areas:

1. *Multimodal and longitudinal integration*: combining genomics, proteomics, neuroimaging, electrophysiology and digital phenotyping across time can capture disease trajectories, improving predictive power and early detection.

2. *Causal and mechanistic modeling*: moving beyond correlation-based models towards causal inference frameworks can identify biomarkers with mechanistic significance, enhancing their translational potential (Kokare and Revathy 2024).

3. *Hybrid human–AI collaboration*: integrating clinician expertise with AI-driven models can enhance interpretability, identify clinically relevant features and facilitate adoption in real-world settings.

4. *Edge computing and real-time monitoring*: advances in mobile and wearable technologies allow continuous collection of digital biomarkers, enabling timely intervention and personalized care (Zheng et al. 2024).

5. *Standardization and reproducibility*: developing universally accepted data standards, preprocessing pipelines and benchmarking datasets will be essential for robust, generalizable biomarker discovery.

By addressing these challenges, computational biomarker discovery can transition from research settings to clinical application, enabling early diagnosis, personalized treatment and improved patient outcomes in neurological and psychiatric disorders (Alves et al. 2022).

6.7. Conclusion

AI has become a game-changer in neurology and psychiatry, enabling earlier disease diagnosis, more accurate prognoses, and personalized treatment for individual patients. Using machine learning, deep learning and combinations of various types of data, scientists will be able to discern complex relationships in genomic, proteomic, neuroimaging, electrophysiological and digital behavioral measurements. These cutting-edge approaches reveal predictive and mechanistic biomarkers that the traditional methods could not previously access. Computational pipelines identify the structural, functional and molecular alterations that agree with the disease progression, onset and treatment response in neurological conditions, including AD, PD, epilepsy and multiple sclerosis. These revelations assist clinicians in keeping track of the disease more precisely and modifying the treatment earlier. Likewise, neuroimaging biomarkers, electrophysiological biomarkers, genetic biomarkers and behavioral biomarkers are revealed through AI-based models in psychiatric disorders (including MDD, schizophrenia, bipolar disorder, anxiety disorders and ASD). These indicators aid in the stratification of patients and enable treatment to be tailored down to a case-by-case basis. Although such gains are made, there are still key challenges that stand out: data may be diverse and noisy; samples are usually small; the models themselves can also be black box; and the ethical issues persist. Standardization, XAI, federated learning and integration of multimodal data over time (among other items) will overcome these hurdles and make computational biomarkers available in everyday clinical practice.

6.8. References

Alves, C.L., Pineda, A.M., Roster, K., Thielemann, C., Rodrigues, F.A. (2022). EEG functional connectivity and deep learning for automatic diagnosis of brain disorders: Alzheimer's disease and schizophrenia. *Journal of Physics: Complexity*, 3(2), 025001.

Asif, S., Wenhui, Y., ur-Rehman, S., ul-ain, Q., Amjad, K., Yueyang, Y., Jinhai, S., Awais, M. (2025). Advancements and prospects of machine learning in medical diagnostics: Unveiling the future of diagnostic precision. *Archives of Computational Methods in Engineering*, 32(2), 853–883.

Billeri, L. and Naro, A. (2021). A narrative review on non-invasive stimulation of the cerebellum in neurological diseases. *Neurological Sciences*, 42(6), 2191–209.

Boes, A.D. (2021). Lesion network mapping: Where do we go from here? *Brain*, 144(1), e5.

Bufano, P., Laurino, M., Said, S., Tognetti, A., Menicucci, D. (2023). Digital phenotyping for monitoring mental disorders: Systematic review. *Journal of Medical Internet Research*, 25, e46778.

Calhoun, V.D., Pearlson, G.D., Sui, J. (2021). Data-driven approaches to neuroimaging biomarkers for neurological and psychiatric disorders: Emerging approaches and examples. *Current Opinion in Neurology*, 34(4), 469–479.

Chan, Y.H., Girish, D., Gupta, S., Xia, J., Kasi, C., He, Y., Wang, C., Rajapakse, J.C. (2025). Discovering robust biomarkers of psychiatric disorders from resting-state functional MRI via graph neural networks: A systematic review. *NeuroImage*, 121422.

Cheung, C.Y., Kong, A.P., Bakhtiar, M. (2025). Individualized connectomic tACS immediately improves oscillatory network with language facilitation in post-stroke aphasia: A feasibility study of a dysfunctome-based targeting approach. *Frontiers in Computational Neuroscience*, 19, 1635497.

Dai, Z.P., Wen, Q., Wu, P., Zhang, Y.N., Fang, C.L., Dai, M.Y., Zhou, H.L., Wang, H., Tang, H., Zhang, S.Q. et al. (2025). γ neuromodulations: Unraveling biomarkers for neurological and psychiatric disorders. *Military Medical Research*, 12(1), 1–21.

Das, J. (2025). Unraveling the brain: A comprehensive exploration of neuroscience's evolution, impact, and future. *Impact, and Future*. doi: 10.2139/ssrn.5439197.

Eslami, T., Mirjalili, V., Fong, A., Laird, A.R., Saeed, F. (2019). ASD-DiagNet: A hybrid learning approach for detection of autism spectrum disorder using fMRI data. *Frontiers in Neuroinformatics*, 13, 70.

García-Gutiérrez, M.S., Navarrete, F., Sala, F., Gasparyan, A., Austrich-Olivares, A., Manzanares, J. (2020). Biomarkers in psychiatry: Concept, definition, types and relevance to the clinical reality. *Frontiers in Psychiatry*, 11, 432.

Glewwe, N., Grissom, N.M., Widge, A.S. (2025). Prefrontal network mechanisms of psychiatric deep brain stimulation. *Journal of Neuroscience*, 45(37), e1944242025. doi: 10.1523/JNEUROSCI.1944-24.2025.

Khaleghi, A., Mohammadi, M.R., Shahi, K., Nasrabadi, A.M. (2022). Computational neuroscience approach to psychiatry: A review on theory-driven approaches. *Clinical Psychopharmacology and Neuroscience*, 20(1), 26.

Kokare, S.S. and Revathy, V.R. (2024). A survey on deep learning for neuroimaging-based brain disorder analysis. In *Machine Learning and Deep Learning in Neuroimaging Data Analysis*, Pillai, A.S. and Menon, B. (eds). CRC Press, Boca Raton.

Lam, S., Arif, M., Song, X., Uhlén, M., Mardinoglu, A. (2022). Machine learning analysis reveals biomarkers for the detection of neurological diseases. *Frontiers in Molecular Neuroscience*, 15, 889728.

Meyler, D., Stimpson, J.P., Peek, M.K. (2007). Health concordance within couples: A systematic review. *Social Science & Medicine*, 64(11), 2297–2310.

Możaryn, J.F. and Szczegielniak, A.R. (2025). Computational psychiatry: A bridge between translation and precision. *International Journal of Neuropsychopharmacology*, 28(Suppl 1), i276–i277.

de Oliveira, G.S., Rodrigues, F.H., Pontes, J.G., Tasic, L. (2025). Artificial intelligence-based methods and omics for mental illness diagnosis: A review. *Bioengineering*, 12(10), 1039.

Park, Y.S., Cosgrove, G.R., Madsen, J.R., Eskandar, E.N., Hochberg, L.R., Cash, S.S., Truccolo, W. (2019). Early detection of human epileptic seizures based on intracortical microelectrode array signals. *IEEE Transactions on Biomedical Engineering*, 67(3), 817–831.

Ricetti, C., Carrara, L., La Torre, D. (2025). The potential of machine learning in diagnosing neurological and psychiatric diseases: A review. *Discover Artificial Intelligence*, 5(1), 105.

Rosca, C.M. and Stancu, A. (2025). A review of neuro-ML breakthroughs in addressing neurological disorders. *Applied Sciences*, 15(10), 5442.

Şerban, M., Toader, C., Covache-Busuioc, R.A. (2025). Brain tumors, AI and psychiatry: Predicting tumor-associated psychiatric syndromes with machine learning and biomarkers. *International Journal of Molecular Sciences*, 26(17), 8114.

Uyanik, H., Sengur, A., Salvi, M., Tan, R.S., Tan, J.H., Acharya, U.R. (2025). Automated detection of neurological and mental health disorders using EEG signals and artificial intelligence: A systematic review. *Wiley Interdisciplinary Reviews: Data Mining and Knowledge Discovery*, 15(1), e70002.

Wang, L., Hu, Y., Jiang, N., Yetisen, A.K. (2024). Biosensors for psychiatric biomarkers in mental health monitoring. *Biosensors and Bioelectronics*, 256, 116242.

Wankhede, N.L., Koppula, S., Umare, P.D., Umare, M.D., Lokhande, S.K., Taksande, B.G., Upaganlawar, A.B., Umekar, M.J., Kopalli, S.R., Kale, M.B. (2025). Neuroimaging biomarkers: A critical review of their role in neurological disease diagnosis and management. *Brain Disorders*, 18, 100222.

Zhang, L., Wang, M., Liu, M., Zhang, D. (2020). A survey on deep learning for neuroimaging-based brain disorder analysis. *Frontiers in Neuroscience*, 14, 779.

Zheng, K., Yu, S., Li, B., Jenssen, R., Chen, B. (2024). Brainib: Interpretable brain network-based psychiatric diagnosis with graph information bottleneck. *IEEE Transactions on Neural Networks and Learning Systems*, 36(7), 13066–13079. doi: 10.1109/TNNLS.2024.3449419.

7

Natural Language Processing for Clinical Narratives and Neurological Case Records

Clinical stories and records of neurological cases have unstructured information that is enriched by how the providers think and what they know about the patients after interacting with them. However, these notes were written in the form of a story, which is why they are hard to analyze automatically, as well as the use of specialized medical terms and numerous abbreviations. Natural language processing (NLP) is an emerging, potent instrument which creates value out of this text. It is capable of converting free-form medical notes into data structures, and automatically summarizing information, and predictive models. This is especially useful in neurology, where patients may have mixed symptoms that cross into different disorders, and the treatment is not acute. Older techniques are being outperformed by machine learning and transformer models in particular, and especially larger language models. Such systems identify minor clinical information, monitor the progress of conditions over time, and in cases where the information is provided, they may combine text and imaging or physiological data. These sophisticated models have enhanced disease phenotyping of stroke, epilepsy, Parkinson's and dementia, when used in yearly records of cases in neurology. They are also useful in assisting decision-making in an emergency context and informing long-term rehabilitation plans. Also, despite the promise, there are still considerable challenges. The assurance of high-quality data, the description of algorithmic decisions, patient privacy and bias prevention have all not yet been resolved. There is a paucity of annotated neurological corpora available, and the notes written by different clinicians are written in varied ways. Such variability lowers the power of existing systems to be applicable in other institutions. Future development relies on the collaborators to create strong, disease-specific resources, integrate neural and symbolic approaches and privacy-saving technology.

Chapter written by Shrikrishna N. BAMNE and Swapna KAMBLE.

7.1. Introduction

The use of clinical narratives is one of the most useful yet least exploited segments of the electronic health record (EHR). Narratives, in contrast to formal data in fields such as lab values or billing codes, reflect the thoughts of clinicians, the history of the patient, the description of minor symptoms and contextual information needed to make a correct diagnosis and treatment (Lefkovitz et al. 2024). Case narratives in neurology provide important information about how the disease occurs, progresses and responds to treatment, because such disorders are usually overlapping or of ambiguous presentation (Pedersen et al. 2020).

However, extensive storytelling documentation is expensive. Free-text records are by their nature not structured with a domain-specific terminology, abbreviations, inconsistencies in typology and style variation among clinicians (Rizzo and Dawson 2025). Additional problems are raised by neurological case records: symptoms change with time, comorbidity creates difficulties in interpretation and fine-grained observations of cognition or motor activity are narrated in language that cannot be readily categorized (Alon et al. 2025). These complexities directly restrict the use of narratives as either a means of analysis on a large scale or as a computational model.

Natural language processing (NLP) provides a way to deal with these shortcomings by converting unstructured texts into structured and machine understandable information. The previous paradigms were based on rule-based systems and curated vocabularies that could be used in limited contexts but were ineffective when implemented in other scenarios (De Rosario et al. 2023). This trend of machine learning (and more recently, deep learning) has significantly enhanced the capacity of NLP systems to make data-driven, context-sensitive processing of clinical narratives. They have potential in neurology, where the details of clinical reasoning in the case notes of a patient are central.

The difference in the clinical relevance of this progress is hard to overestimate. Among the major causes of disability and dependency across the globe are neurological problems that comprise stroke, dementia, Parkinson's disease or epilepsy (Joshi 2025). Longitudinal history of functional status, treatment responses and changing symptomatology is central to their diagnosis and management, and much of this data is contained in unstructured records. NLP can augment neurological research and care provision by making it possible to extract structured variables in an automated way, identify disease-specific phenotypes and create predictive models, creating a better-than-ever chance to enhance the field of study.

The implications of NLP in clinical practices hold relevance for the larger healthcare trends of precision medicine based on data. With the continuing growth in EHR use around the world, the ability to process unstructured text en-masse will continue to be at the heart of clinical decision support, population health management and individual care strategies (Parker and Brush 2025). In the case of neurology, in particular, NLP-based solutions may enable timely identification of disease progression, automatic tracking of cognitive and motor impairment, and enhanced care coordination between multidisciplinary teams.

This chapter examines the NLP value unlocking in clinical narratives and neurological case records. We start breaking down the basics of clinical NLP in terms of understanding its concept and framework and then proceed to its use in the field of neurology. We then revise developments in model architectures, comment on clinical utility and workflow integration and critically examine the challenges and limitations that still persist. Lastly, we point out the future directions, where NLP endeavors to be a validated and transformational instrument in the practice of neurology.

7.2. NLP fundamentals in clinical narratives

NLP is defined as the group of calculation approaches which process, analyze and extract meaning from the human language. In clinical care, clinical narratives, which include progress notes, discharge notes, case reports, etc., hold crucial information, which application fields of structured data lack (Cross et al. 2024). NLP techniques will have to be specialized to tackle domain-related issues to extract this information, such as medical terminology, acronyms, negations and style differences in the story.

Fundamentally, clinical NLP carries out a number of initial functions. The process of tokenization and sentence segmentation divides text into pieces of analysis, namely words or phrases, whereas part-of-speech tagging determines grammatical categories, which subsequently assist with future analysis. More complicated systems are named entity recognition (NER) and relation extraction, which connects entities into meaningful links (e.g. between headache and migraine instead of hypertension). Such approaches transform the raw clinical text into a useful interpretable resource to be used in clinical decision support and research (Pagano et al. 2023).

In the past, the oldest NLP systems have been rule-based computer systems in healthcare. They used manually maintained lexicons, ontologies and heuristics of pattern-matching clinical entities. Standard vocabularies were made available in systems such as the unified medical language system (UMLS), which were used in early text-mining applications (Yang et al. 2024). Rule-based methods could be interpreted and defined, but it would not be long before their limitations were noticed. They needed a lot of domain knowledge to retain, were fragile when tested on new data, and were not easily generalizable to different institutions and clinical subdomains.

Probabilistic models (a conditional random field (CRF) and support vector machine (SVM)) were introduced in the machine learning age. These models substituted manual rules with inference that was based on data. They were taught to categorize or cut text into units depending on annotated corpora, which was good in diverse fields. As an example, an annotated model trained to identify instances of neurological symptoms, such as, for example, tremor or aphasia, was possible given that there were sufficient annotated training cases (Crema et al. 2022). Nevertheless, they were still very reliant on large and high-quality datasets – which continues to be a challenge in clinical NLP due to privacy concerns and the cost of annotation.

The shift to deep learning was a tremendous venture. Recurrent neural networks (RNNs) and their models, including the long short-term memory (LSTM) models, were able to model higher levels of sequential dependency in language. This allowed systems to identify context-sensitive expressions of clinical text (Buchlak et al. 2021). Negation sensitivity was needed to draw the line between no evidence of stroke and evidence of stroke, and the deep learning model was arguably better suited to learning these concepts than the rule-based frameworks.

More recently, transformer architectures have revolutionized NLP by introducing attention mechanisms, which enable the modeling of long-range dependencies and contextual relationships across entire documents. State-of-the-art biomedical NLP systems that are based on pretrained models include BERT, BioBERT and ClinicalBERT, which have been trained on biomedical corpora and can perform well across various clinical NLP problems. They are also particularly useful in the sub-specialties of neurology, where subtle language variations, even the ability to distinguish between mild cognitive impairment and early Alzheimer's disease, are potentially very significant in terms of diagnosis.

NLP basics in healthcare (another essential dimension) is concerned with negation and uncertainty detection. Clinical descriptions tend to be of the type "what is not there" (no seizures observed), and "what is unclear" (possible transient ischemic attack). Income falsehood may also cause mis-extraction. Specialized algorithms such as NegEx and successors are extensively deployed in clinical NLP pipelines to deal with such cases. In the field of neurology, where the diagnostic certainty may gradually develop, to conduct an accurate interpretation of the cases, it is necessary to know the uncertainty.

Besides syntactic and semantic processing, clinical concept normalization transforms extracted entities into standard vocabularies, such as SNOMED CT, ICD-10 or MeSH. This distribution guarantees interoperability and facilitates integration with organized EHR domains. In neurological case records, normalization can also allow the researcher to trace references in the narrative related to symptoms, such as shaking or trembling, to the standardized concepts that describe the concept of Parkinsonian tremor, which, in turn, can increase consistency with the overall data collection.

7.3. Applications in neurology and case records

The history of applying NLP to neurological records has grown significantly in recent times, since clinicians have to be able to extract valuable information in bulk unstructured notes. Neurological conditions are difficult due to the slow development of symptoms and their affective overlaps, and they need long-term follow-up. Converting free-text into structured information allows NLP to enhance disease surveillance, support personalized care, and facilitate research into disease mechanisms and patient outcomes (Breithaupt et al. 2025).

7.3.1. *Stroke documentation and prognosis*

Stroke is one of the most common neurological crises. Documentation is extremely crucial, as there are tight therapeutic windows. In cases where structured fields are not available, NLP has the ability to extract stroke severity scores such as that of the NIHSS based on clinical notes. Time-to-treatment markers, which enable retrospective guideline compliance checking, also get located by automated systems (Yeung et al. 2023). In addition to the acute phase, longitudinal records of recovery and rehabs and revivals are examined to forecast the outcomes in the long-term. These applications demonstrate the transformation of NLP by making the habitual documentation a quality assessment and prognosis tool.

7.3.2. *Dementia and cognitive disorders*

Dementia care is based on narrative records where clinicians explain behavioral changes in subtle cognitive, behavioral and functional aspects. NLP is able to identify early indicators of impairment in the primary-care records, through which timely referrals to have formal assessments conducted are made (Hernandez-Boussard et al. 2020). Follow-up notes and case reports will give clues to disease progression including memory loss, language deterioration or executive impairment, which could go undetected in structured tests. With narrative descriptions, NLP-based phenotyping makes the distinction between Alzheimer's, frontotemporal dementia and other subtypes. Such tools are able to track the progress and assess treatment effectiveness during clinical trials.

7.3.3. *Epilepsy case records*

During epilepsy, clinical accounts are the records regarding epileptic seizures, their causes and the reaction to treatment. NLP has the ability to automatically identify the frequency, type and severity of patient seizures, and correlate them with medication history and EEG outcomes (Jui and Rivas 2024). These systems enable a vast amount of research on the effectiveness of treatments with a lower amount of manual work being carried out by the clinicians. NLP also assists in developing seizure diaries based on the notes that provides patients and providers with an automated means of measuring the outcomes over time.

7.3.4. *Parkinson's disease and movement disorders*

Decades later, there are neurological conditions that involve movements within the body called Parkinson's and movement disorders. Parkinson's, and similar movement disorders, have varied motor and non-motor symptoms, which have commonly been reported qualitatively. NLP identifies mentions of tremor, rigidity, gait problems and non-motor signs, such as sleep problems or mood problems (Huang et al. 2024). The resulting features can be used in automated phenotyping, to predict disease progression and/or track treatment response. When NLP outcomes are coupled with structured data, i.e. medication dosages with neuroimaging, researchers create models predicting individual patterns. These methods bring the importance of narrative data to the management of chronic neurological conditions.

7.3.5. *Uncommon and uncharacteristic neurological disorders*

Extreme neurological disorders are also examined by NLP. Rarely occurring syndromes are mined with case reports and case series, typically the primary source of evidence, to uncover clinical presentation, diagnostic and treatment patterns. Examples include NLP-based literature mining. This has revealed connections between uncommon genetic mutations and clinical manifestation, which is useful for precision medicine in neurogenetics (Li et al. 2022). This demonstrates that NLP can be used as a research instrument and as a clarification connecting the isolated case reports with the more clinical knowledge.

Neurological disorder	NLP application focus	Extracted information	Clinical/research utility
Strokes	Extraction of severity scores and treatment markers	NIHSS score, time-to-treatment, rehabilitation notes	Enables quality assessment, prognosis and compliance tracking
Dementia and cognitive disorders	Early identification and monitoring	Memory loss, behavioral and language decline	Assists in early detection and subtype phenotyping (e.g. Alzheimer's vs. FTD)
Epilepsy	Automated seizure event extraction	Frequency, type, severity, treatment response	Supports seizure diary automation and treatment optimization
Parkinson's and movement disorders	Symptom tracking and disease phenotyping	Tremor, rigidity, gait, non-motor symptoms	Predicts progression and supports personalized therapy
Rare/uncharacteristic disorders	Literature and case mining	Clinical–genetic linkages, uncommon phenotypes	Enables discovery of novel associations and supports precision medicine

Table 7.1. *Major applications of NLP in neurological disorders*

7.4. Advances in model architectures

The fast progress of NLP systems has had a significant impact on the possibility of analyzing the clinical narratives. Rule-based systems and shallow machine learning models, in turn, were the first steps towards traditional methods, as they were constrained by the number of features that had to be crafted manually and the failure to generalize beyond these features. The shift to deep learning and, more recently, to transformer-based models and large language models (LLMs) has increased the range of clinical uses of NLP significantly, particularly in the field of neurology (Sarker et al. 2021).

7.4.1. *Transformer models in clinical NLP*

The concept of transformer architectures, proposed in the context of the so-called attention mechanism, changed NLP by enabling models to focus on long-range dependencies between text readings in a text on a document scale, rather than processing the text sequentially. In the clinical field, ClinicalBERT, BioBERT and BlueBert have demonstrated better performance in tasks such as named-entity recognition and relation extraction, as well as clinical text classification (Shankar et al. 2025). These models acquire contextual embeddings, which is essential in neurology to know how to differentiate slight linguistic variations. Considering the nuances between a contextually interpreted meaning between a probable transient ischemic attack and definite ischemic stroke, is an example of a task that transformer-based models do better than their predecessors.

7.4.2. *Large language models (LLMs)*

LLMs have pushed these abilities even further. Architectures based on GPT are able to do zero-shot or few-shot learning models, which means that they do not require large amounts of annotated data. Domain-adapted clinical LLMs can also perform the former, which means that they also do not require large amounts of annotated data. This is particularly necessary in neurology where large-labeled corpora are not highly available. Based on general biomedical text pre-training and smaller neurology-specific dataset fine-tuning, the performance of LLMs on specific tasks, such as the ability to detect signs of dementia progression or to write summaries of seizure case notes in formatted language, is high (Malviya et al. 2025). Furthermore, interactive applications, such as a question–answering system, can be driven with the assistance of LLMs to assist clinicians live, retrieving and summarizing case records to find the necessary information.

7.4.3. *Neurological multimodal NLP*

Information other than the text, for example, neuroimaging, electrophysiology or wearable sensor data, is frequently combined with neurological practice. Recent studies have examined multimodal NLP systems which combine textual data with an image or time-series data to form a more comprehensive view of a patient's condition (Norori et al. 2021). As an illustration, the combination of narrative descriptions of the impaired motor capacities with gait sensor data enhances the quality of the Parkinson's disease progression models. On the same note, the data obtained through the application of radiology reports and MRI images helps in the automatic identification of stroke subtypes. These multimodal systems go beyond text mining and coexist with the holistic approach to neurological diagnosis and treatment.

7.4.4. *Explainability and trustworthiness*

In combination with the improvement of performance, the development of model architectures has led to the initiative to improve interpretability. Modules of attention maps built with the help of transformers, as well as LLM explanation tools, can identify the phrases or sentences that a model pays the most attention to. Such openness is paramount in the field of neurology; the stakes of treatment here are high, and clinical professionals have to take action on information generated by AI.

As an example, if a model forecasts early cognitive impairment, clinicians should comprehend whether the choice was made on the basis of documented language limitations, behavior change or comorbid issues that are outlined in the record.

7.5. Clinical Utility: diagnosis, prognosis and treatment support

NLP has the potential to help in clinical decision-making in the real world as well as extract insights, which is the eventual worth of this technology in the field of neurology. NLP systems are liaised within developing messages into actionable knowledge between the diagnosis and prognosis stages and treatment planning. These apps directly solve the fundamental issues of neurology, including heterogeneity of the disease, the insidiousness of its manifestations and the absence of individual approaches to care (Kuzucu et al. 2024).

7.5.1. *Diagnostic support*

There are frequent instances where the neurological disorders might necessitate subtle interpretation of clinical observations that are written in physician notes. NLP improves the diagnostic accuracy because the extraction and organization of the data are done systematically.

As an example, with NLP algorithms run on the records of the emergency department, potential stroke cases can be recognized in advance, and patients will receive timely thrombolytic treatment. Automatic recognition systems can detect features, such as language deficits, gait abnormalities, or tremors in outpatients, and map them to likely diagnoses. Although NLP does not substitute clinical judgment, it offers decision support by outlining patterns that might not have been developed otherwise, particularly in a hectic clinical setting (Ueda et al. 2024).

7.5.2. *Prognostic modeling*

Prognostication in neurology has a bad reputation as being exceptionally difficult because disease progressions can vary. NLP makes it possible to model predictions based on the mining of longitudinal case records of disease progress. Observations of increasing falls or diminished facial expression in Parkinson's disease can be used as precursors of deterioration in motor skills. On the same note, the transitions between mildly impaired cognition and dementia may be predicted using narrative accounts of memory decline or behavioral alterations. Including time data, NLP is used in dynamic prognostic models that are used to guide patient counseling and care planning. Clinical trials based on the risk of quick progression may also stratify patients with such systems to provide clinical trials that are more efficient and relevant (Le Glaz et al. 2021).

7.5.3. *Monitoring and response evaluation of the treatment*

Neurology treatment is often associated with long-term monitoring, the clinical notes of which include qualitative assessments of treatment response. NLP tools derive information about medication adherence, side effects and treatment results in the form of structured indicators in these narratives. In the case of epilepsy, automatic seizure frequency–extraction of follow-up notes can facilitate the objective measurement of the antiepileptic drugs. Progress notes regarding functional gains in stroke rehabilitation may be summed to determine the response to physical and occupational therapy. There is less manual review of charts in these systems, and this will enable clinicians to access a large number of patients more efficiently.

7.5.4. *Clinical decision support systems (CDSS)*

Clinical decision support systems (CDSS) are the computer programs that help clinicians to make clinical decisions when they are delivering care. As a component of EHRs, NLP gets integrated into CDSS. Such systems include warnings about high-risk patients, recommending follow-up investigations or creating a summary of pertinent clinical history in the course of follow-up. Cases of suspected stroke or status epilepticus are given priority in NLP-powered CDSS in the field of neurology to guarantee the provision of timely interventions. They provide continuity of care, too, in that they can generate short summaries of long case histories, particularly when dealing with patients with chronic neurological issues and the need to offer them multidisciplinary care.

7.5.5. *Patient engagement and communication*

In addition to clinician-facing communication, patient communication is facilitated with the help of NLP-based systems. The artificial production of lay summaries based on clinical notes can help patients and caregivers to gain a better insight into the diagnoses and the treatment plan. In neurological patients, especially those with cognitive-impairment, adherence and shared decision-making can only be achieved through clear communication. NLP fills the chasm between the complicated medical papers and understandability for the patients.

7.6. Integration with EHR and clinical workflows

Implementation of NLP in the field of neurology requires effective functioning of the model in addition to the integration of clinical settings. EHRs are the key center of patient data, so they are intuitive when it comes to the integration of NLP-based instruments. Integration guarantees that insights, predictive capabilities and the decision support capabilities extracted are made readily accessible in the current workflow of clinicians, so that they do not disrupt their usual workflows and are adopted to full advantage (Guo et al. 2024).

7.6.1. *Embedding NLP in EHR systems*

EHRs today can record structured and unstructured data, although the latter aspect has the tendency to prevail in neurological care. With NLP pipelines embedded into the EHR system, real-time structuring of free-text entries may be configured. As a neurologist records a visit, NLP is capable of extracting and classifying mentions of symptoms (e.g. tremor, aphasia), with one stylized terminology, and filling structured fields automatically, without further specialized intervention. This helps to decrease the documentation workload and enhance data quality to be used in downstream analysis.

Integration is also used to facilitate automated summarization tools that can reduce the long case histories into brief summaries. Neurology patients have multifaceted, longitudinal histories across numerous encounters and disciplines. However, the lack of critical information is made obvious to a patient by automated summaries that NLP has created. Those summaries could include prior imaging results, seizure history or reactions to medications.

7.6.2. *Workflow optimization*

In addition to documentation, NLP can also streamline clinical work processes through triage and priority. NLP may be used to scan the incoming notes to identify the possible stroke cases, and attention may be given to them in emergency situations. Owing to the low response rates of follow-up in outpatient clinics, NLP tools may be used to detect patients who are late to receive follow-up or present symptoms of disease progression to proactively treat them. Such workflow improvements are efficient in ensuring patient safety standards are high.

7.6.3. *Interoperability and multidisciplinary care*

There is a tendency towards cross-functional cooperation in the context of neurological care, including neurosurgery, psychiatry, rehabilitation and primary care. Systems of NLP-enhanced EHR support this coordination through the provision of standard documentation rules and exchange of cross-specialty information. An example of such features, that may be shared with rehabilitation teams to facilitate continuity of care, are those extracted by looking at the neurology notes (functional status or cognitive decline) (Joshi 2025). Interoperability is particularly important in the case of patients with long-term neurological conditions, where interrupted documentation tends to inhibit care quality.

7.6.4. *Barriers to adoption*

Integration is still difficult in spite of these advantages. Technical obstacles comprise variability among vendors of EHR systems, computational needs of giant NLP network models and real-time performance requirements. Adoption is also affected by organizational issues, including, but not limited to, clinician training, redesigning workflow and alignment of the requirements of the regulations. These barriers need very close cooperation between clinicians and health system administrators and developers.

7.7. Challenges: bias, privacy, data scarcity and interpretability

NLP has enormous potential in the field of neurology but there are numerous obstacles in the practical clinical implementation. Such hindrances are technical, ethical, organizational and societal. It is important to overcome them in order to ensure that NLP becomes a reliable and fair instrument in the treatment of neurological patients (Hadar and Moura 2025).

7.7.1. *Bottlenecks in data scarcity/annotation*

Another of the most urgent constraints will be addressed by the limited number of annotated neurological corpora. In contrast to other fields, such as oncology or radiology, where curated large datasets exist, neurology is not well represented in publicly available corpora. This is partly due to the lack of ease in neurological recording. Minor differences in language may be significant in terms of diagnosis. Such data can only be annotated with specific knowledge of neurologists and is therefore resource-intensive and expensive. This leads to the usage of relatively small datasets in many neurology NLP systems, which may restrict the model generalizability. Transfer learning and domain adaptation have been beneficial but the scarcity of large, standardized corpora has been a bottleneck to improvement.

7.7.2. *Privacy and data security*

Clinical narratives include some of the most vulnerable patient information. They are usually comprised of a personal history, cognitive test and psychiatric observations. When free-text data is exchanged across institutions, there is an increased risk of re-identifying the patient. Privacy laws, for example, HIPAA and GDPR, have very strict de-identification standards that would distort original text and lower the utility in training NLP. Federated learning methods as well as differential privacy can provide these solutions, whereby models would be able to use distributed data without being directly shared. There are, however, technical and organizational complications associated with such strategies, particularly when resources are limited in healthcare systems.

7.7.3. *Bias and fairness*

Bias in the NLP models is a key issue. Demographic and institutional bias in clinical practice often have an impact on training data. When record keeping of cases is biased towards women or minorities, trained models can still promote differences in advice in the diagnosis or treatment recommendation. The practices of documentation also vary between institutions, which introduces systematic bias in the deployment of models in other institutions.

To fix bias, conscious actions should be taken in terms of dataset curation, fairness–conscious model training and continuous auditing to allow equitable performance between groups of patients.

7.7.4. *Interpretability and trust*

Clinicians have to learn to believe NLP results, especially in cases where this is a determinant in making high-stakes diagnosis, such as stroke or prompting the start of dementia treatment. Transformer models and deep learning can be black boxes that have low transparency. Visualizations of attention, feature attribution techniques and hybrid neuro-symbolic process representations where data-driven models and explicit clinical knowledge are learned, have been used in an attempt to clarify the interpretation. Where patient conditions cannot be easily categorized and are complex, NLP systems rely on an explanation that is clear and clinically meaningful.

7.7.5. *Barriers to the organization and implementation*

Organizational issues are a barrier to adoption beyond technical and ethical issues. Implementing NLP in current workflows needs to include changing the practice of documentation, educating clinicians and making it compatible with EHR systems. Technical solutions might be embraced slowly due to resistance to change and the fears of extra documentation load, even in situations when there is a technical solution. Effective implementation requires effective cooperation of clinicians, informaticians and health administrators in designing NLPs which are usable and clinically relevant (Kundi et al. 2023).

7.8. Future perspectives

7.8.1. *Multimodal multilingual integration*

New NLP systems will integrate clinical records with images, recording brain waves and electrodes installed in the body. A combination of text and numbers will provide a more comprehensive perspective of a patient and enhance predictions concerning the development of a disease. Creating multilingual NLP models will also enable such tools to benefit individuals around the globe, limit the lapses in clinical understandings and carry out international studies (Mehrabi et al. 2021).

7.8.2. *Advanced model adaptation and continual learning*

Constant learning enables NLP models to adapt to other medical knowledge and the evolving styles of documentation without losing previous knowledge. Neurology has a high turnover of conditions and treatments; thus, the relevance of incremental learning models does not decrease in this area. Domain adaptation assists in the utilization of pretrained models, even when a lab has limited labeled data, thus facilitating large-scale usage.

7.8.3. *Ethical and responsible AI*

As NLP becomes deeply inculcated into care matters, matters of ethics should be in the frontline. Fairness checks, transparent processes and accountability systems are examples of responsible AI frameworks that will help to ensure that models do not increase the health disparity. Federated learning and homomorphic encryption are some of the techniques that allow hospitals to completely train jointly without jeopardizing patient information. Such safeguards will benefit, unimpeded by AI safeguards, neurology especially, where there are scores of vulnerable groups.

7.8.4. *Collaborative research and open science*

Open science and collaborative research go hand-in-hand with these activities. The future of healthcare development depends on the collaboration of clinicians, data scientists, informaticians and ethicists. Open-source tools and annotated corpora allow new concepts to be developed faster, making the community create better-built, stronger and more generalizable NLP systems. The collaborative systems also allow benchmark experiment and reproducibility to convert the breakthroughs in the field of neurology NLP to the actual clinical advantages.

7.9. Conclusion

NLP is now an influential means of extracting the treasure in the clinical narrative and neurology case history. These unstructured documents hold the in-depth reasoning, continuously observed information and patient-specific information, which are usually lacking in structured EHR data. Converting free-text narratives to be structured and readable by machines, NLP enhances the benefits of diagnostic assistance, supports successful prognostic models and assists in tracking the response to treatment in neurologic treatment. New model architectures, including transformer-based systems, LLMs and multimodal frameworks increase the capability of NLP in addressing complex clinical text. Such models find the elusive contextual information, combine information of different sources and give actionable insights that reflect directly on patient care. NLP helps in real-time decision-making when incorporated into EHR systems and clinical processes, promotes collaboration between various specialties, as well as reduces the work burden of manual chart review. What will follow is an improved and quality neurological care experience. Notwithstanding these gains, some challenges still exist. Issues such as scarce data, privacy considerations, bias and the necessity of explainable models remain a problem. They can only be overcome with interdisciplinary collaboration, proper ethical management and the development of NLP systems which are sound, scalable and just. In the future, NLP in combination with multimodal data, continuous learning and precision medicine is likely to enhance patient care, accelerate the research process and transform the protocol of delivering neurological practice.

7.10. References

Alon, Y., Naimi, E., Levin, C., Videl, H., Saban, M. (2025). Leveraging natural language processing to elucidate real-world clinical decision-making paradigms: A proof of concept study. *Journal of Biomedical Informatics*, 166, 104829.

Breithaupt, A.G., Tang, A., Miller, B.L., Pinheiro-Chagas, P. (2025). Integrating generative artificial intelligence in ADRD: A framework for streamlining diagnosis and care in neurodegenerative diseases. arXiv preprint arXiv:2502.06842.

Buchlak, Q.D., Esmaili, N., Bennett, C., Farrokhi, F. (2021). Natural language processing applications in the clinical neurosciences: A machine learning augmented systematic review. In *Machine Learning in Clinical Neuroscience: Foundations and Applications*, Staartjes, V.E., Regli, L., Serra, C. (eds). Springer, Cham.

Crema, C., Attardi, G., Sartiano, D., Redolfi, A. (2022). Natural language processing in clinical neuroscience and psychiatry: A review. *Frontiers in Psychiatry*, 13, 946387.

Cross, J.L., Choma, M.A., Onofrey, J.A. (2024). Bias in medical AI: Implications for clinical decision-making. *PLOS Digital Health*, 3(11), e0000651.

De Rosario, H., Pitarch-Corresa, S., Pedrosa, I., Vidal-Pedrós, M., de Otto-López, B., García-Mieres, H., Álvarez-Rodríguez, L. (2023). Applications of natural language processing for the management of stroke disorders: Scoping review. *JMIR Medical Informatics*, 11, e48693.

Guo, Z., Lai, A., Thygesen, J.H., Farrington, J., Keen, T., Li, K. (2024). Large language models for mental health applications: Systematic review. *JMIR Mental Health*, 11(1), e57400.

Hadar, P.N. and Moura, L.M. (2025). Clinical applications of artificial intelligence in neurology practice. *CONTINUUM: Lifelong Learning in Neurology*, 31(2), 583–600.

Hernandez-Boussard, T., Bozkurt, S., Ioannidis, J.P., Shah, N.H. (2020). MINIMAR (MINimum Information for Medical AI Reporting): Developing reporting standards for artificial intelligence in health care. *Journal of the American Medical Informatics Association*, 27(12), 2011–2015.

Huang, Y., Guo, J., Chen, W.H., Lin, H.Y., Tang, H., Wang, F., Xu, H., Bian, J. (2024). A scoping review of fair machine learning techniques when using real-world data. *Journal of Biomedical Informatics*, 151, 104622.

Joshi, H. (2025). Natural language processing of electronic health records for predicting Alzheimer's disease. In *Deep Generative Models for Integrative Analysis of Alzheimer's Biomarkers*, Kumar, A., Kumar, S.R., Gayathri, N., Srivel, R., C, D. (eds). IGI Global, Hershey, PA, 141–174.

Jui, T.D. and Rivas, P. (2024). Fairness issues, current approaches, and challenges in machine learning models. *International Journal of Machine Learning and Cybernetics*, 15(8), 3095–3125.

Kundi, B., El Morr, C., Gorman, R., Dua, E. (2023). Artificial intelligence and bias: A scoping review. In *AI and Society*, El Morr, C. (ed.). CRC Press, Boca Raton.

Kuzucu, S., Cheong, J., Gunes, H., Kalkan, S. (2024). Uncertainty as a fairness measure. *Journal of Artificial Intelligence Research*, 81, 307–335.

Le Glaz, A., Haralambous, Y., Kim-Dufor, D.H., Lenca, P., Billot, R., Ryan, T.C., Marsh, J., Devylder, J., Walter, M., Berrouiguet, S. et al. (2021). Machine learning and natural language processing in mental health: Systematic review. *Journal of Medical Internet Research*, 23(5), e15708.

Lefkovitz, I., Walsh, S., Blank, L.J., Jetté, N., Kummer, B.R. (2024). Direct clinical applications of natural language processing in common neurological disorders: Scoping review. *JMIR Neurotechnology*, 3(1):e51822.

Li, I., Pan, J., Goldwasser, J., Verma, N., Wong, W.P., Nuzumlalı, M.Y., Rosand, B., Li, Y., Zhang, M., Chang, D. et al. (2022). Neural natural language processing for unstructured data in electronic health records: A review. *Computer Science Review*, 46, 100511.

Malviya, R., Kumar, S., Solanke, A.S., Goyal, P., Chauhan, K. (eds) (2025). *Artificial Intelligence in Neurological Disorders: Management, Diagnosis and Treatment.* John Wiley & Sons, New York.

Mehrabi, N., Morstatter, F., Saxena, N., Lerman, K., Galstyan, A. (2021). A survey on bias and fairness in machine learning. *ACM Computing Surveys (CSUR)*, 54(6), 1–35.

Norori, N., Hu, Q., Aellen, F.M., Faraci, F.D., Tzovara, A. (2021). Addressing bias in big data and AI for health care: A call for open science. *Patterns*, 2(10), 100347.

Pagano, T.P., Loureiro, R.B., Lisboa, F.V., Peixoto, R.M., Guimarães, G.A., Cruz, G.O., Araujo, M.M., Santos, L.L., Cruz, M.A., Oliveira, E.L. et al. (2023). Bias and unfairness in machine learning models: A systematic review on datasets, tools, fairness metrics, and identification and mitigation methods. *Big Data and Cognitive Computing*, 7(1), 15.

Parker, T.M. and Brush, B. (2025). An overview of artificial intelligence in neurology. *Seminars in Neurology*.

Pedersen, M., Verspoor, K., Jenkinson, M., Law, M., Abbott, D.F., Jackson, G.D. (2020). Artificial intelligence for clinical decision support in neurology. *Brain Communications*, 2(2), fcaa096.

Rizzo, M. and Dawson, J.D. (2025). AI in neurology: Everything, everywhere, all at once Part 1: Principles and practice. *Annals of Neurology*, 98(2), 211–230.

Sarker, A., Al-Garadi, M.A., Yang, Y.C., Choi, J., Quyyumi, A.A., Martin, G.S. (2021). Defining patient-oriented natural language processing: A new paradigm for research and development to facilitate adoption and use by medical experts. *JMIR Medical Informatics*, 9(9), e18471.

Shankar, R., Bundele, A., Mukhopadhyay, A. (2025). Natural language processing of electronic health records for early detection of cognitive decline: A systematic review. *npj Digital Medicine*, 8(1), 133.

Ueda, D., Kakinuma, T., Fujita, S., Kamagata, K., Fushimi, Y., Ito, R., Matsui, Y., Nozaki, T., Nakaura, T., Fujima, N. et al. (2024). Fairness of artificial intelligence in healthcare: Review and recommendations. *Japanese Journal of Radiology*, 42(1), 3–15.

Yang, Y., Lin, M., Zhao, H., Peng, Y., Huang, F., Lu, Z. (2024). A survey of recent methods for addressing AI fairness and bias in biomedicine. *Journal of Biomedical Informatics*, 154, 104646.

Yeung, J.A., Wang, Y.Y., Kraljevic, Z., Teo, J.T. (2023). Artificial intelligence (AI) for neurologists: Do digital neurones dream of electric sheep? *Practical Neurology*, 23(6), 476–488.

8

AI-Integrated Wearable Technologies for Continuous Neurological Monitoring

Wearables with AI have transformed the way we perform continuous monitoring of neurological systems. It enables early diagnosis, individualized therapy and improved results for the patients. Conventional neurological examinations rely on infrequent visits to the clinic and reports made by patients. Such approaches tend to overlook short (or even minor) incidences that may be an indication of a major disorder. Present-day wearable technology has enhanced biosensors that continuously monitor and capture signals, such as EEG, ECG, EMG, motion, speech and sleep patterns. The interpretation of these data streams with AI algorithms makes real-time analytics, anomaly detection and predictive modeling more accurate than standard diagnostics. Epilepsy, Parkinson's disease, Alzheimer's disease, multiple sclerosis, traumatic brain injury and post-stroke rehabilitation are already monitored by wearable-AI systems. Machine learning models acquire the baseline of every patient, detect variation with high accuracy and assist the clinician in making evidence-based choices. With AI, there is also the possibility of remote care since huge multimodal datasets may be transformed into actionable clinical information and relieve the pressure on hospitals. Nonetheless, the mentioned aspects such as data privacy, algorithm bias, lack of interpretability, power consumption and regulatory challenges are yet to be tackled. Future developments will include fluid cloud-edge integration, small multi-sensory regularly packaged, explainable AI and personalized electronic medication. This chapter summarizes the advancements in the area of continuous neurological monitoring by using AI-driven wearable technology, highlights the clinical applications, obstacles and future development of this technology, and shows that the technology can revolutionize the field of neurology.

8.1. Introduction

The significance of public health problems is massive, since neurological diseases are among the largest global public health problems, with a significant

---

Chapter written by Swati JAGTAP and Ashish N. PATIL

disability burden, death burden and high healthcare expenses. Epilepsy, Parkinson's, Alzheimer's, multiple sclerosis (MS), stroke and traumatic brain injuries, etc., are some of the conditions that plague hundreds of millions of lives. These conditions may be difficult to manage long term and may necessitate continual monitoring (Shin et al. 2022). Traditional or conventional neurological evaluations are dependent on hospital-based examinations, neuroimaging and episodic visits to the clinic. These approaches have drawbacks because of their sporadic nature, high cost and reliance on patient self-reporting, which does not always reflect transient or subtle symptoms. Consequently, warning symptoms of neurological degeneration are often overlooked, which contributes to the creation of interventions and worse results (Lim et al. 2025).

Wearable technologies have become a strong means to bridge this gap. Wearables have biosensors to record a wide range of physiological and behavioral cues, such as brain activity, muscle activity, heartbeat, movement and speech dynamics. These tools allow the real-time application of neurophysiologic conditions to be monitored in real activities and not in artificial laboratory health facilities. They therefore produce high-resolution, longitudinal data that shed more light on disease pathogenesis and the degree of changes in symptoms on a daily basis (Japaridze et al. 2023).

The real transformative metric of wearables is linked to its incorporation with artificial intelligence (AI). Deep learning (DL) and machine learning (ML) can facilitate automated processing of large streams of biosignals to reveal previously unknown patterns. The algorithms in AI can be used to detect anomalies in real time, categorize states of diseases and even anticipate neurological events that may happen in the future, such as a seizure or tremor. Hence, there is a change between the reactive, symptom-centered care to proactive, predictive and individualized neurological health management (Heremans et al. 2025).

Wearables with AI implementation are applicable to several neurological fields. In epilepsy, AI models are useful to determine subtle pre-ictal conditions, which may signal to the patient and their caregivers that they are going to have a seizure. In the case of Parkinson's disease (PD), smartwatches can measure the intensity of tremors, gait issues and motor variability, and change the treatment regimen using motion sensors. Speech and behavior analysis are emulated via wearables with AI, used in the work on Alzheimer's disease (AD) and dementia to indicate early cognitive impairment. These applications demonstrate that continuous care and AI analytics provide the greatest chance to revolutionize neurological care (Hizem et al. 2025).

Although these benefits are achieved, there are still serious problems. Data privacy concerns, interpretability of the algorithms, regulatory acceptance and energy-efficient design of devices are the challenges that need to be overcome to ensure the widespread clinical acceptance of AI-based wearables. In addition, generalizability of various AI algorithms in the context of different groups of patients remains a challenge in the majority of cases, as most of these models are trained using narrow samples. Ethical issues, particularly the management of sensitive brain-related information also bring in another dimension of complexity.

This chapter synthesizes, in detail, the recent contributions to the development of AI-based wearable technologies to accomplish uninterrupted neurological surveillance. It starts with a summary of wearable sensing modalities and AI algorithms, then proceeds to discuss clinical applications in diverse fields of clinical importance for major neurological diseases. The chapter continues by discussing the system architectures that support real-time analytics and multimodal integration, and will then discuss important challenges in the form of data security, bias in algorithms and regulatory challenges. Lastly, it talks about the future of explainable AI (XAI), the integration of brain–computer interfaces and the customization of digital therapeutics. This chapter signifies how the AI-driven wearables revolutionize the shift toward more predictive, personalized and patient-centered neurological care.

8.2. AI in wearable neurological monitoring

The inculcation of AI into wearable neurological monitoring systems is a sign of a new time of accuracy in health technology. Conventional sensors may demand such a manual interpretation of the biosignals and, on the contrary, the AI-based wearables are auto-scalable and have adaptable analytics that can make real-time sense of continuous signals. The systems discover patterns, predict results and produce actionable insights, which are otherwise unreachable to clinicians or patients through the use of ML and DL algorithms (Li et al. 2022).

8.2.1. *Wearable sensor modalities*

Multimodal biosensors are common in neurological wearables. Among the most significant types of monitoring of brain electrical activity are electroencephalography (EEG) sensors, which provide an opportunity to identify neural oscillations of abnormal characteristics in case of seizures, impaired cognitive functions or sleep disorders. EMG sensors can be used to provide information on muscle activation which is valuable in monitoring neuromuscular conditions and motor dysfunction in diseases such as Parkinson's and MS. Smartwatches or wristbands can measure the dynamics of movement by including accelerators and gyroscopes on the device to record gait pattern, tremors and postural instability. Also, wearable photoplethysmography (PPG) sensors and electrocardiovascular dynamics (ECG) sensors measure cardiovascular dynamics that are, in most cases, an interaction with neurological health (AbuAlrob and Mesraoua 2024).

Other than these physiological indicators, wearables are being enhanced to record behavioral and cognitive indicators. An illustration of this is how speech recognition devices built into wearable microphones can determine speech fluency, pauses and prosody, which are preliminary signs of cognitive impairment. Equally, actigraphy or EEG head-based sleep tracking is an instrumental indicator of several disorders associated with insomnia, REM sleep disorders and narcolepsy, among others, which have strong connections to the dysfunction of the nervous system (Wang and Jing 2025).

8.2.2. *AI in data processing*

The wearable devices used in life have generated a lot of complex and voluminous data, which require the use of AI elements in processing and analysis. Support vector machines (SVMs), random forests and k-nearest neighbors are all common ideas in traditional approaches to ML that have been used in the classification of motor states, seizure detection and differentiating between normal and pathological data. As DL continues to grow, convolutional neural networks (CNNs) and recurrent neural networks (RNNs) have become particularly important as they are able to automatically discover spatiotemporal features within raw biosignals (Ding et al. 2022).

CNNs can especially perform a better degradation of hierarchical features in EEG or EMG data, which can be used to accurately classify neurological states. RNNs, in particular, long short-term memory (LSTM) networks, are particularly effective in dealing with sequential data such as time-series signals, and can therefore be applied in predictions, such as in seizure prediction or gait cycle prediction. Hybrid models which integrate CNNs with LSTMs are also much better as they will capture the space and time aspects of the neurological information. Also, unsupervised and semi-supervised methods of learning are under development to solve the small set of labeled data, so that AI systems can learn more effectively across patient populations (Bonanno et al. 2025).

8.2.3. *Real-time monitoring and edge AI*

An important benefit of the AI-based wearables is that they can be monitored in real time. Conventional methods usually involve transmitting the data to centralized servers, which creates delays and increases privacy concerns. New developments in edge AI, where algorithms are applied to wearable devices or to the nearby gateways, can be used to provide much faster, much safer and less energy-intensive analytics. This is important in neurological applications where they must be able to provide feedback instantly, for example, seizure detection or to prevent falls.

As an illustration, smartwatches with neural networks installed on their edges will be able to identify tremors or unusual gait patterns within milliseconds, and issue alerts or treatment. Equally, wearable EEG headbands with inside-built AI processors have the capability of classifying sleep stages on the device, eliminating the need to connect cloud servers and enhancing user confidence. Edge AI also supports hybrid architectures, where by lightweight models can be used to respond to any query immediately, but more complex analyses can be done remotely at scale on bountiful data over a longer time period (Li et al. 2022).

8.3. Clinical applications

8.3.1. *Epilepsy*

Wearables that can detect symptoms of epilepsy are one of the most widely researched neurological monitors. Conventional diagnosis and treatment is based on infrequent intermittent EEG recordings in controlled settings, which frequently overlook cases of spontaneous seizures. AI-powered wearable devices do not have this issue since they allow continuous ambulatory monitoring.

EEG headbands, wrist-worn accelerators and electrodermal activity (EDA) detectors are used to detect seizure patterns that are abnormal in physiological and motor activities. To learn the distinction between seizure and non-epileptic events in these data streams, AI models (especially convolutional and RNNs) are expected to handle these streams (Dabnichki and Pang 2024). Research has demonstrated that AI multimodal models that integrate EEG and motion data capacities can identify seizures with more than 90% accuracy and have less false alarms.

In addition to detection, AI predictive models are promising in making the predictions of seizures several minutes or hours prior. Through pre-ictal EEG readings, cardiovascular alterations or even minor behavioral indications, such systems can offer the patient the necessary time to move to a secure place or administer rescue medication.

In illustration one, DL algorithms used on wearable EEG have demonstrated emerging predictiveness in the pilot study, with an accuracy of above 80% (Ghadi et al. 2025). These predictive systems symbolize a paradigm shift in the management of epilepsy, and bring about its management to a proactive form.

8.3.2. *Parkinson's disease*

Parkinson's disease (PD) has both motor symptoms which include tremors, rigidity, bradykinesia and gait impairments, and non-motor symptoms which evolve over time. Old-fashioned clinical examinations are intermittent and subjective, and they are not able to detect daily variability. Continuous objective monitoring is provided through wearable sensors that apply AI.

The motion data are collected using smartwatches and inertial measurement units (IMUs) fitted with gyroscopes and accelerators. This data is analyzed by AI in order to determine the magnitude of tremor, gait abnormalities and the severity of dyskinesia. Such digital biomarkers allow clinicians to track motor variations with enhanced precision compared to the traditional scales such as the Unified Parkinson's Disease Rating Scale (UPDRS). The latest AI applications are capable of accurately distinguishing between medication on and off (Elfouly and Alouani 2025).

Beyond motor symptoms, AI-driven speech analysis from wearable microphones or smartphone-based applications can detect vocal changes associated with PD progression. Combined with movement data, multimodal AI systems can provide a holistic view of disease burden. Importantly, real-time monitoring allows dynamic adjustment of therapies, such as fine-tuning deep brain stimulation parameters or optimizing medication schedules (Srinivasan and Dangayach 2025).

8.3.3. *Alzheimer's disease and dementia*

Alzheimer's disease (AD) and any other dementia is hard to trace since mental deterioration occurs at a slow pace and is easily eluded during on-call visits. AI-based wearables are becoming ever more popular as tools that will be able to track the disease and discover the initial signs of it.

Biomarkers of speech and language are particularly promising. Wearables and smartphone-based devices are capable of capturing speech. These are features which are analyzed by AI, which finds words with pauses, the complexity of sentences and the natural flow of speech. Research indicates that these signs are very much comparable to early cognitive loss (Gutman et al. 2024).

Sleep-trackers are also more informative, due to the fact that sleep issues tend to manifest themselves at an early stage in AD. Taking actigraphy and EEG data, AI can be used to identify anomalies in sleep structure organization, which is an indicator of cognitive impairments. Wearables will also have motion sensors that look out for wandering or less activity, which are important behavioral indicators of an aggravation of dementia (Huang et al. 2025).

8.3.4. *Multiple sclerosis*

Multiple sclerosis (MS) is a long-term or chronic condition that impairs the insulation around the nerves, causing outbursts and deterioration of disability. Due to the necessity of observing the changes that do not manifest themselves immediately, it is important to continue monitoring the process. The standard methods of monitoring, such as periodic MRIs and doctor appointments, cannot be regarded as sufficient.

Movement, fatigue and mobility can be measured objectively using wearable devices based on AI principles. Inertial sensor gait data is a good example. The AI analyzes such information on small issues that a clinician may overlook. These symptoms can be used to forecast the possibility of relapse or the effectiveness of a treatment. EMG signals can also be analyzed using AI in order to identify neuromuscular changes that monitor disease progression (Rizzuto et al. 2025).

8.3.5. *Stroke and rehabilitation*

The primary cause of disability is stroke, and recovery normally requires a long and intensive treatment. Wearable sensors with AI are becoming popular in assisting in controlling the acute stage of stroke or tracking rehabilitation.

During the initial phases of treatment, early deterioration of neurology will be identified through the EEG and movement sensors. AI interprets such signals and relays the information to the doctors. The gadgets used in rehab detect the movements of patients during treatment, and AI assesses their strides and discipline in the course. The objective data is useful to the patients and therapists, and assists home rehabilitation (Shaeri et al. 2022).

Most recent advancements include exoskeletons and rehabilitation technology based on robots that read wearable signals and AI. As the patient is making progress, they increase or decrease the level of the therapy dynamically, to enhance the plasticity of the brain and improve recovery.

Also, speech-monitoring wearables are under testing in stroke patients with aphasia who see AI monitoring the progression of their language improvement in the months following the stroke (Kasawala and Mouli 2025).

8.3.6. *Traumatic brain injury*

Traumatic brain injury (TBI) poses challenges due to its heterogeneous symptoms and unpredictable recovery patterns. Wearable technologies, particularly those capturing EEG, motion and cardiovascular data, are being developed to monitor patients in real-world settings.

AI algorithms can detect abnormal neural oscillations associated with post-traumatic seizures or cognitive dysfunction. In sports-related concussion management, wearable headbands and mouthguards with embedded accelerometers record impact forces, while AI models predict concussion likelihood based on biomechanical and physiological data. This allows timely removal of athletes from play, reducing the risk of secondary injury (Ahmed 2023). Table 8.1 shows the application and clinical impact of AI-integrated wearable technologies in neurological monitoring.

Neurological disorder	Primary wearable sensors	AI/ML techniques used	Clinical applications/ outcomes	Advantages over conventional methods
Epilepsy	EEG headbands, accelerometers, EDA sensors	CNNs, RNNs, hybrid CNN–LSTM	Seizure detection and prediction; differentiation of epileptic vs. non-epileptic events	Continuous monitoring, early seizure warnings, > 90% detection accuracy
Parkinson's disease	IMUs, accelerometers, gyroscopes, microphones	SVMs, random forests, deep neural networks	Tremor and gait analysis, dyskinesia quantification, speech monitoring	Objective motor/non-motor assessment; therapy optimization
Alzheimer's disease and dementia	Speech/sleep trackers, motion sensors	NLP models, CNNs, unsupervised ML	Speech and sleep-based cognitive decline detection	Early detection of cognitive impairment; passive, real-world data collection
Multiple sclerosis (MS)	EMG, IMU, gait sensors	Decision trees, CNNs	Mobility and fatigue monitoring; relapse prediction	Objective quantification of progression; remote assessment

Neurological disorder	Primary wearable sensors	AI/ML techniques used	Clinical applications/ outcomes	Advantages over conventional methods
Stroke and rehabilitation	Motion sensors, EEG, exoskeletons, EMG	Reinforcement learning, LSTM, hybrid AI models	Motor recovery tracking, therapy adaptation, aphasia rehabilitation	Personalized rehab feedback; improved recovery rates
Traumatic brain injury (TBI)	EEG, accelerometers, cardiovascular sensors	Predictive DL models, gradient boosting	Impact detection, cognitive dysfunction analysis, concussion prediction	Early intervention and prevention of secondary injuries
Cross-cutting applications	Multimodal (EEG + motion + speech + ECG)	Multimodal fusion, explainable AI (XAI), federated learning	Real-time anomaly detection, disease forecasting, patient-specific modeling	Holistic monitoring, data privacy protection, real-world integration

Table 8.1. *AI-integrated wearable technologies in neurological monitoring: applications and clinical impact*

8.4. System architecture and data integration

Effective wearable neuromonitoring based on the AI relies not only on sensors and algorithms, but also on the system architecture which may make continuous data collection, processing and analysis possible. A well thought-out architecture links the sensors, data pipelines, compute platforms and clinical decision tools together in a seamless manner. The new trends revolve around the integration of multiple types of data, balancing edge and cloud resources, patient-oriented digital native environments (Adão Martins et al. 2021).

8.4.1. *Data acquisition and preprocessing*

Wearable devices are able to capture many types of biosignals, including neural activation, muscle reactions, motion properties and cardiovascular measurements. The raw signals typically have noise due to the interference of the environment and sensor drift or movement of the patient. This is done during the simple preprocessing stages, such as filtering, artifact removal and normalization on the device level or local (edge) level to enhance quality before transmitting data.

Clean EEG and EMG signals are essential in neurological monitoring, as they may hide valuable clinical data because blinks, muscular activities and movements may cause the EEG signals to mask. The use of adaptive filters and unsupervised learning has become the norm. They are now used to identify and remove unwanted noise using AI-driven methods. These techniques increase the accuracy of the future analysis and eliminate manual selection of prolonged datasets among clinicians (Rauck et al. 2022).

8.4.2. *Feature extraction and AI pipelines*

After the process of preprocessing, biosignals are subjected to feature extraction and AI analysis. Traditional solutions are based on manually designed features, such as EEG frequency bands, tremor magnitudes in accelerometer data or formants in speech analysis. These characteristics are then fed into ML classifiers, which differentiate between normal and pathological conditions.

DL has changed feature extraction to automated learning of raw signals only. CNNs are spatial networks, whereas RNNs are time-dependent networks. These strengths are combined by hybrid CNN-LSTM architectures, and they are well fitted to dynamic neurological processes, such as seizure onset or gait cycles (Adão Martins et al. 2021).

8.4.3. *Multimodal sensor fusion*

Neurological disorders manifest across multiple domains – electrical, motor, cognitive and behavioral – making multimodal data fusion a cornerstone of advanced monitoring systems. Fusion can occur at several levels:

– Data-level fusion integrates raw signals from multiple sensors, enabling simultaneous analysis of EEG, accelerometer and speech data.

– Feature-level fusion combines engineered or learned features from different modalities to enhance classification accuracy.

– Decision-level fusion aggregates predictions from separate models, providing robust consensus outputs.

For example, seizure detection accuracy improves significantly when EEG features are combined with electrodermal and accelerometry data, reducing false positives. Similarly, in PD, integrating gait metrics with speech biomarkers provides a more holistic assessment of motor and non-motor symptoms (Rauck et al. 2022).

8.4.4. *Edge–cloud collaboration*

Balancing edge and cloud computing is also one of the critical design factors in system architecture. Edge AI supports small models applied on wearables or local hubs to provide real-time processing within a small amount of latency. This is necessary in time-sensitive applications such as the prediction of seizures. But the edge devices will be constrained in memory, processing ability and battery life.

Scalable storage and processing functions provided by cloud computing allow advanced analytics, retraining models and long-term integration of data. Hybrid edge–cloud is becoming increasingly widespread. For example, a wearable could perform basic classification in the background of the device and then forward the unprocessed or halfway-processed data to the cloud to be further analyzed. These frameworks are comprehensive and insightful to neurological monitoring (Fang et al. 2025).

8.4.5. *Digital twins in neurology*

The concept of digital twins, which is a virtual representation of a patient that mirrors its neurological condition in real time, is a new trend in system integration. The combination of data collected from wearable devices and AI can replicate the course of a disease, anticipate the course of events and evaluate potential treatment options with the help of digital twins. A case example is stroke rehabilitation, where the digital twin of a motor functioning of a patient forecasts the recovery routes and adjusts therapy plans. This method is still in the experimental stage, but it could deliver age-specific and predictive neurology (Adão Martins et al. 2021).

8.4.6. *Security, privacy and interoperability*

Data privacy and interoperability are issues that system architectures have to take into consideration. Neurological information is very delicate. They also entail safe transmission protocols, encryption and adherence to medical laws such as the HIPAA and GDPR. A privacy-saving solution such as federated learning, which is focused on training AI models on devices without raw data exchange, is gaining momentum.

Another important requirement is interoperability. Wearables should be perfectly compatible with electronic health records (EHRs), hospital information systems and telemedicine systems. It is necessary to standardize data formats and communication to make wearable-generated insights useful in clinical practice (Rauck et al. 2022).

8.5. Challenges and limitations

8.5.1. *Data privacy and security*

One of the most sensitive categories of personal health data is neurological, particularly, EEG and cognitive biomarkers. Accessing them or using them in the wrong way may be a huge infringement of patient privacy and autonomy. Wearable devices traditionally transmit data wirelessly and retain it in the cloud, which makes it susceptible to vulnerabilities such as data breaches, hacking and third-party attacks.

Legal protection can be provided by laws such as the U.S. HIPAA and the European GDPR, and the maintenance of the real-time systems in distributed form remains challenging.

Innovative technologies such as federated learning allow AI models to be trained on data stored on local machines without any further communication of the raw signals to a central server, which is a promising solution to privacy protection and a preservation of model performance (Tegon et al. 2025). However, these strategies create additional challenges such as the increase of communication expenses and the necessity of ensuring fairness of the diverse devices.

8.5.2. *Algorithmic bias and generalizability*

The quality and diversity of training data is crucial to the AI models. Current AI systems that are wearable are often constructed using small homogeneous datasets that cannot reflect the full diversity of the patients.

As an example, the seizure detection engines may be effective with one group of people but not with another due to the differing shapes of the seizures, co-morbidities or ways of life. Similarly, gait-analysis devices usually do not generalize across ages, ethnic origins or disease stages.

In biased training data, model performance is not balanced, and this casts questions of morality and undermines trust in a clinical environment. To address this, it requires considerable, multi-center total data, which covers a representative range of patient characteristics. Generalization can also be enhanced with the help of transfer-learning and domain-adaptation techniques that reuse knowledge on similar datasets (Meier et al. 2025).

8.5.3. *Interpretability and clinical trust*

Clinicians tend to be reluctant to implement AI-based systems due to the fact that most DL models are black boxes. Although such algorithms can be predictive with a high degree of accuracy, their results are not easily interpretable, and in particular, it is a serious issue that such algorithms can be used to make high-stakes neurological decisions, including predicting the onset of seizures or assessing stroke recovery.

XAI technologies are being developed: attention mechanisms, saliency mapping, feature-attribution approaches, etc., to increase transparency. XAI can generate confidence in clinicians and contribute to the use of AI tools as a regular practice by identifying which aspects of a prediction or signal segments make the biggest difference (Asgher et al. 2023). Nonetheless, it is not easy to currently balance interpretability and performance.

8.5.4. *Energy efficiency and wearability*

Wearable devices must operate continuously while maintaining a low-profile form factor; however, real-time AI processing is computationally intensive and power demanding. Due to these energy constraints, fairly simple models can run on the device, particularly edge AI models. The issue becomes bigger when multimodal systems have to deal with EEG, movement, words and heart signals simultaneously.

In order to address these problems, scholars resort to the following methods: model compression, quantization and low-power inference hardware tuning. Custom-wearable neuromorphic processors and new neuromorphic processors are also promising. Other than the usage of power, comfort and convenience of use are also important. Easy to manage or heavy gadgets discourage patients from using them, nullifying the use of continuous monitoring. Hence, the devices must be lightweight, flexible and easy on the eye to ensure that users are entertained with time (Tegon et al. 2025).

8.5.5. *Regulatory and ethical considerations*

The legal environment that defines AI-connected wearables is still in a piecemeal condition and under continuous change. Medical equipment has yet to demonstrate its safety, effectiveness and dependability by means of rigorous clinical trials. However, the conventional regulatory models do not cope with AI systems that are self-educated and self-evolving, once deployed. Regulators have to somehow give approval to these dynamic algorithms without jeopardizing safety.

Ethical issues do not stop with regulation. Constant surveillance raises the question of surveillance, autonomy and informed consent. The patients may be uncomfortable with the aspect of non-stop data gathering, particularly the ones that focus on cognitive or behavioral measurements. An essential step in establishing trust is being clear about how data will be used and the risks involved in data use, as well as the benefits. Besides, it is important to make sure it can be equally accessible, as the existence of advanced wearables may create healthcare disparities when it is accessible only to the wealthiest groups (Meier et al. 2025).

8.5.6. *Integration with clinical practice*

Successful adoption depends on the integration of wearable data into existing healthcare systems, even in the case that technical and regulatory issues are addressed. There is already data overload on clinicians. The incorporation of continuous streams generated by wearables may not make things easier, but may complicate them (Asgher et al. 2023). Clarity in visualization tools, decision support tools and a smooth connection with EHRs, on the part of wearable insights, should stop them from being overwhelmed.

It is also important that healthcare professionals can be trained to use and interpret AI results. Without an appropriate education or alignment of the working processes, the potential of the technology will remain unexploited.

8.6. Future directions

8.6.1. *Personalized and adaptive neurology*

One of the key trends is the shift to personalized neurological monitoring, in which AI models will adjust to the specifics of the physiology of a patient, their life and the evolution of the disease. These adaptive AI systems are continuously updated using actual patient data (such as real-world data) as opposed to the static models, which are constructed using generalized datasets. This enables daily re-direction of seizure levels in epilepsy, customized tremor identification in Parkinson's and personalized forecasts of cognitive decline in dementia.

Reinforcement learning and transfer learning will become more important in wearable devices so that they can have personalized models without requiring extensive volumes of labeled data. They enhance the clinical relevance and patient interaction, thus increasing the therapeutic outcomes by providing personalized insights (Cai et al. 2022).

8.6.2. *Explainable and trustworthy AI*

The new generation of wearable systems should prioritize explainability and clinical trust. DL models are very powerful, and they are usually criticized to be black boxes. The systems that will be introduced in the future will include XAI methods that provide clinicians with clear and interpretable information on the reasons why a single prediction was made. They may, for example, indicate certain EEG waveforms which caused a seizure prediction, or indicate gait phenomena, which raises the risk of falls, in assessment.

Explainability will not only enhance clinician confidence, but also facilitate regulatory approval, as transparent systems are easier to validate for safety and efficacy. Trustworthy AI frameworks will also emphasize fairness, ensuring equitable performance across diverse patient populations (Liao et al. 2025).

8.6.3. *Integration with brain–computer interfaces*

Wearable AI devices and brain–computer interfaces (BCIs) have a promising future together. BCIs allow the brain to communicate directly to VUCA. In the event of having AI-driven wearables, they can provide closed-loop therapy.

As an example, a wearable BCI can identify pre-seizure (pre-ictal) indications in epilepsy and stimulate specific parts of the neurons to prevent seizures. It is able to tune deep-brain stimulation features in real time in relation to motor data, for PD. In stroke rehabilitation, it is able to enhance motor recovery by strengthening the neural plasticity using adaptive feedback (Valerio et al. 2025).

A natural and smooth connection of wearables and BCIs is a step toward neuroadaptive systems-technologies with the ability to monitor and intervene in the work of the brain in real time (Path 2021).

8.7. Conclusion

The combination of AI and wearable technology is transforming our approach to the monitoring of neurological status. These systems allow us to capture sensitive, transient and complicated signals in the brain, which were difficult to detect previously due to the linkage of brief check-ups by clinicians with our daily life. Wearables are no longer just mere data gathering tools, but multimodal sensors and adaptive ML, with real-time analytics, which allow them to act as active, personalized, tools. They are able to pre-direct clinicians as well as patients. The strength of AI-enhanced wearables can be shown in the clinical use cases of epilepsy, PD, AD, MS, stroke and TBI. They are capable of forecasting seizures, monitoring motor changes, identifying early signs of cognitive deterioration and enhancing rehabilitation plans. The improvements contribute to safety and quality of life, and also provide the doctors with more in-depth, data-driven information compared to standard tests. Precision neurology is central to remote care, predictive analytics and digital biomarkers, making AI wearables the core of precision neurology. Yet, challenges persist. Privacy, prejudices, explainability, the exercise of power and safety regulations should be addressed with caution to guarantee riskless and reasonable implementation. Future success depends on the establishment of trustful, open systems that would integrate with current healthcare ecosystems very well. With help and collaboration among the engineers, clinicians, policymakers and patients, the hurdles will be overcome.

8.8. References

AbuAlrob, M.A. and Mesraoua, B. (2024). Harnessing artificial intelligence for the diagnosis and treatment of neurological emergencies: A comprehensive review of recent advances and future directions. *Frontiers in Neurology*, 15, 1485799.

Adão Martins, N.R., Annaheim, S., Spengler, C.M., Rossi, R.M. (2021). Fatigue monitoring through wearables: A state-of-the-art review. *Frontiers in Physiology*, 12, 790292.

Ahmed, I. (2023). AI-based smart textile wearables for remote health surveillance and critical emergency alerts: A systematic literature review. *American Journal of Scholarly Research and Innovation*, 2(2). doi: 10.63125/ceqapd08.

Asgher, U., Ayaz, Y., Taiar, R. (2023). Advances in artificial intelligence (AI) in brain computer interface (BCI) and Industry 4.0 for human machine interaction (HMI). *Frontiers in Human Neuroscience*, 17, 1320536.

Bonanno, M., Ielo, A., De Pasquale, P., Celesti, A., De Nunzio, A.M., Quartarone, A., Calabrò, R.S. (2025). Use of wearable sensors to assess fall risk in neurological disorders: Systematic review. *JMIR mHealth and uHealth*, 13, e67265.

Cai, S., Li, H., Wu, Q., Liu, J., Zhang, Y. (2022). Motor imagery decoding in the presence of distraction using graph sequence neural networks. *IEEE Transactions on Neural Systems and Rehabilitation Engineering*, 30, 1716–1726.

Dabnichki, P. and Pang, T.Y. (2024). Wearable sensors and motion analysis for neurological patient support. *Biosensors*, 14(12), 628.

Ding, S., Wu, D., Zhao, L., Li, X. (eds) (2022). Frontier of smart healthcare engineering management. In *Smart Healthcare Engineering Management and Risk Analytics*. Springer, Singapore, 21–55.

Elfouly, T. and Alouani, A. (2025). A comprehensive survey on wearable computing for mental and physical health monitoring. *Electronics*, 14(17), 3443.

Fang, S.J., Yin, Z.D., Cai, Q., Li, L.F., Zheng, P., Chen, L. (2025). Harnessing artificial intelligence for brain disease: Advances in diagnosis, drug discovery, and closed-loop therapeutics. *Frontiers in Neurology*, 16, 1615523.

Ghadi, Y.Y., Shah, S.F., Waheed, W., Mazhar, T., Ahmad, W., Saeed, M.M., Hamam, H. (2025). Integration of wearable technology and artificial intelligence in digital health for remote patient care. *Journal of Cloud Computing*, 14(1), 39.

Gutman, B., Shmilovitch, A.H., Aran, D., Shelly, S. (2024). Twenty-five years of AI in neurology: The journey of predictive medicine and biological breakthroughs. *JMIR Neurotechnology*, 3(1), e59556.

Heremans, E.R., Devulder, A., Borzée, P., Vandenberghe, R., De Winter, F.L., Vandenbulcke, M., Van Den Bossche, M., Buyse, B., Testelmans, D., Van Paesschen, W. et al. (2025). Wearable sleep recording augmented by artificial intelligence for Alzheimer's disease screening. *npj Aging*, 11(1), 34.

Hizem, M., Aoueileyine, M.O., Belhaouari, S.B., El Omri, A., Bouallegue, R. (2025). Sustainable E-Health: Energy-efficient tiny, AI for epileptic seizure detection via EEG. *Biomedical Engineering and Computational Biology*, 16. doi: 10.1177/11795972241283101.

Huang, M., Hu, C., Xu, B., Huang, X., Gao, X., Ding, Z., Guo, S. (2025). Wireless EEG monitoring system with wearable self-powered flexible sensors. *Chemical Engineering Journal*, 519, 165446.

Japaridze, G., Loeckx, D., Buckinx, T., Armand Larsen, S., Proost, R., Jansen, K., MacMullin, P., Paiva, N., Kasradze, S., Rotenberg, A. et al. (2023). Automated detection of absence seizures using a wearable electroencephalographic device: A phase 3 validation study and feasibility of automated behavioral testing. *Epilepsia*, 64, S40–S46.

Kasawala, E. and Mouli, S. (2025). Dual-mode visual system for brain–computer interfaces: Integrating SSVEP and P300 responses. *Sensors*, 25(6), 1802.

Li, L., Wang, D., Pan, H., Huang, L., Sun, X., He, C., Wei, Q. (2022). Non-invasive vagus nerve stimulation in cerebral stroke: Current status and future perspectives. *Frontiers in Neuroscience*, 16, 820665.

Liao, Y., Tan, G., Zhang, H. (2025). Surface electromyography combined with artificial intelligence in predicting neuromuscular falls in the elderly: A narrative review of present applications and future perspectives. *Healthcare*, 13(10), 1204.

Lim, M.J., Lo, J.Y., Tan, Y.Y., Lin, H.Y., Wang, Y.H., Tan, D., Wang, E., Naing, M.Y., Ng, J.J., Jefree, R.A. et al. (2025). The state-of-the-art of invasive brain–computer interfaces in humans: A systematic review and individual patient meta-analysis. *Journal of Neural Engineering*, 22(2). doi: 10.1088/1741-2552/adb88e.

Meier, F., Spacone, G., Frey, S., Benini, L., Cossettini, A. (2025). A parallel ultra-low power silent speech interface based on a wearable, fully-dry EMG neckband. *arXiv preprint*. doi: 10.48550/arXiv.2509.21964

Path, P. (2021). Previous issues. *Annals of Coloproctology*, 37(1), S1–S3.

Rauck, R., Loudermilk, E., Paez, J., Bojrab, L., Noles, J., Turley, T., Ibrahim, M., Patwardhan, A., Scowcroft, J., Przkora, R. et al. (2022). 0045/#626 Artificial intelligence-driven closed-loop SCS: Early patient feedback on personalized therapy recommendations from a digital-health assistant: Track 3: Vagus nerve stimulation/tools to inform patient care. *Neuromodulation: Technology at the Neural Interface*, 25(7), S72–S73.

Rizzuto, D.S., Herrema, H.G., Hu, Z., Utin, D., Kahn, J., Ho, C., Smiles, A., Gross, R.E., Lega, B.C., Das, S.R. et al. (2025). A wireless, 60-channel, AI-enabled neurostimulation platform. *Brain Stimulation*. doi: 10.1016/j.brs.2025.103013.

Shaeri, M., Afzal, A., Shoaran, M. (2022). Challenges and opportunities of edge AI for next-generation implantable BMIs. In *2022 IEEE 4th International Conference on Artificial Intelligence Circuits and Systems (AICAS)*. 190–193.

Shin, J.H., Kwon, J., Kim, J.U., Ryu, H., Ok, J., Joon Kwon, S., Park, H., Kim, T.I. (2022). Wearable EEG electronics for a Brain–AI closed-loop system to enhance autonomous machine decision-making. *npj Flexible Electronics*, 6(1), 32.

Srinivasan, V. and Dangayach, N.S. (2025). Transport of the neurocritical care patient. *Current Treatment Options in Neurology*, 27(1), 32.

Tegon, A., Ingolfsson, T.M., Wang, X., Benini, L., Li, Y. (2025). FEMBA: Efficient and scalable EEG analysis with a bidirectional Mamba Foundation model. *arXiv preprint*. doi: 10.48550/arXiv.2502.06438.

Valerio, J.E., Vera, G.D., Gomez, M.P., Zumaeta, J., Alvarez-Pinzon, A.M. (2025). Advancing early identification of clinical trials in neurosurgical interventions for Parkinson's disease: The critical role of AI-driven platforms and technological innovation. *Preprints*, 15, 494. doi: 10.20944/preprints202503.0054.v1.

Wang, C. and Jing, W. (2025). Artificial intelligence in electroencephalography analysis for epilepsy diagnosis and management. *Frontiers in Neurology*, 16, 1615120.

9

Epilepsy Forecasting and Seizure Prediction Through AI Algorithms

Epilepsy is one of the most prevalent neurological diseases in the world. It is characterized by numerous sudden unpredictable seizures which hugely impair a person's quality of life. Even though medications and surgeries have improved, not all individuals respond to treatment. This highlights the need for new approaches to predict responses and minimize adverse effects. Artificial intelligence (AI) has become a groundbreaking device, one that can predict seizures and control epilepsy. The computer models applied in AI read brain signals and patient markers specific to an individual. Through analysis of EEG, brain scan and other physiological objects, AI is able to identify mechanics that manifest themselves even prior to the onset of a seizure. This allows physicians to develop individual prediction agents. Convolutional and recurrent neural networks, along with machine and deep learning methods, have been extremely successful at picking up the irregularities in timing dynamics in EEG data. These tools exceed rudimentary threshold alarms. They are real time and can be connected with wearable devices and mobile health applications. Explainable AI can be used to make clinicians trust the models by revealing their decision-making process. Doctors are assured about the use of prediction as they understand the motive of making the prediction. Through federated learning, different hospitals can share knowledge without any exposure of patient information. This model manages the issue of privacy and maintains confined information. Once prediction algorithms have been implemented into closed-loop neuromodulation devices, they can not only predict an oncoming seizure but also activate timely treatments. Such a combination of brain science and computer intelligence allows patients to gain greater control over some of the emotional and medical burdens of epilepsy. Further development of the work will improve the accuracy of algorithms, render the technology more accessible and result in actually personalized, proactive epilepsy treatment.

Chapter written by Ashwini R. GARGATE and Komal M. JUJAR.

9.1. Introduction

Epilepsy is a long-term neurological disease that causes morbidity to over 50 million individuals across the world. It is also one of the most prevalent brain disorders known by the World Health Organization (WHO). The disease is characterized by spontaneous, unprovoked seizures that are a result of abnormal, coordinate neuron discharges that interfere with the normal functioning of the brain (Kerr et al. 2024). Besides the acute physical effects of seizures, epilepsy has been shown to have major psychological, social and economic consequences; these decrease the quality of life of the affected patients and their caregivers. The unpredictability of seizures has been one of the key challenges in the treatment of epilepsy, which has led to anxiety and thus restricted daily activities, as well as the risk of being injured or dying (Stirling et al. 2021).

Antiepileptic drugs (AEDs) are used to treat most patients, with approximately 70% of them being controlled with medication. Approximately a third of the patients, however, are drug-resistant and continue to suffer seizures, despite optimal medical care. Surgery, vagus nerve stimulation and ketogenic diets are other options that can be applied to such patients; however, they cannot solve the issue of the unpredictability of seizures (Khan et al. 2025). This gap has created the need to study predictive techniques in seizures in order to anticipate them early and enable patients to prepare, avert unsafe conditions or activate responding therapies.

Seizure prediction can now be achieved using computational neuroscience. The presence of underlying patterns in EEG and other physiological indicators insidious enough to give warning of seizures can be identified using artificial intelligence (AI), particularly machine learning (ML) and deep learning (DL). In comparison with conventional statistical tools, AI processes size and high-dimensional data, a nonlinear relationship of time series and intricate signal dynamics. This would help to transform the concept of seizure prediction into a viable clinical instrument (Yu et al. 2025).

An AI-based prediction forms its objective on the identification of pre-ictal state (the change in brain activity that happens some minutes to hours before a seizure). Early detection of this condition will enable individualized notifications and active treatment. Practically, the predictive system may be integrated with wearables or implanted neurostimulators to issue early alarms or stimulate therapies to place epilepsies into a proactive mode, rather than a reactive mode. The greater effect involves a higher level of patient autonomy, reduced cases of injuries due to seizures, and reduced emergency care and hospitalization costs.

Challenges still exist. Heterogeneity of the data, variability of patients, false positives and interpretability of the model prevent clinical use. The other issues that need to be solved include the privacy of data, regulatory acceptance and ethics. Nevertheless, the combination of neuroengineering, AI and digital health is accelerating the development of reliable seizure prediction.

In this chapter, existing AI algorithms that are used to predict epilepsy are considered. It talks about key developments in ML and DL models, multimodal integration of data, wearables and explainable AI (XAI) in clinical practices. The remaining challenges are also reviewed, and further steps in the implementation of predictive algorithms in the daily practice of epilepsy are provided. Combining these findings, this chapter aims to demonstrate how AI-based predictions can change the work with epilepsy and positively influence millions of people around the globe.

9.2. Pathophysiology and challenges of seizure prediction

Epilepsy is a condition of neuronal excitation and network coordination. When excitatory and inhibitory signals are dissuaded, this is known as a seizure. This ergonomic imbalance causes abnormal and hypersynchronous discharges, which diffuse around cortical and sub-cortical regions (Tveit et al. 2023). Alterations of ion channels, release of neurotransmitters and synaptic plasticity on a cellular basis contribute to this imbalance. Genetic mutations, brain damage and infections, as well as developmental errors, are all factors that can initiate the process of epileptogenesis – the transformation of a normal brain to an epileptic one. Seizures are hard to predict because these causes vary with individuals.

9.2.1. *Pre-ictal traffic jam and variability*

Seizures can be predicted using the pre-ictal condition, the period that immediately precedes a seizure and exhibits slight variations in brain activity. It has been demonstrated, through EEG and iEEG, that this condition may start several minutes to hours prior to a seizure (Saadoon et al. 2025). The common pre-ictal changes can include an increase in spectral power, the modification of the phase locking and the alteration of network connectivity. However, these indicators do not occur prior to all of the seizures. The duration of the pre-ictal window is also not constant in all individuals and may vary with time. This is because there is a discrepancy when making predictions using algorithms.

9.2.2. *Difficulties with the biomarker identification*

The identification of good pre-ictal biomarkers is not easy due to a number of reasons. First, EEG signals are noisy. The obscure neural variability that we require is concealed in movements, eye movements and noise in the environment. Second, the network of the brain is very dynamic. Thresholds to seizures may vary with sleep, stress, drugs or the circadian rhythm (Hasija et al. 2025). Third, inter-ictal spikes, which are abnormal discharges occurring between seizures, may be misinterpreted as pre-ictal activity and will give false positives. Differentiation between these states is a challenging issue to both clinicians and AI systems.

9.2.3. *Patient-specific variability*

There are many epilepsy syndromes. Each of these has its neuro-physiological fingerprint of temporal-lobe epilepsy, generalized epilepsy and focal cortical dysplasia. Due to this fact, a predictor that may be practical for one individual does not necessarily work for another. As an illustration, the algorithm that is trained on the data of one patient cannot work well with a different patient, and scaling of the forecasting systems is restricted. This cross-patient sensitivity emphasizes the importance of adaptive models that are individual and continuously learn using the personal data of a patient.

9.2.4. *Ethical and regulatory issues*

AI-based seizure forecasting tools present ethical and regulatory concerns. Privacy legislation must safeguard patient information to be used in training the models, and the long-term monitoring should be agreed with. Additionally, regulatory approval is in the form of accuracy plus safety, usability and clinical benefit. These challenges have the ability to delay the process of researching approved medical devices.

9.3. AI in epilepsy forecasting: an overview

The use of AI is rapidly gaining strength in the healthcare field, particularly in the predictive field of epilepsy. While the goal of traditional seizure detection is to detect an actual seizure just in time, forecasting is meant to foresee a seizure several minutes to hours in advance. This would necessitate sophisticated calculation software to detect nonlinearities of brain behavior that are difficult to notice through other methods – which AI excels at (Yang et al. 2024).

9.3.1. *From statistical models to AI-driven forecasting*

Preliminary models of seizure prediction performed statistical analysis of EEG features including spectral power, amplitude and indices of synchronization. These techniques provided useful information, but the precision was restricted since they were reliant on manually created features and presupposing that the signal was stationary.

The current AI algorithms, such as machine learning (ML) and deep learning (DL), are programs that are taught by patterns that distinguish automatically between raw or minimally processed data. Through large data processing and predicting complicated processes, AI algorithms outperform the more traditional methods and are more accurate in prediction (Brinkmann et al. 2021).

9.3.2. *AI algorithms that are used*

Several methods have been used in seizure forecasting using AI:

– *Supervised ML*: support vector machine (SVM), random forests (RF) and logistic regression models are algorithms that label EEG samples of pre-ictal and inter-ictal materials. These models tend to require a lot of feature engineering; however, they are interpretable and have a low execution time.

– *Unsupervised learning*: seizure-prone state detection and clustering systems are also capable of identifying them without labeling, which is useful in situations where there is not enough labeling information about patients.

– *DL architectures*: CNNs and RNNs, such as long short-term memory (LSTM) networks, have revolutionized the prediction of the seizure process by extracting spatial and time-related patterns in the EEG signals automatically. CNNs focus on spatial representations among electrodes, and RNNs follow the sequential relations among the time-series data (Miron and Meisel 2024). The performance is further improved with the use of hybrid architectures, which incorporate these approaches.

9.3.3. *The main benefits of AI-based solutions*

AI forecasting creates various advantages that are not found in conventional forecasting techniques. To start with, AI systems are patient-friendly as they adjust into an individual pattern, developing detailed models that enhance with the process of constant learning. Second, such models are capable of incorporating multimodal information regarding EEG, neuroimaging, heart rate variability and wearable sensors, and prediction is more reliable and applicable. Third, AI can be deployed in real time, and its algorithms can be tailored to low-power wearable devices, so new opportunities to constantly monitor patients emerge, which could be used in the non-hospital future.

9.3.4. *Restrictions and continued hindrances*

Although there has been progress, there is still a large challenge regarding epilepsy research, which provides little annotated data on which to train AI models; they require large quantities of data, patients vary a lot and long records are not very common. There is the risk of overfitting, particularly when dealing with small datasets. Besides, the black-box quality of most systems based on DL poses a challenge to interpretability, which is demanded by clinicians and regulators. To fill this gap, XAI techniques are being created to highlight the aspects that shape the predictions, thus making them more transparent.

9.4. Machine learning approaches for seizure prediction

ML has established itself as a fundamental part of the development of seizure prediction. It bridges the gap between the traditional methods of statistics and more advanced DL models that prevail in current studies. Due to their ability to identify the existence of small patterns in complex data, ML algorithms are particularly effective at the analysis of electroencephalography (EEG) signals, neuroimaging and other physiological indicators which are important to epilepsy (Raj et al. 2024). These models are then trained using pre-productive and inter-productive portions of data that can be used to classify or give an approximation of the risk of a seizure happening.

9.4.1. *Unifying machine learning via feature engineering*

The effectiveness of the ML-based seizure prediction depends on the effective feature extraction pipeline. EEG data are high-dimensional and non-stationary, and raw data therefore has to be extracted into useful descriptors. This is constrained by the typical spectral power of delta, theta, alpha, beta and gamma band, measures of phase synchrony, entropy and nonlinear dynamics including fractal dimensions (Mourad et al. 2025). Time-domain-based features such as variance, Hjorth parameters, etc., are also common. The choice of the appropriate features directly affects the performance of the classifiers. Principal component analysis (PCA) and linear discriminant analysis (LDA) are two dimensionality-reduction procedures that are regularly used to filter out the noise and retain the most discriminating data.

9.4.2. *Classical algorithms of machine learning*

Some ML possibilities have been demonstrated to be useful in predicting seizures:

– *Support vector machines (SVMs)*: SVMs are recommended when they work with high-dimensional data and they construct hyperplanes to distinguish between pre-ictal and inter-ictal classes with the greatest margin. Nonlinear boundaries are possible by use of Kernel tricks to increase accuracy.

– *Random forests (RFs)*: these are the collections of decision trees, which are trained on randomly selected subsets of features and are resistant to overfitting as well as multifaceted interactions, and are thus useful in seizure prediction

– *k-nearest neighbors (kNN)*: kNN use nearest neighbors in the feature-space to assign a label. Though quite simple, they are able to work efficiently with well-thought-out features, but are computationally costly on large data points.

– *Online tools*: naïve Bayes and logistic regression: both are probabilistic models with an easily interpretable result and are used as a baseline or hybrids with other sophisticated algorithms.

The algorithms are so efficient that they can be deployed on devices smaller than a hand, or wearable, but they rely on manually developed features, so they cannot be generalized (Koirala et al. 2025).

9.4.3. *Patient-specific versus generalized models*

One of the central discussions in ML-based seizure prediction is whether it is better to model them more specifically to individual patients or to create generic models that can be applicable across populations. Patient-specific models, which are trained with the information of an individual patient, are often better than generic models since they are able to match important biomarkers of seizures unique to a particular person. However, training them would require lengthy EEG recordings, which may not always be available. Generalized models aim to find universal pre-ictal signatures, but are not good at being reliable with diverse patients. The combination of methods between generalized and fine-tuning on single data with transfer learning or retraining incrementally represents a hopeful trade-off (Wu et al. 2021).

9.4.4. *Handling imbalanced data*

Seizure prediction datasets are not balanced as there are seizures that are quite uncommon when contrasted to the length of the inter-ictal duration. This imbalance may favor the majority category of algorithms, making them less sensitive to the onset of seizures. Typical solutions involve oversampling of minority examples such as the synthetic minority oversampling technique

(SMOTE), cost-sensitive learning which punishes misclassifications and ensemble ones which trade global performance off.

9.5. Deep learning and neural network models

Although classical ML has provided helpful insight on the prediction of seizures, it is prone to relying on manual feature engineering and cannot handle high-dimensional and non-stationary data. DL has altered that, whereby it learns via raw signals or insignificantly processed ones. DL models have large datasets as well as hierarchical representations to predict seizures.

9.5.1. *Advantages of deep learning over traditional ML*

In contrast to ML approaches, which generate the job-specific features with the use of hand cues, DL generates discriminative representations automatically and operates at various levels of abstraction. This is exceptionally useful when analyzing EEG data, in which patterns of epileptic seizures are conceived in complex spatial–temporal influences. DL models are nonlinear dependency models, cross-channel correlations and long-range temporal sequences, which are essential in the model of the pre-ictal state (Gurmessa and Jimma 2025). Hardware advancements and open data have also increased the use of DL in studies of epilepsy.

9.5.2. *Convolutional neural networks (CNNs)*

CNNs are superior in processing spatially structured data, and they are popular with seizure forecasting. CNN architectures are a natural fit for EEG recordings, which have electrode arrays. EEG can be converted to time frequency images (spectrograms or wavelet transforms), and the 2-D CNNs find spatial features associated with the occurrence of a seizure, whereas the 1-D CNNs use raw EEG sequences directly. These models usually perform better than the classical feature-based prediction, particularly when predicting patients.

9.5.3. *Recurrent neural networks (RNNs) and LSTM models*

Using temporal dynamics is important when learning about the development of seizures. This can be performed well by RNNs, but especially LSTMs that deal with long-term dependencies as compared to the normal RNNs. LSTMs train time-dependent connections between EEG segments, which includes the multi-minute pre-ictal period of time. BiLSTMs or bidirectional LSTMs enhance the level of accuracy by allowing the past and future context of a sequence (Keikhosrokiani et al. 2024).

9.5.4. *Autoencoders and generative models*

Variational autoencoders (VAEs) are trained to find small latent features of EEG data; they can identify abnormalities in the inter-ictal activity, which are indicative of pre-ictal activity. Generative adversarial networks (GANs) are provided as data augmentation, which produces believable synthetic EEG against the problem of small pre-ictal samples. These techniques are used to correct the imbalance of classes and enhance the strength of the model.

AI/computational approach	**Input data modalities**	**Core features/ processing methods**	**Applications in seizure prediction**	**Key advantages/ outcomes**
Traditional machine learning (SVM, RF, kNN, LR)	EEG, iEEG, ECG	Spectral power, phase synchrony, entropy, Hjorth parameters	Classification of pre-ictal versus inter-ictal states	Simple implementation, interpretable models, suitable for wearable deployment
Deep learning (CNN, RNN, LSTM, BiLSTM)	EEG (raw/spectrogram)	Spatial–temporal pattern learning, automatic feature extraction	Seizure onset forecasting; long-term EEG pattern recognition	High accuracy (> 90%), learns complex nonlinear relationships
Hybrid CNN–LSTM Models	EEG + physiological signals	Combined spatial and temporal feature learning	Short- and long-term seizure risk estimation	Improved performance and generalization; adaptable to patient-specific patterns
Generative models (VAE, GANs)	EEG (limited datasets)	Latent feature learning, synthetic data generation	Data augmentation; anomaly detection of pre-ictal activity	Reduces data imbalance; improves robustness of training
Multimodal integration (EEG + ECG + motion + neuroimaging)	EEG, MRI, HRV, accelerometry	Data/feature/ decision-level fusion	Comprehensive seizure forecasting; context-aware models	Higher sensitivity, fewer false positives

Edge/wearable AI systems	Wearable EEG, smartwatches, EDA sensors	On-device processing; real-time anomaly detection	Continuous monitoring and real-time forecasting	Low latency; privacy-preserving, patient-centric care
Explainable AI (XAI) and federated learning	Distributed clinical data	Attention maps, SHAP, local feature attribution	Clinician-interpretable predictions; cross-site model training	Trustworthy, privacy-compliant, regulatory-ready solutions

Table 9.1. *Artificial intelligence techniques for seizure prediction and forecasting in epilepsy*

9.6. Multimodal data integration for seizure forecasting

Epilepsy diagnosis and the prediction of seizures have been mainly based on EEG. Seizures are, however, not a phenomenon that is purely brain-based. They are a product of complicated processes between neural systems, cardiovascular systems, metabolic systems and behavioral systems.

9.6.1. *Multimodal data integration*

Multimodal data integration, a combination of EEG and complementary physiological and neuroimaging data, is an enlightening approach that may be exploited to improve the reliability, robustness and clinical usefulness of seizure prediction (Halimeh et al. 2025). This can be done by combining various data streams to form more extensive signatures of the pre-ictal state; in comparison, single-modality methods can have higher predictive accuracy with AI algorithms.

9.6.2. *EEG as the primary modality*

EEG is still the gold standard in predicting epileptic seizures since it directly measures the activity of the cortices using electrical activity. Scalp EEG and intracranial EEG (iEEG) can both provide rich temporal resolution, which allows real-time observation of brain dynamics in transition. Scalp EEG is noninvasive and easy to use, but has poor spatial resolution, and is susceptible to noise and artifact contamination. iEEG has a high signal fidelity and spatial resolution, but it is a more invasive procedure that can only be used on a population of study patients. Multimodal frameworks are also meant to supplement EEG by the use of additional physiological signals to counteract these limitations.

9.6.3. *Neuroimaging modalities*

The structural and functional neuroimaging systems contain great information on epileptogenic networks. MRI has been shown to have structural abnormalities regarding cortical dysplasia or sclerosis of the hippocampus. The fMRI is used to record hemodynamic activity associated with epileptic activity. Further spotting of metabolic changes in seizure-prone areas can be achieved through positron emission tomography (PET) and single-photon emission computed tomography (SPECT). Neuroimaging modalities are generally not well adapted to continuous monitoring, although when combined with EEG data in the process of training a model, this approach assists AI algorithms in identifying patient-specific anatomical and functional biomarkers and enhances personalization of forecasting models (Carmo et al. 2024).

9.6.4. *Integration strategies*

The problem of multimodal forecasting is to effectively combine heterogeneous data which differ in terms of time and space density. Fusion strategies include:

– *Early fusion*: joining raw features across a number of modalities prior to the training of the model.

– *Intermediate fusion*: run each modality through distinct feature–extraction postulates and then find a unification at an intermediate representation.

– *Late fusion*: fusion between the independent model outputs using ensemble or voting models.

The DL models with multimodal convolutional and recurrent networks demonstrate high ability in the synthesis of such varied signals. The attention systems also increase the performance by prioritizing each channel based on its predictive importance.

9.6.5. *Benefits and challenges*

Multimodal combination is more sensitive and less false, and also provides more resilience to noise or artifact in one data stream. It also provides more clinical information by emphasizing systemic and environmental factors that contribute to the risk of seizures. However, challenges remain. Multimodal databases are challenging to gather in a synchronized manner. Patient adherence to various monitoring devices is hard to achieve. This is caused by data heterogeneity, which imposes technical problems of model alignment and generalizability. In addition, there is a higher level of data collection, and this brings privacy and ethical issues that need to be regulated and ensured by safe infrastructure (AbuAlrob et al. 2025).

9.7. Wearable devices and real-time forecasting

The uncertainty surrounding seizures could readily threaten epileptic patients, reduce their autonomy and increase risk of injury. The specified issues can be addressed with the help of real-time seizure forecasting, which provides appropriate notifications in time, complemented by timely and efficient safety measures. The wearable devices are on the frontline, starting with EEG headsets, then smart watch and biosensor patches, which can analyze physiological signals when they arrive using AI (Otu et al. 2025).

9.7.1. *Wearable EEG systems*

The advances that miniature, wireless EEG devices have gone through have dramatically advanced such that brain monitoring can be continuous, without the need to be in the clinic. These wearables put much emphasis on portability, comfort and long-term usage, which other versions of bulky hospital systems do not consider. Dry electrodes, reduction in channels and wireless transmission are some of the features that enhance patient compliance. They record the same pre-seizure brain activity as conventional EEG, but its in-built AI processes data in situ, reducing latency and removing electronic computers. One of the major issues is the tradeoff between signal quality and wearability because the number of electrodes will complicate spatial resolution.

9.7.2. *Physiological wearables other than EEG*

Wearable technology also tracks changes in the system related to the risk of seizures. Fitness trackers and smartwatches measure heart rate, heart rate variation (HRV), electrodermal activities and movement. The autonomic modifications that are usually triggered by seizures include tachycardia, which can be detected in advance or at the time of seizure occurrence. Gyroscopes and accelerometers on wearables record motor activity caused by seizures, which become contextualized to predict algorithmically. Multi-sensor systems, which integrate EEG with cardiovascular, and motion recordings have further potential for pinpointing extensive real-time intuitions (Chiang et al. 2022).

9.7.3. *Edge computing and real*

Multimodal data transmission in real time to external servers causes delays and privacy issues. More recent wearables have started to incorporate edge computing and have AI algorithms integrated into the device. This enables real-time forecasts with a low level of latency and reduced dependence on cloud computing resources (Cui et al. 2023). Authorities are researching energy-efficient and neuromorphic hardware to maximize performance with low power allocation.

9.7.4. *Problems and future perspectives*

Wearable forecasting systems have a number of challenges, despite recent advancement. In fact, it is hard to keep the signal quality constant, particularly with ambulatory EEG, as electrodes can fall off, and noise or movement artifacts can ruin data. Data security and privacy are of high concern as the gadgets acquire sensitive body information. Regulatory approvals of wearables and standardization are still an ongoing issue (Rathod and Naik 2022). It seems possible that future directions are related to multi-sensor integration, the development of the low-powered AI chips and XAI features to enhance transparency. Through these developments, wearable real-time prognostic systems will be integrated into the management of individualized epilepsy (Vieira et al. 2023).

9.8. Privacy, ethics and data challenges

The use of AI-powered seizure prediction applications provokes significant privacy, ethical and data issues. Although ML and DL have increased accuracy in prediction, the gathering, storing and processing of sensitive patient information presents more challenges than technical problems (Amrani et al. 2024).

9.8.1. *Data privacy concerns*

The process of forecasting a seizure is based on the ongoing gathering of physiological and behavioral information: EEG, heart rate, motion activity, sleep and stress data, and other contextual data. This would be a major breach of privacy: any unauthorized transmission would deprive someone of sensitive health information. It is necessary to comply with laws of data protection such as the U.S. HIPAA and the EU GDPR. Mobile apps and wearable devices should encrypt and transmit data through secure methods and anonymize patient data.

9.8.2. *Ethical considerations*

AI-based seizure forecasting entails a number of ethical problems:

– Accuracy matters. False positives may trigger unnecessary anxieties, restrict normal lives or lead to incorrect treatment, whereas false negatives may endanger patients.

– Equitable access is key. The socio-economic disparities may restrict the use of wearables, continuous EEG or AI environments, and become a contributor to health inequity.

– Informed consent and patient autonomy are vital. Users need to know what data is being collected, the functionality of the AI and the interpretation of predictions. Limitations to algorithms used in forecasting should be transparent, ensuring that dependence is not put on automated forecasting (Wang and Jing 2025).

9.8.3. *Regulatory and legal problems*

Seizure forecasting devices that use AI should meet the requirements of medical gadgets, information security and software-as-a-combined-medical-gadget (SaMD) standards. Regulators have been requiring transparency of their algorithm, representation using a diverse population and a complete description of how models have been updated. It is not clear who should be held legally accountable for making incorrect predictions; this is because manufacturers, clinicians and patients should know where their liability starts and ends.

9.9. Future directions in AI-driven seizure forecasting

Seizure forecasting through AI has already evolved rapidly, and aspects such as prediction accuracy, clinical application and patient value are yet to be enhanced. The future will involve more advanced algorithms, integration of multimodal data, patient-specific model customization and deeper incorporation of these tools into healthcare systems (King-Stephens 2024).

9.9.1. *Categorized and adaptation model*

Personalization will be key. The models will be trained to each patient and the brain and behavioral data, and the adaptive learning will enable it to keep updating as new data becomes available. This method is better than general-use models since it measures the variations between and among patients, increasing sensitivity and reducing false alarms. Predictions will become even more topical with the addition of lifestyle data, adherence to medication and circadian rhythms.

9.9.2. *Multimodal systems and sensory modality*

The next generation of monitors will include EEG, imaging biomarkers and autonomic outputs, as well as environmental information in one predictive system. Biosensors attached to the wearable will record heart, metabolic and motion signals with high accuracy and low latency. These data will be run on edge AI and cloud servers, providing real-time and continuous forecasting and actionable alerts to patients and clinicians.

9.9.3. *Explainable and clinically trustworthy AI*

In more complicated models, explainability is a prerequisite to clinical uptake. A detailed new architecture will involve decipherable architectures, attention scripts and graphic instruments so that clinicians can observe why a model makes a choice. Elucidated AI will facilitate collaborative decision-making, legal compliance and patient trust, and will help to bridge the gap between algorithm outputs and clinical responses (Mansilla et al. 2024).

9.10. Conclusion

The prediction of epilepsy and seizures has emerged as a rapidly developing area, which is supported with neurophysiology, AI and digital health applications. The spontaneous quality of the seizures has been a thorn in the side of patients and other clinicians with regard to safety and quality of life, as well as treatment regimen. ML and DL models could identify pre-ictal biomarkers, early warning patterns in EEG and other physiological measurements, and allow patient-specific real-time prediction, which is changing in-patient care practices from reactive to proactive. Wearable devices, multimodal sensors and edge computing can now provide continuous monitoring in day-to-day life. XAI enhances effective transparency, which provides doctors and patients with comprehensible explanations of predictions. Privacy approaches such as federated learning allow teams to safely learn with data deployed in a distributed manner, and trade progress off with ethics. However, problems of data heterogeneity, false positives, regulatory impediments and unequal access remain. Ongoing research would concentrate on personalized adaptive models, closed-loop therapeutic system integration and lean multimodal data pipelines, which will further enhance the precision of the prediction and patient empowerment, and decrease the pressure on the health system.

9.11. References

AbuAlrob, M.A., Itbaisha, A., Mesraoua, B. (2025). Unlocking new frontiers in epilepsy through AI: From seizure prediction to personalized medicine. *Epilepsy & Behavior*, 166, 110327.

Amrani, G., Adadi, A., Berrada, M. (2024). Explainable deep learning for enhanced epilepsy monitoring and diagnosis: A review. In *International Conference on Advanced Intelligent Systems for Sustainable Development*, 17 December, 117–131. Springer, Cham.

Brinkmann, B.H., Karoly, P.J., Nurse, E.S., Dumanis, S.B., Nasseri, M., Viana, P.F., Schulze-Bonhage, A., Freestone, D.R., Worrell, G., Richardson, M.P. et al. (2021). Seizure diaries and forecasting with wearables: Epilepsy monitoring outside the clinic. *Frontiers in Neurology*, 12, 690404.

Carmo, A.S., Abreu, M., Baptista, M.F., de Oliveira Carvalho, M., Peralta, A.R., Fred, A., Bentes, C., da Silva, H.P. (2024). Automated algorithms for seizure forecast: A systematic review and meta-analysis. *Journal of Neurology*, 271(10), 6573–6587.

Chiang, S., Baud, M.O., Worrell, G.A., Rao, V.R. (2022). Seizure forecasting and detection: Computational models, machine learning, and translation into devices. *Frontiers in Neurology*, 13, 874070.

Cui, J., Balzekas, I., Nurse, E., Viana, P., Gregg, N., Karoly, P., Stirling, R.E., Worrell, G., Richardson, M.P., Freestone, D.R. et al. (2023). Perceived seizure risk in epilepsy: Chronic electronic surveys with and without concurrent electroencephalography. *Epilepsia*, 64(9), 2421–2433.

Gurmessa, D.K. and Jimma, W. (2025). A comprehensive evaluation of interpretable artificial intelligence for epileptic seizure diagnosis using an electroencephalogram: A systematic review. *Digital Health*, 11, 20552076251325411.

Halimeh, M., Jackson, M., Loddenkemper, T., Meisel, C. (2025). Training size predictably improves machine learning-based epileptic seizure forecasting from wearables. *Neuroscience Informatics*, 5(1), 100184.

Hasija, T., Kuschel, M., Jackson, M., Dailey, S., Menne, H., Reinsberger, C., Vieluf, S., Loddenkemper, T. (2025). Improving wearable-based seizure prediction by feature fusion using an explainable growing network. *Artificial Intelligence in Medicine*, 103228.

Keikhosrokiani, P., Isomursu, M., Uusimaa, J., Kortelainen, J. (2024). A sustainable artificial-intelligence-augmented digital care pathway for epilepsy: Automating seizure tracking based on electroencephalogram data using artificial intelligence. *Digital Health*, 10, 20552076241287356.

Kerr, W.T., McFarlane, K.N., Figueiredo Pucci, G. (2024). The present and future of seizure detection, prediction, and forecasting with machine learning, including the future impact on clinical trials. *Frontiers in Neurology*, 15, 1425490.

Khan, F.A., Umar, Z., Jolfaei, A., Tariq, M. (2025). Explainable AI for epileptic seizure detection in Internet of Medical Things. *Digital Communications and Networks*, 11(3), 587–593.

King-Stephens, D. (2024). AI and EEG: Should EEGers RIP (rest in peace)? *Epilepsy Currents*, 24(2), 111–113.

Koirala, N., Adhikari, S.R., Adhikari, M., Yadav, T., Anwar, A.R., Ciolac, D., Shrestha, B., Adhikari, I., Khanal, B., Muthuraman, M. (2025). Assistive artificial intelligence in epilepsy and its impact on epilepsy care in low- and middle-income countries. *Brain Sciences*, 15(5), 481.

Mansilla, D., Tveit, J., Aurlien, H., Avigdor, T., Ros-Castello, V., Ho, A., Abdallah, C., Gotman, J., Beniczky, S., Frauscher, B. (2024). Generalizability of electroencephalographic interpretation using artificial intelligence: An external validation study. *Epilepsia*, 65(10), 3028–3037.

Miron, G. and Meisel, C. (2024). Seizure forecasting based on AI-supported analysis of multidien and circadian cycles in EEG and non-EEG long-term datasets. *Clinical Epileptology*, 37(4), 278–281.

Mourad, R., Diab, A., Merhi, Z., Khalil, M., Jeannès, R.L. (2025). Machine and deep learning methods for epileptic seizure recognition using EEG data: A systematic review. *Brain Research*, 1864, 149797.

Otu, W., Khan, M.U., Javed, H.T., Sheikh, I.S. (2025). Artificial intelligence in epilepsy education. *Advanced Neurology*, 4(3), 16–28.

Raj, D., Jeevan, A.J., Rafeeque, R., Rhishitha, T.S., Akshay, S., Merry, K.P. (2024). Enhancing seizure detection through deep learning-based wearable devices. In *2024 International Conference on Integrated Circuits, Communication, and Computing Systems (ICIC3S)*, 8 June, 1–6. IEEE.

Rathod, P. and Naik, S. (2022). Review on epilepsy detection with explainable artificial intelligence. In *2022 10th International Conference on Emerging Trends in Engineering and Technology-Signal and Information Processing (ICETET-SIP-22)*, 29 April, 1–6. IEEE.

Saadoon, Y.A., Khalil, M., Battikh, D. (2025). Machine and deep learning-based seizure prediction: A scoping review on the use of temporal and spectral features. *Applied Sciences*, 15(11), 6279.

Stirling, R.E., Grayden, D.B., D'Souza, W., Cook, M.J., Nurse, E., Freestone, D.R., Payne, D.E., Brinkmann, B.H., Pal Attia, T., Viana, P.F. et al. (2021). Forecasting seizure likelihood with wearable technology. *Frontiers in Neurology*, 12, 704060.

Tian, F., Yang, J., Zhao, S., Sawan, M. (2021). A new neuromorphic computing approach for epileptic seizure prediction. In *2021 IEEE International Symposium on Circuits and Systems (ISCAS)*, 22 May, 1–5.

Tveit, J., Aurlien, H., Plis, S., Calhoun, V.D., Tatum, W.O., Schomer, D.L., Arntsen, V., Cox, F., Fahoum, F., Gallentine, W.B. et al. (2023). Automated interpretation of clinical electroencephalograms using artificial intelligence. *JAMA Neurology*, 80(8), 805–812.

Vieira, J.C., Guedes, L.A., Santos, M.R., Sanchez-Gendriz, I. (2023). Using explainable artificial intelligence to obtain efficient seizure-detection models based on electroencephalography signals. *Sensors*, 23(24), 9871.

Wang, C. and Jing, W. (2025). Artificial intelligence in electroencephalography analysis for epilepsy diagnosis and management. *Frontiers in Neurology*, 16, 1615120.

Wu, D., Shi, Y., Wang, Z., Yang, J., Sawan, M. (2021). C2SP-Net: Joint compression and classification network for epilepsy seizure prediction. arXiv preprint, arXiv:2110.13674.

Yang, H., Mueller, J., Eberlein, M., Kalousios, S., Leonhardt, G., Duun-Henriksen, J., Kjaer, T., Tetzlaff, R. (2024). Seizure forecasting with ultra long-term EEG signals. *Clinical Neurophysiology*, 167, 211–220.

Yu, H., Mu, Q., Liu, C., Wang, S., Sun, J. (2025). Technical system of electroencephalography-based brain-computer interface: Advances, applications, and challenges. *Neural Regeneration Research*, 10, 4103.

Zou, Z., Chen, B., Xiao, D., Tang, F., Li, X. (2024). Accuracy of machine learning in detecting pediatric epileptic seizures: Systematic review and meta-analysis. *Journal of Medical Internet Research*, 26, e55986.

10

Intelligent Robotic Systems for Neurorehabilitation and Assistive Care

Smart artificial intelligence (AI) robots are now turning into revolutionary devices in neurorehabilitation and in offering a helping hand. They offer innovative remedies to the increasing global burden of neurological disorders and disabilities. The prevalence of conditions such as strokes, spinal cord injuries, Parkinson's disease and cerebral palsy is on the rise, so the need for innovative rehabilitation techniques that are not limited to traditional therapy is growing. Intelligent robotics involves state-of-the-art sensing, machine learning (ML), AI and adaptive control to provide customized, and fine and constant interventions, based on the needs of each patient. Instead of using conventional methods of rehabilitation, which consumes resources and is restricted by the availability of the therapist, robotic platforms allow high-intensity and repetitive training, and training that is specific to a task. This kind of training is necessary in enhancing neuroplasticity and functional recovery. Such systems provide their extension into the assistive domain, including mobility, communication and daily activities of the individuals with chronic impairment. Some of the major advances include exoskeletons for gait training and robotic-assisted rehabilitation devices. Additionally, wearable sensors, cloud-based analytics and tele-rehabilitation platforms can increase access to wearable sensors. It is also capable of remote monitoring and ongoing care. Nevertheless, despite the major development, there are still obstacles. These are affordability of the system, its capacity to meet different types of patients, its safety assurance and ethical concerns of autonomy and confidentiality of the data.

In this chapter, we critically discuss the principles, paradigms and new trends of intelligent robotic systems in neurorehabilitation and assistive care. It brings to the forefront recent progress, clinical evidence and problems and research in order to establish patient-centered, friendly and sustainable rehabilitation eco-systems.

Chapter written by Debabrata SAHANA and Atul Namdev PAWAR.

10.1. Introduction

Some of the leading causes of disability in the world include neurological disorders and injuries. They increase health expenses and reduce life quality. Strokes, spinal cord injuries, traumatic brain injuries, Parkinson's disease and multiple sclerosis are some of the common conditions requiring a significant duration of care (Zhang et al. 2025). Conventional therapy (e.g. physiotherapy) and occupational therapy have a weak point due to the number of therapists, adherence of patients to the programs and the necessity of repetitive and intensive exercise, stimulating the brain to restructure (Carnevale et al. 2025).

The manipulation of robots used in overcoming these challenges is being developed through robot systems using artificial intelligence (AI), machine learning (ML), sensors and control theory. They are able to help patients perform repetitive actions as well as adapt to the needs of every patient. They frequently do better than traditional forms of practice, since they provide narrow, brutal and sustained practice. By including brain–computer interfaces, cloud computing and wearables, these robots can be used to serve patients outside of the clinic as well as at home or via tele-rehabilitation (Alshami et al. 2025).

This chapter summarizes the design concepts and present-day and future trends of intelligent robotics in neurorehabilitation and the assistive care of people in general. It follows the history of the emergence of rehabilitation technology, examines practical applications and speculates on how robotics can assist individuals to lead normal lives. Of equal importance are the critical barriers discussed, including cost, availability, safety, ethical considerations and the need for extensive clinical testing. The chapter summarizes the recent developments and demonstrates how intelligent robotics can transform the future of neurorehabilitation and the ways of establishing a more effective care ecosystem.

10.2. Principles of intelligent robotic systems

10.2.1. *Human–robot interaction (HRI)*

One of the fundamental principles of intelligent robotics is the safe and natural interaction of humans and robots. Rehabilitation robots must attract people with possible motor, sensory or cognitive deficiencies. In order to do this, they must have highly responsive and adapting interfaces. There is a need to sense multimodally. Force sensors, motion capture, EMG, EEG and IMUs make it possible to detect small-scale movements and muscle reactions, as well as motor intent from the robot. This sensing enables the robot to give out proportional and timely help. For example, EMG-driven exoskeletons can detect residual muscle activity in stroke patients and provide support only when needed, thereby encouraging voluntary effort and promoting neuroplasticity (Lingampally et al. 2024).

10.2.2. *Task-specific and repetitive training*

Neurorehabilitation relies heavily on neuroplasticity, which is promoted through intensive, task-specific and repetitive practice. Robotic systems excel in delivering consistent and precise repetitions of functional tasks such as reaching, grasping or walking. Unlike traditional therapy, which can be limited by therapist fatigue or time constraints, robots enable high-frequency, high-intensity interventions that are tailored to the patient's recovery stage. End-effector and exoskeleton devices are commonly used to guide limb movements along physiologically accurate trajectories, ensuring proper joint kinematics and minimizing compensatory strategies (Nicora et al. 2025).

10.2.3. *Adaptive control and personalization*

Intelligent robotic systems have a characteristic of adaptability. The patients are different in terms of skills, exhaustion and progression; hence, the robot should dynamically adjust to their needs. The support can be changed dynamically by using adaptive control algorithms, which are typically driven by ML or reinforcement learning (RL). As an example, a robotic arm can be presented by providing complete aid to a patient with severe hemiparesis and gradually lessen aid as the motor performance of this patient is restored. Therapy scheduling, difficulty scaling and feedback methods are also subject to personalization, which makes the interventions remain motivating and efficient (Rad and Brisan 2025).

10.2.4. *Safety and compliance*

Safety is the most important factor when dealing with vulnerable people. Compliant actuators, soft padding and impedance control are used by intelligent robots to minimize possible injuries. They constantly track forces, torque and joint angles and, in case of unstable situations, the system halts or varies the movement immediately. This defining principle of safety is required in home-based rehabilitation or in cases of unsupervised usage, where the supervision of therapists can be reduced.

10.2.5. *Multimodal integration*

Contemporary intelligent robots are designed in such a way that they can be controlled in collaboration with other technologies to enhance therapy.

Brain–computer interfaces or BCI allow patients to operate machines by their brain signals. This comes in handy, especially in individuals who are severely paralyzed. The AR and VR platforms build on the immersive spaces that encourage patients and provide real-time feedback on performance. Physical changes monitored by wearable biosensors include the heart rate, fatigue of the muscles and their oxygen levels. They enable the workload to automatically increase. The combination of various forms of technology offers a patient-centered comprehensive solution that helps with both mobility and thinking.

10.3. Robotics in neurorehabilitation

10.3.1. *Upper-limb rehabilitation*

Impairment of the upper limb is common following a stroke, traumatic brain injury or spinal cord injury and may lead to significant challenges in the patient's day-to-day activities. Traditional therapy is based on labor-intensive and repetitive exercises which cannot be easily sustained throughout the process of rehabilitation (Hobbs and Artemiadis 2020). Organized, rigorous training to restore arm and hand functions is provided by robotic systems, which include end effector systems (including MIT-Manus) and exoskeletons (including Armeo and MyoPro).

Devices based on exoskeletons mimic the movement of the human joints allowing shoulder, elbow, wrist and finger movement to be accurately controlled. The anaerobic bench can be programmed to an active-assisted mode, an active-resistive mode or a totally passive mode, depending on the patient's abilities. The newer improvements now incorporate electromyographic (EMG) signals to detect an intention of the patient and provide corresponding aid (Yuan et al. 2021).

The other trend, which gains momentum, is the integration of virtual and augmented reality (VR/AR) with robotic training. VR-based robots can direct the patients into engaging conditions and encourage participation, as well as track the motor performance. As an example, interaction between Armeo and VR activities has enhanced motor performance compared to robotic therapy (Karami et al. 2024).

10.3.2. *Lower-limb rehabilitation and gait training*

Patients who have suffered a stroke, a spinal cord injury or Parkinson's disease prioritize restoring their mobility. Rehabilitation robots designed to work with the lower limbs through the treadmill can be in turn split into treadmill-based gait typers (e.g. Lokomat and gait trainer GT) and wearable exoskeletons (e.g. EksoGT, ReWalk and HAL).

The equipment is used to support a gait training program using treadmill-based machines to support the body weight of a patient during natural walking with varying robotic support. With the help of such systems, gait cycles can be intensively repeated, and patient safety can be ensured (Guatibonza et al. 2024).

Conversely, wearable robotic exoskeletons not only provide overground walking, but also allow patients to train locomotion in the real world, not only in the clinic. They enable patients to walk in more natural and real-world environments (Ezra Tsur and Elkana 2024).

Gait rehabilitation has been improved through the implementation of intelligent control strategies. Adaptive algorithms have the ability to adjust the gait speed, the length of the strides and the joint torque with regard to the fatigue or the recovery level of the patient. Sensor combination (e.g. inertial measurement units and pressure sensors) will be used to give real-time information about the quality of gait. According to clinical studies, the walking endurance, balance and independence improve after the assistance of an exoskeleton (Brown and Xie 2024).

10.3.3. *Cognitive rehabilitation*

Cognitive impairment frequently accompanies neurological disorders, reducing independence and quality of life. Socially assistive robots (SARs) are increasingly used for cognitive rehabilitation, providing companionship, structured interactions and memory exercises. Unlike physical rehabilitation robots, SARs focus on stimulating cognitive engagement and emotional well-being (McDermott et al. 2024).

There are therapeutic seal robots such as PARO and a humanoid robot called Pepper, which have been applied to patients who have dementia and Alzheimer's disease, as well as those with post-elemental cognitive issues. These robots assist patients to recall, practice attention and socialize, hence reducing loneliness. Since they process natural language with the help of AI, they are capable of having meaningful conversations with each patient, establishing a therapeutic relationship with them (Vaida et al. 2025).

Adoption of cognitive training in addition to the motor rehabilitation is yet another promising line. The existence of robot systems involving serious games and VR platforms involves the combination of the movement and the thinking portion of the recovery simultaneously, which facilitates the more comprehensive experience of healing (Calabrò et al. 2021). The combined approaches are particularly applicable to stroke survivors that have physical and cognitive challenges.

10.4. Assistive robotics for daily living

10.4.1. *Mobility assistance*

Paralysis is one of the most disabling consequences of neurological diseases, which include strokes, spinal cord injuries or multiple sclerosis. Mobility assistive robots include powered wheelchairs, robotic walkers and wearable exoskeletons. In contrast to purely rehabilitative systems, they can be applied to support employees on a long-term basis (Aprile et al. 2020).

AI-based software is becoming popular in robotic wheelchairs. These allow for the detection of obstacles, planning the path and autonomously controlling the environment in complex areas. Indicatively, powered wheelchairs, categorized as AI use cameras and LiDAR sensors, maneuver safely in indoor and outdoor environments. Balance and adaptive gait assistance are also available on the robotic walkers, particularly when they are used with older adults with neurodegenerative symptoms.

ReWalk and Indego wearable exoskeletons are now used as a long-term assistive mobility device. They allow the users who have suffered a spinal cord injury to walk on the ground. In addition to the physical advantages, the devices enhance psychological health and minimize secondary morbidity such as cardiovascular deterioration and osteoporosis (Arthanat et al. 2020).

10.4.2. *Communication and social interaction*

Individuals with a compromised nervous system usually have problems with communication and speech, and this curtails their ability to socially participate. The gap can be addressed with the assistance of speech syntheses, natural language processors and gesture recognition through the help of assistive robots.

The humanoid robots such as Pepper and NAO provide interactive communicative capabilities, particularly with persons who have aphasia or neurodegenerative ailments (Fareh et al. 2023).

In addition to real-time communication, SARs enhance emotional health, making them less lonely and depressed. They are able to initiate conversation, remind patients to take medications, engage patients in games or do therapy exercises with them. They are particularly needed in nursing homes, where social isolation is a problem.

10.4.3. *Home-care integration*

One of the current trends of assistive robotics' official functions is incorporating it into smart homes. Home robots may be used to assist in the day-to-day chores of feeding, changing clothes or picking things up. Care-Obot and the human support robot (HSR) made by Toyota are service robots that are able to clean the house, pick up objects from the floor, respond to voice commands and carry out simple household caregiving activities (Falzarano et al. 2019).

Linking such robots to Internet of Things (IoT) systems will increase their capabilities. The sensors, appliances and wearable devices relay information to the robot and monitor vital signs, a fall and real-time communication with the caregivers or the medical workers. The outcome is a more comprehensive vision of the assistive care in which assistive robots will serve as companions and clinical monitors.

10.5. Technological paradigms and enablers

10.5.1. *ML and AI*

An intelligent robotic system will rely on ML and AI. The ML algorithms make predictions about user intentions, optimize training procedures and personalize interventions in real time by processing vast amounts of data, namely, patient movements, physiological indicators and therapy results (Vaida et al. 2025).

As an example, RL can be used in the control of exoskeletons, whereby the robots can learn to apply the best assist levels of patient effort and support. Deep learning (DL) works with EEG and EMG records, which are accurate during identifying the motor intent required to carry out rehabilitation activities. As AI applications do, these AI-driven solutions enhance the customization of therapy intensity and difficulty to the pace of individual accomplishment.

10.5.2. *Brain–computer interfaces (BCIs)*

BCIs represent one of the most transformative enablers of intelligent robotics. By translating neural signals directly into control commands, BCIs allow patients with severe motor impairments to operate robotic devices. Noninvasive BCIs using EEG are most common, although invasive techniques offer higher accuracy.

In neurorehabilitation, BCIs can detect motor imagery (e.g. imagining hand movements) and trigger robotic arms to perform the intended action. This strengthens brain–muscle connectivity and supports neuroplasticity (McDermott et al. 2024).

10.5.3. *Wearable sensors*

Wearable sensors provide real-time information, which improves the reactivity of robots. Exoskeletons or wearable orthoses include common gait pattern, limb motion and balance capture devices called IMUs, accelerometers, gyroscopes and pressure sensors.

The embedded real-time information allows robots to change assistance in real time to make sure that therapy is safe and effective. Oxygen-saturation monitors, heart-rate meters and muscle-activation sensors are wearable physiological sensors that can provide clinicians with information about patient fatigue and provide the opportunity to dynamically process the workload (Fasano et al. 2025).

10.5.4. *IoT and cloud-based integration*

IoT and cloud computing provide not only robotic rehabilitation but also have the opportunity to be integrated into a broader context of a clinic. The IoT-based robots can simply interface with the smart home appliances, hospital information system and caregiver platform in a seamless continuum of care.

Remote monitoring, tele-rehabilitation and patient progress insights are cloud-based systems that allow patients to be analyzed using data (Warutkar et al. 2022). As an illustration, therapists will be able to adjust training regimes remotely, whereas AI will finish its calculations using aggregated data to improve interventions toward various patient groups. This does particularly well in carrying rehabilitation services to under-served and rural areas.

10.6. Clinical evidence and applications

Intelligent robotic systems have continued to be more widely implemented in neurorehabilitation and assistive care in the past decade due to increasing evidence. They demonstrate not only therapeutic, but also practicable viability in regard to a wide variety of neurological disorders, including strokes, spinal cord injuries, traumatic brain injuries, Parkinson's disease and neurodegenerative diseases.

10.6.1. *Evidence in upper-limb rehabilitation*

Impairment of upper limbs is a frequently observed after-effect of stroke and other neurological conditions, which frequently limits self-sufficiency in day-to-day activities. In clinical studies, robotic-assisted upper-limb therapy is always associated with the improvement of motor activity and the increase in the level of activities of daily living. The implementation of gadgets such as MIT-Manus, Armeo and MyoPro has undergone a lot of research on the randomized controlled trials. These works demonstrate a high level of improvement in Fugl-Meyer assessment (FMA) scores, which are the signs of an improvement in motor recovery (Feingold-Polak et al. 2021).

Also, robotic therapy with the use of virtual reality (VR) or physical activities in the form of games improves patient engagement and compliance. VR-enhanced robotic therapy allows the patient to repeat movements more often, with better quality motion and to remain motivated, all of which are related to higher neuroplasticity. Nonetheless, it has been suggested that robot therapy should start immediately after a stroke to increase the recovery of motor senescence, but there is no indication of the time and frequency of their application.

10.6.2. *Evidence in lower-limb and gait training*

Wearable exoskeletons and robotic gait trainers have been integrated as a regular rehabilitative device in the lower limbs. The clinical trials performed in the use of treadmill-based technologies, such as Lokomat and G-EO System, as well as on overground exoskeletons, including ReWalk and Ekso, demonstrate that patients walk faster, with additional step symmetry and endurance (Hirt et al. 2021).

Secondary health benefits are also provided through robot gait training. This decreases spasticity, increases cardiovascular fitness and reduces the occurrence of pressure ulcers since patients are able to be more upright. The studies suggested that robot-aided gait training combined with the regular physiotherapy is more effective than each one alone. Adaptive control systems change the support according to the condition of the performance of the patient and the level of their fatigue. Such systems provide a safer training process, promote active engagement and assist the patient with the highest level of functional improvements.

10.6.3. *Evidence in cognitive and social rehabilitation*

It is depicted that SARS and cognitive rehabilitation platforms play increasingly greater roles in enhancing cognitive function and psychosocial well-being. Researchers which involve the use of robots, including PARO, Pepper and NAO, alongside individuals with dementia, or who have undergone a stroke, have lower rates of anxiety, depression and loneliness. These robots contribute to an improved level of memory recall, attention and involvement into organized cognitive tasks as well (Zhang et al. 2023).

Recent studies give added value to the combination of cognitive and motor rehab. Serious games and both VR and robotic motor training platforms involve both body and brain simultaneously. Initial experiments suggest increases in executive capability, attention and working memory as well as motor restoration. This is because the full functional reintegration can be accelerated with fully integrated robotic interventions.

10.6.4. *Evidence in home-based and long-term use*

Smart robots are at an ever-increasing use in the home environment. Research indicates that they are possible and patients are contented. IoT-enabled devices allow the clinicians to follow the patients remotely and customize rehab plans, eliminating the necessity of having them regularly visit the clinic. Home-based robotic therapy has the benefit of keeping the patient on a constant treatment regimen, enhancing their independence and reducing the cost of recurring in-clinic treatment. These benefits mostly help in the short to medium term but researchers are exploring both long-term findings, functional independence as well as improvements in quality of life. All in all, present-day clinical evidence confirms the intelligent robotic systems as a promising supplement to the traditional treatment, which has the potential to revolutionize not only inpatient but also community neurorehabilitation. Table 10.1 shows a list of applications of AI-based robotic systems in the field of neurorehabilitation and assistive care.

Application domain	Representative robotic systems/devices	AI/computational techniques	Primary functional goals	Clinical/functional outcomes
Upper-limb rehabilitation	MIT-Manus, Armeo, MyoPro	Adaptive control, EMG-based intent detection; RL	Facilitate repetitive, task-specific arm and hand movement; promote neuroplasticity	Improved Fugl-Meyer scores; enhanced motor coordination and muscle activation
Lower-limb and gait training	Lokomat, EksoGT, ReWalk, HAL	Adaptive gait algorithms; sensor fusion (IMU + pressure sensors)	Re-learn walking patterns, gait symmetry, balance restoration	Increased gait speed, endurance and postural control

Cognitive and social rehabilitation	PARO, Pepper, NAO	NLP, emotion recognition, RL	Cognitive stimulation, emotional engagement, social interaction	Reduced anxiety and depression; improved memory and attention
Assistive mobility and daily living	ReWalk, Indego, Care-O-bot, Toyota HSR	Path planning (AI vision), obstacle detection, autonomous navigation	Long-term mobility, home assistance, environmental interaction	Enhanced autonomy, improved quality of life for users with SCI or neurodegeneration
Brain–computer interface (BCI)-controlled systems	EEG-based robotic arms, exoskeletons	Motor imagery decoding, DL classifiers	Enable control through neural signals; promote brain–muscle reconnection	Increased cortical activation; improved voluntary control in paralyzed patients
IoT and cloud-based rehabilitation platforms	Cloud-connected exoskeletons, tele-rehabilitation systems	Predictive analytics, Cloud ML models	Remote monitoring, adaptive therapy scheduling	Improved accessibility, continuity of care, reduced cost
Soft and hybrid robotic systems	Soft exosuits, FES-integrated robotics	Biomimetic control, hybrid neuroprosthetic modeling	Enhance comfort and natural movement through soft materials and FES synergy	Increased therapy adherence, reduced fatigue, better functional recovery
Tele-robotics and remote care	IoT-enabled home robots, smart wheelchairs	AI-based supervision, remote RL	Home-based, clinician-supervised rehabilitation and assistance	Expanded access to care, reduced hospital visits

Table 10.1. *AI-integrated robotic systems in neurorehabilitation and assistive care*

10.7. Challenges and limitations

Although intelligent neurorehabilitation and assistive care robots have achieved a considerable amount of progress, these tools are still restricted by a lot of technical, clinical, economic and ethical issues that constrain the prevalence and the overall effects of the technology.

10.7.1. *Cost, affordability and reimbursement*

The barrier that exists to both the institutions and the patients is high initial expenditure and continuous maintenance. State-of-the-art exoskeletons, robotic gait trainers and multi-sensor suites are too expensive to be purchased in small clinics and homes. Robotic therapies are unevenly reimbursed in many healthcare systems, making it difficult to predict, as this delays the process of adoption (Nizamis et al. 2021). There are no clear reimbursement channels, and cost–benefit data have proven that these technologies can be expanded beyond pilot projects.

10.7.2. *Quality of the evidence and long-term outcomes*

There is a great number of randomized controlled trials and pilot studies demonstrating that robotic therapy has short-term effect benefits, yet there are few long-term data. The variation in studies includes design, size of the samples, selection of patients and outcomes and, as such, it is difficult to make certain conclusions regarding the overall effectiveness. To confirm persistence of functional gains and cost-effectiveness, large, multicenter, standardized protocol trials with longer follow-up are required (Nizamis et al. 2021).

10.7.3. *Safety, robustness and human factors*

Safety issues would involve over-help that may result in learnt helplessness, skin lacerations when constantly in contact, improper use of force or even failure of the device when it is in use. It is difficult to guarantee the strength of the real-world application, which can be in different body sizes, spastic, involuntary movements and at home (Vaida et al. 2023). The weight of a device, the difficulty in putting the device on or removing it and general usability of a device have strong effects on acceptance and routine use. Regulatory schemes demand stringent safety tests and could increase the time to market and expenses.

10.7.4. *Interoperability and standardization*

Proprietary hardware and software are frequently used in robotic systems, and interoperability between devices, sensors and clinical data systems is not always clear. The absence of universally accepted data formats and outcome measures limit data aggregation between centers to perform meta-analyses and to incorporate robotics in electronic health records. To promote comparative effectiveness of research and clinical decision-making, standardization activities are required (Vaida et al. 2023).

10.7.5. *Adapting to patient diversity*

Neurological populations are extremely diverse: the age, comorbidities, lesion location, severity and psychosocial factors influence rehabilitation processes. It is open-ended to design algorithms that are able to generalize across this diversity without much retraining. Trained ML models that are based on small datasets are prone to bias and likely not to work in under-represented patient groups, unless it is actively mitigated during development and validation.

10.8. Emerging trends and future directions

Neurorehabilitation and assistive care intelligent robotic systems are a rapidly evolving field. This development is being driven by a new technology, enhanced clinical knowledge and increased need of patient-centered and home-based solutions. They are looking to a day in the future when rehabilitation, as well as assistive devices, are more powerful, flexible and available as a normal aspect of life.

10.8.1. *Soft robotics and biomimetic design*

The conventional hard-bodied exoskeletons and the robot devices, though practical, are generally cumbersome and uncomfortable to wear and hence cannot be used over a long period of time. One of the changes is soft robotics. This obeys and is compliant with flexible materials simulating the movement of muscles and tendons (Sumner et al. 2023). They are less uncomfortable and less prone to injuries and more versatile in terms of complex, multi-joint movements. The biomimetic designs can be highly effective with children, aged individuals and individuals who are disabled or have weak bones. The next-generation of soft robots can be designed to have modular components, whereby it can be adapted to anatomies and functions of each patient.

10.8.2. *Hybrid neuroprosthetic systems*

Robotics in conjunction with functional electrical stimulation (FES) is emerging as a powerful treatment method. Hybrid neuroprosthetic systems are used to target both nervous and musculoskeletal systems, enhancing the motor recovery in complementary ways. As an illustration, an exoskeleton which promotes FES in addition to guiding limb motions can stimulate muscle contractions and provide enhancements in brain plasticity and accelerated functional improvements. Initial experiments indicate that hybrid systems are effective as opposed to either robotics or FES in upper-limb and gait rehabilitation. They constitute a new step in the development of devices of the next generation (Tzepkenlis et al. 2025).

10.8.3. *Personalized and adaptive therapies*

Rehabilitation robotics of the future will be concerned with extremely personalized treatments. Patient information, including their movements, physiological indicators, brain activity and performance, will be used broadly to adapt therapy in real time by using AI algorithms. Predictive models will predict the fatigue, plateaus or the recovery trajectory and enable robots to control the difficulty level of tasks, assistance level, as well as scheduling. This individualization enhances the efficacy, involvement, compliance and long-term outcomes. Home and clinical settings will be connected through cloud-based services, which will allow continuous monitoring and control.

10.8.4. *Tele-robotics and remote care*

Robot-based tele-rehabilitation coupled with IoT will expand the use of robots in remote or underserved regions. Through supervised therapy, patients are able to complete their therapy at home, and the clinicians observe progress and adjust interventions remotely. This minimizes travel expenses, saves money and ensures that therapy remains the same to individuals who have difficulty moving around or those who have chronic illnesses. The new tele-robot solutions introduce video feedback, sensor monitoring and AI decision support opportunities to enhance the safety and efficiency.

10.9. Conclusion

Neurorehabilitation as well as assistive care are being transformed by intelligent robotic systems. They combine accuracy, elasticity and customization to generate new, more forceful solutions. These systems combine high-tech sensing systems, ML systems, brain–computer interfaces and simulation environments. They combine to provide therapy, which is accurate and specific to an individual to enhance motor, cognitive and day-to-day functions. Cases of clinical trials confirm that they are effective in recovery of upper and lower limbs, gait training and in maintaining mental lightness in patients. Assistive robots also provide individuals with long-term disabilities with a higher level of independence and improved quality of life. Although this is moving rapidly, there are still lots of obstacles. The field is not developed to the full extent because of cost, access, safety and nonexistence of standard rules, as well as ethical concerns. These barriers have to be overcome by a team effort. All stakeholders (engineers, clinicians, policymakers and patients) should collaborate to ensure that deployment is just, reliable and effective to everyone. New trends are even better. Care is also becoming more patient-centered and highly accessible with the help of soft robotics, hybrid neuroprosthetics, personalized adaptive therapies and tele-robotics. As for universal care, with the development of the field, robots may substitute the reactive and clinic-only strategy with a proactive, ongoing care ecosystem. Its aim is continuous rehabilitation. These innovations can help improve the healthcare service delivery to people with various neurological conditions, improve functional recovery, autonomy and quality of life.

10.10. References

Alshami, A., Nashwan, A., AlDardour, A., Qusini, A. (2025). Artificial intelligence in rehabilitation: A narrative review on advancing patient care. *Rehabilitación*, 59(2), 100911.

Aprile, I., Guardati, G., Cipollini, V., Papadopoulou, D., Mastrorosa, A., Castelli, L., Monteleone, S., Redolfi, A., Galeri, S., Germanotta, M. (2020). Robotic rehabilitation: An opportunity to improve cognitive functions in subjects with stroke. An explorative study. *Frontiers in Neurology*, 11, 588285.

Arthanat, S., Begum, M., Gu, T., LaRoche, D.P., Xu, D., Zhang, N. (2020). Caregiver perspectives on a smart home-based socially assistive robot for individuals with Alzheimer's disease and related dementia. *Disability and Rehabilitation: Assistive Technology*, 15(7), 789–798.

Brown, D.F. and Xie, S.Q. (2024). Effectiveness of intelligent control strategies in robot-assisted rehabilitation: A systematic review. *IEEE Transactions on Neural Systems and Rehabilitation Engineering*, 32, 1828–1840.

Calabrò, R.S., Sorrentino, G., Cassio, A., Mazzoli, D., Andrenelli, E., Bizzarini, E., Campanini, I., Carmignano, S.M., Cerulli, S., Chisari, C. et al. (2021). Robotic-assisted gait rehabilitation following stroke: A systematic review of current guidelines and practical clinical recommendations. *European Journal of Physical and Rehabilitation Medicine*, 57(3), 460–471.

Carnevale, A., Raso, A., Antonacci, C., Mancini, L., Corradini, A., Ceccaroli, A., Casciaro, C., Candela, V., de Sire, A., D'Hooghe, P. et al. (2025). Exploring the impact of socially assistive robots in rehabilitation scenarios. *Bioengineering*, 12(2), 204.

Ezra Tsur, E. and Elkana, O. (2024). Intelligent robotics in pediatric cooperative neurorehabilitation: A review. *Robotics*, 13(3), 49.

Falzarano, V., Marini, F., Morasso, P., Zenzeri, J. (2019). Devices and protocols for upper limb robot-assisted rehabilitation of children with neuromotor disorders. *Applied Sciences*, 9(13), 2689.

Fareh, R., Elsabe, A., Baziyad, M., Kawser, T., Brahmi, B., Rahman, M.H. (2023). Will your next therapist be a robot?: A review of the advancements in robotic upper extremity rehabilitation. *Sensors*, 23(11), 5054.

Fasano, A., Mauro, M.C., Beani, E., Nicora, G., Germanotta, M., Falchini, F., Pavan, A., Habib, V., Quaglini, S., Sgandurra, G. et al. (2025). Towards the identification of patients' needs for promoting robotics and allied digital technologies in rehabilitation: A systematic review. *Healthcare*, 13(7), 828.

Feingold-Polak, R., Barzel, O., Levy-Tzedek, S. (2021). A robot goes to rehab: A novel gamified system for long-term stroke rehabilitation using a socially assistive robot: Methodology and usability testing. *Journal of Neuroengineering and Rehabilitation*, 18(1), 122.

Guatibonza, A., Solaque, L., Velasco, A., Peñuela, L. (2024). Assistive robotics for upper limb physical rehabilitation: A systematic review and future prospects. *Chinese Journal of Mechanical Engineering*, 37(1), 69.

Hirt, J., Ballhausen, N., Hering, A., Kliegel, M., Beer, T., Meyer, G. (2021). Social robot interventions for people with dementia: A systematic review on effects and quality of reporting. *Journal of Alzheimer's Disease*, 79(2), 773–792.

Hobbs, B. and Artemiadis, P. (2020). A review of robot-assisted lower-limb stroke therapy: Unexplored paths and future directions in gait rehabilitation. *Frontiers in Neurorobotics*, 14, 19.

Karami, V., Yaffe, M.J., Gore, G., Moon, A., Rahimi, S.A. (2024). Socially assistive robots for patients with Alzheimer's disease: A scoping review. *Archives of Gerontology and Geriatrics*, 123, 105409.

Lingampally, P.K., Ramanathan, K.C., Shanmugam, R., Cepova, L., Salunkhe, S. (2024). Wearable assistive rehabilitation robotic devices: A comprehensive review. *Machines*, 12(6), 415.

McDermott, E.R., DeFoor, M.T., Dekker, T.J., DePhillipo, N.N. (2024). Artificial intelligence in rehabilitation. In *Artificial Intelligence in Orthopaedic Surgery Made Easy*, Familiari, F., Galasso, O., Gasparini, G. (eds). Springer, Cham, 197–204.

Nicora, G., Pe, S., Santangelo, G., Billeci, L., Aprile, I.G., Germanotta, M., Bellazzi, R., Parimbelli, E., Quaglini, S. (2025). Systematic review of AI/ML applications in multi-domain robotic rehabilitation: Trends, gaps, and future directions. *Journal of NeuroEngineering and Rehabilitation*, 22(1), 79.

Nizamis, K., Athanasiou, A., Almpani, S., Dimitrousis, C., Astaras, A. (2021). Converging robotic technologies in targeted neural rehabilitation: A review of emerging solutions and challenges. *Sensors*, 21(6), 2084.

Rad, O.L. and Brisan, C. (2025). Control algorithms in robot-assisted rehabilitation: A systematic review. *Applied Sciences*, 15(16), 9184.

Sumner, J., Lim, H.W., Chong, L.S., Bundele, A., Mukhopadhyay, A., Kayambu, G. (2023). Artificial intelligence in physical rehabilitation: A systematic review. *Artificial Intelligence in Medicine*, 146, 102693.

Tzepkenlis, A., Camardella, C., Germanotta, M., Aprile, I.G., Mauro, M.C., Leonardis, D., Frisoli, A. (2025). Systematic data management for effective AI-driven decision support systems in robotic rehabilitation. *Scientific Reports*, 15(1), 27835.

Vaida, C., Rus, G., Lupu, D., Gherman, B., Tucan, P., Horvath, D., Machado, J., Pîslă, D. (2023). Assessment of different biosignals with potential benefits in robotic assisted neuromotor rehabilitation. In *International Conference on e-Health and Bioengineering*. Springer, Cham, 86–94.

Vaida, C., Rus, G., Pisla, D. (2025). A sensor-based classification for neuromotor robot-assisted rehabilitation. *Bioengineering*, 12(3), 287.

Warutkar, V., Dadgal, R., Mangulkar, U.R. (2022). Use of robotics in gait rehabilitation following stroke: A review. *Cureus*, 14(11), e31075.

Yuan, F., Klavon, E., Liu, Z., Lopez, R.P., Zhao, X. (2021). A systematic review of robotic rehabilitation for cognitive training. *Frontiers in Robotics and AI*, 8, 605715.

Zhang, Y., Liu, X., Qiao, X., Fan, Y. (2023). Characteristics and emerging trends in research on rehabilitation robots from 2001 to 2020: Bibliometric study. *Journal of Medical Internet Research*, 25, e42901.

Zhang, J.Z., Chen, J., Liu, X.L., Yan, L.B., Xu, S.M. (2025). Effectiveness of intelligent robotic-assisted training system combined with repetitive facilitative exercise on upper limb motor function after stroke: A randomized controlled trial. *BMC Sports Science, Medicine and Rehabilitation*, 17, 178.

11

Personalized Medicine in Multiple Sclerosis Through AI-Driven Analytics

Multiple sclerosis (MS) is a neurodegenerative, chronic and immune-mediated disease. It presents a great variety of clinical manifestations, erratic courses and responses to treatment. This is complex, which makes it difficult to develop effective customized management strategies. The latest developments in artificial intelligence (AI) and data-driven analytics provide an opportunity to customize medical intervention based on each patient, beyond population-wide medical interventions. The variety and quantity of data that AI algorithms can combine and process (examples include neuroimaging, genetics, clinical records, biomarkers and patient-reported outcomes) can be used to create a predictive model that aids in diagnosis, prognosis and treatment planning. Machine learning (ML), deep learning (DL) and natural language processing (NLP) can help clinical professionals to identify subtle disease patterns, find the most appropriate treatment and forecast disease activity more precisely. The potential of AI-enhanced decision-support systems to surveil real-world data through wearable sensors and mobile health applications in order to vary the therapy also demonstrates some potential and can be applied practically. Incorporating big data using electronic health records and multi-centric clinical trials allows these models to become increasingly enhanced so that individualized MS care can be updated in line with the latest evidence. Yet, challenges still exist. Data standardization, interpretability of the algorithms, ethical concerns and equitable access must be resolved before clinical uses can be increased.

This chapter will review the role of AI-driven analytics in motivating the development of personalized medicine in MS. It discusses the existing applications, new innovations and the obstacles which restrict clinical translation. AI can potentially revolutionize the process of MS care to be a personal, individualized treatment process by integrating computational intelligence with clinical neuroscience.

Chapter written by Chaitnya GODBOLE and Shrikant Rangrao KADAM.

11.1. Introduction

Multiple sclerosis (MS) is an immune mediated, chronic disorder of the central nervous system (CNS). It has a global prevalence of about 2.8–3 million individuals, and its prevalence is on the increase in both developed and developing nations. MS entails inflammation, loss of myelin and axonal degeneration that usually result in long-term neurological disability and high socioeconomic cost (Naji et al. 2023). This disease most commonly starts in young adults, affecting women unequally, and manifests itself in various subtypes: relapsing-remitting MS (RRMS), primary progressive MS (PPMS) and secondary progressive MS (SPMS) (Ganjgahi et al. 2025).

MS is difficult to manage due to its heterogeneity. Chronic conditions vary among patients in their disease activity, radiographical presentation, response to therapy and prognosis, and therefore, a one-size-fits-all approach may not be effective. Treatment disease-modifying therapies (DMTs) have demonstrated better results, with a reduced rate of relapse and a slowed disability without equal response in all patients (Nabizadeh et al. 2023). Others have side effects or resistance, which highlights the importance of individual medicine, in which every individual patient has been adjusted to medical care according to their biology and clinical profile.

Artificial intelligence (AI) and machine learning (ML) are already new forces that can be used to enhance personalization in MS care. Compared to conventional statistics, AI is able to integrate high-dimensional and multimodal data, including neuroimaging, genetics, proteomics, immune markers and patient reports in the real world, to discover concealed disease patterns and construct anticipatory frameworks to diagnose, forecast and optimally treat patients (Patil et al. 2025).

With these technologies, clinicians can shift to precision care strategies that are both effective in therapeutic care and increase the quality of life by early detection and proactive management, and adaptive treatment courses.

This chapter examines the role of AI-based analytics in the development of personalized medicine in MS. It discusses the heterogeneity of diseases, the use of AI in disease diagnosis, prognosis, treatment choice and patient monitoring, and points out the challenges associated with its application, such as ethical issues, data standardization and clinical application. Lastly, it provides future directions in terms of translating computational intelligence in practice in daily MS care, with an eminent place for AI in changing treatment to treat-each-patient care.

11.2. Overview of multiple sclerosis and the need for personalization

MS is a complicated disease, which entails neuroinflammation, myelin loss and neurodegeneration. Its course is unpredictable. There are those who experience regular relapses and an accelerated deterioration, and there are those who are mildly active with prolonged periods of calmness (Chen et al. 2023). Patients and doctors have a difficult time when it comes to making decisions about this treatment because of this uncertainty.

The most common forms of multiple sclerosis (MS) are relapsing–remitting MS (RRMS), which accounts for about 85% of initial diagnoses, and the progressive types, including primary progressive MS (PPMS) and secondary progressive MS (SPMS). All of the subtypes have a different pathophysiological pattern, but overlaps are numerous, so it can be difficult to identify the unique classification (Mouazen et al. 2025). The symptoms can include dysfunction of the senses, issues with vision, feelings of weakness, motor issues and cognitive problems, which differ among individuals, as well as changes in an individual.

This heterogeneity demonstrates the inefficiency of universal treatment strategies. DMTs vary in terms of their mechanisms of action, effectiveness, safety and tolerability. There are patients that respond to first-line injectable therapy, whereas others require the use of high-efficacy monoclonal antibodies in the management of the disease (Villar-Delfino et al. 2025). Other health conditions, genetics, environmental exposures and lifestyle habits are influencing factors when treating an illness, which is why individual approaches must be implemented.

Personalized medicine is expected to be something more than the generalized protocols and to develop patient-specific treatment flows. It involves a fusion of a wide variety of data (clinical history, imaging, biomarkers, genomics and patient-reported outcomes) to create a comprehensive representation of the risk and probable response of the disease. Traditional approaches are unable to synthesize and analyze such complicated data, which leaves a gap that can be addressed by AI and ML. To extract hidden patterns, the technologies have the capability of analyzing high-dimensional data to deliver actionable insights (Praet et al. 2024).

11.3. AI in MS diagnosis and early detection

It can be noted that accurate and timely diagnosis of MS is a significant clinical issue, since the disease manifests itself in so many different forms and can be mistaken with other neurological disorders. The McDonald criteria that fuse clinical findings with MRI results combined with CSF analysis have traditionally been used by doctors (Gupta et al. 2025). These criteria are not ideal: early lesions may be nonspecific and atypical, and may look like the neuromyelitis optical spectrum disorder (NMOSD), small vessel ischemic disorder or inflammatory neuropathies. A wrong diagnosis may slow down the commencement of disease-modifying treatment (DMTs) and cause irreparable neurological effects.

AI provides the means of enhancing the accuracy of diagnosis through the application of ML and deep learning (DL) algorithms to multimodal data. The AI models are capable of processing myriad MRI scans to identify patterns of suspected lesions, and even identify MS lesions compared to the ones wrought by other diseases. Convolutional neural networks (CNNs) have demonstrated high bias in white-matter lesion detection, and differentiating MS and NMOSD or cerebrovascular disease (Jayasinghe 2024).

In addition to lesion detection, AI is capable of identifying early signs of radiologic damage such as cortical demyelination and atrophy changes in the brain, which could be overlooked by the classical analysis results.

Clinical information integration aids more in accuracy of diagnosis. Certain algorithms of natural language processing (NLP) can be used to filter electronic health records (EHRs) to extract structured information in unstructured clinical notes. This enables automatic identification of MS phenotypes in the early stages and clusters of symptoms (Mottaghi-Dastjerdi and Soltany-Rezaee-Rad 2024). Such systems can assist clinicians in referring patients to specialists earlier, by identifying those with initial indications of MS.

Inter-observer variability is also minimized by AI. Human radiologists usually differ when detecting and interpreting lesions, particularly in doubtful cases. AI tools would offer objective and reproducible analyses, which are considered to be more consistent across centers. Moreover, the MRI is auto-analyzed, which reduces the load of the radiologist and accelerates the process of making a diagnosis.

Although there are these promises, diagnostic AI tools continue to be problematic, and these problems need to be resolved before they can be fully incorporated into clinical practice. These need large and annotated datasets to train; they should perform well in a variety of imaging platforms, and they are required to be interpretable. Nevertheless, AI in MS diagnosis remains an important move in the direction of personalized medicine as it will allow timely and more correct diagnoses to be made that directly affect future results (Chen et al. 2025).

11.4. AI-driven prognostic modeling in MS

11.4.1. *Relapse prediction*

Relapses are one of the common features of relapsing remitting MS (RRMS) and can have a significant impact on the outcomes of patients. Traditional prediction of relapse depends on clinical history and MRI results, but these factors are not enough to externalize the underlying disease activity. Longitudinal MRI datasets have been trained by ML models to detect subtle radiological alterations which predict relapses. In comparison to human judgment, these algorithms are sensitive to the formation of new lesions and inflammatory activity, and enable a clinician to predict relapses and adjust therapy to them (Ali et al. 2024).

11.4.2. *Disability progression*

Disability is also cumulative and is commonly measured in the Expanded Disability Status Scale (EDSS); this is different among the patients. AI-based methodical frameworks simulate physical and mental deficit trajectories by assembling vast clinical trial and registry information. Applications of DL frameworks, such as the use of multimodal inputs such as MRI-based measures of brain atrophy, cerebrospinal fluid (CSF) biomarkers and genetic profiles to predict long-term disability outcomes have been demonstrated (Johnson et al. 2021). Due to the benefits of such models helping clinicians to counsel patients or direct the intensity of therapy, it is important to determine who is at a high risk of aggressive disease.

11.4.3. *Treatment response forecasting*

Another important prognostic feature is the prediction of response to particular DMTs. Some patients are stable on first-line treatment, while others may be subjected to exponential results from stronger monoclonal antibodies.

The predictors of the treatment response are identified with AI analytics, which use real-world evidence, imaging markers and immunological data. ML models under supervision can forecast which patients may be responsive to B-cell-depleting therapy and which patients may be responsive to oral agents (Voigt et al. 2021). These lessons can help make those therapy choices more specific, without exposing patients to useless or unnecessary toxic therapy.

11.4.4. *Longitudinal disease modeling*

Longitudinal AI reimbursements can be applied to further developments of prognostic models through continuous learning of changing patient data. These models render forecasts continuously to modify accompaniments of serial MRI scans, recurrent biomarker tests and wearable data as the illness advances. Algorithms of reinforcement learning are also helpful in this regard because they update predictions dynamically, which is a nonlinear process of MS progression (Jonna and Natarajan 2025). Adaptive modeling gives a more actualized representation of the patient outcomes, which makes it possible to approach the management strategies proactively.

11.5. Personalized treatment strategies through AI analytics

11.5.1. *Therapy selection*

The traditional models of treatment frequently involve step-up therapy, where the initial therapy will involve the use of lower-efficacy drugs, which will subsequently be followed by high-efficiency drugs in case the disease activity continues. But there is also accumulating evidence that new aggressive disease course patients can be helped by instituting powerful therapies earlier in life, and the results that may emerge would be better.

AI analytics can help in this change by sorting patients based on the perceived treatment response. For example, under supervised ML, models that have been trained to use real-world data will be able to recognize subpopulations that have a high likelihood of responding to particular drug groups, including B-cell depleting therapies and sphingosine-1-phosphate (S1P) receptor modulators (Dara et al. 2025). These predictive tools enable the clinicians to find the right drug, and match it to the right patient at the right time.

11.5.2. *Switching and optimization of treatment*

Most patients need to switch their treatment switch, despite optimal initial treatment because of break-through disease activity and side effects. The timing of the switch and the type of therapy to use is still a major clinical challenge that can be predicted with difficulty. AI algorithms may be able to pore through longitudinal clinical and imaging data to become aware of the minor signs of a failure in treatment sooner than the traditional approach. As an example, predictive models of dynamic MRI lesions and recurrence rate can inform us about an untimely response prior to clinical disability (Uddin et al. 2025). The incorporation of such models in decision-support systems contributes to the proactive adjustment of the treatment systems, which lessens the chance of permanent development of the disease.

11.5.3. *Safety and risk management*

Although high-efficacy DMTs provide a strong level of disease control, they involve the risk of opportunistic infections, cardiovascular problems or malignancy. Pharmacovigilance systems based on AI can track adverse event reporting, EHRs and patient registries, and anticipate individual risk. An example is the method of clustering lab findings and immune system biomarkers without supervision, which may pinpoint trends in laboratory results and immune system signals that suggest any kind of complication such as progressive multifocal leukoencephalopathy (PML) (Gashi et al. 2024). The insights will enable the clinicians to tailor monitoring plans, reducing risk but maximizing therapeutic results.

11.5.4. *Accurate dose and adherence assistance*

Other than the choice of the drug, AI can help to optimize therapy dosing and adherence. DL algorithms are in development to simulate the pharmacodynamics and pharmacokinetics of patients, and it is expected that they will yield the best dosing schedule, dependent on genetics, metabolism and immune response.

In the same spirit, digital health apps combined with wearable devices and mobiles enable the collection of adherence data by offering real-time feedback and AI-generated reminders to uphold medication adherence. This guarantees the consistency of therapeutic efficacy so as to not be compromised by low adherence, which is a daily problem facing the management of chronic diseases.

11.5.5. *Patient-centered treatment personalization*

Notably, personalized treatment is not restricted to biological markers only. AI-powered patient engagement platforms combine clinical outcomes with patient-reported outcomes of fatigue, cognition and quality of life. Holistic care plans can be developed by integrating these subjective perceptions and objective biomarkers that have a strong focus on disease management and patient health (Amin et al. 2024). This paradigm move of personalization regarding patients is coherent with the general trend of precision medicine in chronic neurological diseases.

11.6. Integration of multi-omics and biomarkers

The advent of multi-omics technologies – including genomics, transcriptomics, proteomics, metabolomics and epigenomics – has revolutionized our understanding of complex diseases such as MS. These datasets capture complementary aspects of disease biology, from genetic predisposition to dynamic changes in protein expression and metabolic activity. However, the sheer volume and complexity of omics data present a major challenge for traditional analysis methods. AI and ML offer robust tools to integrate multi-omics data, enabling the identification of personalized disease signatures and therapeutic targets (Aslam et al. 2022).

11.6.1. *Genomics and genetic risk profiling*

There are significant genetic components in the risk of MS. Mutations in HLA-DRB1 and other immunogenic genes increase the risk. Genome-wide association data by way of genome-wide association studies can be analyzed using AI algorithms to reveal a complex relationship between risk alleles, which results in creating individualized genetic information that can be used to explain the onset and progression of diseases. It is also possible to use machine-learned models to predict the probability of a patient requiring a certain therapy, which can be used by clinicians to select the best treatments at an earlier stage (Ramezanian et al. 2025).

11.6.2. *Proteomics and biomarker discovery*

The examination of proteins in the CSF and plasma provides an insight into MS activity and immune disorders. AI-based techniques of clustering and pattern recognition identify slight modifications in the number of proteins, which are related to the risk of relapse, progression of the disease or efficacy of a treatment. Such methods not only discover new biomarkers, but are also predictive and enhance the accuracy of individual treatment programs (Wang and Tang 2025).

11.6.3. *Metabolomics and immune profiling*

Metabolomic profiling is followed as the changing activity of the metabolic pathways modulating inflammation and damaging the nervous system. With the help of AI models, combining metabolite data with immune markers, researchers will be able to specify metabolic signatures of patients in relation to active disease or upcoming relapse. As an example, controlled learning algorithms may integrate the levels of cytokines, the concentration of metabolites and the results of MRI to predict future clinical flare-ups, enabling the active management of treatment to proceed in advance (Creagh et al. 2022).

11.6.4. *Multi-omics fusion and forecasting*

The most significant advantage of AI in multi-omics is that it combines various forms of data. DL networks, which include autoencoders and multimodal networks, combine genomic, proteomic, metabolomic and clinical data to create disease maps. With the help of these models, we can get personalized risk measures, identify the most optimal treatment paths and facilitate continuous predictions. AI-based multi-omics applications are trained to continuously optimize their individual treatment models as the condition evolves by consuming longitudinal data.

11.7. Role of neuroimaging and computer vision

11.7.1. *Automated lesion detection*

The current state of the art in automated lesion segmentation in MS is now convolutional neural networks (CNNs). These neural net systems have been shown to detect and demarcate white matter and cortical lesions on MRI images highly comparable to the accuracy of expert neuroradiologists. Changes in lesion load over a period of time can also be traced with the help of AI-based segmentation, providing clinicians with an accurate means of monitoring disease activity and responding to changes in therapy in a timely manner (Afzal et al. 2022).

11.7.2. *Brain and spinal cord atrophy at measurement*

Neurodegeneration in MS is usually manifested in brain and spinal cord atrophy. AI algorithms quantify such changes in volume with serial MRI scans, which provide objective indicators of disease progression. The AI can identify the signs of neurodegenerative processes, which could manifest themselves earlier than a clinical disability, and can therefore be used to support proactive treatment strategies by identifying atrophy early in its progression (Yousef et al. 2024).

11.7.3. *Radiomic predictive modeling and feature extraction*

Radiomics is the procedure that pays out a high-scale collection of quantitative characteristics of medical pictures, including texture, shape and intensity. These signatures are studied by AI models that anticipate disease subtype, the risk of relapse and the way a patient is going to respond to treatment. As an illustration,

ML classifiers that use MRI radiomic images are capable of distinguishing between the relapsing–remitting and progressive types of MS, and the decision can result in an accurate diagnosis and optimal therapy option (Yousef et al. 2024).

11.7.4. *Completion with multimodal data*

AI in imaging can be used predictively and is complemented by other sources of information, including genomics, proteomics and clinical evaluations to increase its predictive power. Multi-computational models combine structural and functional visualization characteristics along with biological indicators, producing thorough patient reports. Precision medicine in MS can be achieved with these built-in AI tools that give personalized risk scores on disease activity, disability progression and treatment response (Guo et al. 2023).

11.8. AI-powered monitoring and patient engagement

11.8.1. *Wearable devices and remote monitoring*

Wearable sensors, including accelerometers, gyroscopes and smartwatches, can track mobility, gait abnormalities, tremors and activity levels in real time. AI algorithms process these high-dimensional datasets to detect subtle changes indicative of disease progression or impending relapse. For example, ML models can identify deviations in step count, stride symmetry or upper-limb dexterity, alerting clinicians to potential exacerbations before they manifest clinically (Naskar et al. 2025).

11.8.2. *Mobile health platforms*

Mobile health (mHealth) applications allow patients to report symptoms, track fatigue, cognitive changes and medication adherence. NLP and supervised learning algorithms can analyze these unstructured patient-reported outcomes to detect emerging trends or predict relapse risk. The integration of mHealth data with EHRs enables AI-driven decision-support systems to provide individualized recommendations, optimize treatment schedules and enhance patient engagement (Antar et al. 2023).

11.8.3. *Real-time predictive analytics*

AI-powered predictive analytics combine wearable and mHealth data with historical clinical and imaging records to generate real-time risk scores. These models can forecast relapses, detect early signs of functional decline and recommend interventions, enabling preemptive adjustments to therapy. Reinforcement learning algorithms allow models to adapt dynamically, refining predictions as new patient data become available, thereby enhancing personalization and accuracy (Antar et al. 2023).

11.8.4. *Patient-centered engagement*

Individualized tracking makes patients empowered because they are provided with practical facts about their health. Learning tools, reminders and customized feedback offered through AI-driven platforms are used to facilitate adherence and self-management. Representing the dynamics of mobility, fatigue or cognitive functions will allow patients to know how being ill will change their lives, and will encourage patients to adhere to treatment protocols. Such a patient-centered approach would be coherent with precision medicine, which focuses not only on the biological personalization, but also behavioral and lifestyle adaptation (Naji et al. 2023). Table 11.1 shows AI applications and clinical utility in personalized MS care.

Domain	AI technique/model	Data source/modality	Primary objective/function	Clinical utility/outcome
Diagnosis and early detection	Convolutional neural networks (CNNs)	MRI, CSF, clinical data	Automated lesion detection and classification (MS vs. NMOSD)	Early diagnosis, reduced observer variability
Diagnosis and early detection	Natural language processing (NLP)	Electronic health records (EHRs), clinical notes	Extraction of unstructured data for phenotype identification	Accelerates early referral and clinical decision-making
Prognosis	Supervised machine learning (SVM, random forests)	Longitudinal MRI, biomarkers	Relapse and disability progression prediction	Enables proactive treatment modification
Prognosis	Deep learning (LSTM, autoencoders)	Multi-modal longitudinal data	Continuous modeling of disease activity	Improves forecasting accuracy for relapse timing
Treatment response prediction	Ensemble ML Models	Imaging, immune markers, real-world registry data	Forecast patient response to specific DMTs	Supports personalized DMT selection and therapy optimization

Domain	AI technique/model	Data source/modality	Primary objective/function	Clinical utility/outcome
Treatment optimization	Reinforcement learning (RL)	Clinical, pharmacogenomic and adherence data	Adaptive optimization of therapy switching and dosing	Minimizes side effects and enhances therapeutic outcomes
Biomarker discovery	Clustering and pattern recognition	Proteomics, metabolomics, CSF biomarkers	Identify relapse and progression-related protein/metabolite signatures	Improves accuracy of disease activity tracking
Multi-omics integration	Multimodal deep networks (autoencoders, GNNs)	Genomics, proteomics, metabolomics, imaging	Fusion of biological and clinical data for risk stratification	Enables precision-based treatment planning
Neuroimaging analytics	Radiomics and CNNs	MRI (T1/T2/FLAIR), DTI, fMRI	Lesion detection, brain atrophy measurement	Quantifies disease activity and progression objectively
Digital monitoring and engagement	Mobile AI platforms and wearables	Accelerometer, smartphone, PROs	Track gait, fatigue, cognition and relapse signals	Enhances patient engagement and self-management

Table 11.1. *AI applications and clinical utility in personalized multiple sclerosis care*

11.9. Challenges, ethical concerns and limitations

11.9.1. *Information quality and workability*

AI uses massive datasets that are clean. The data in the case of MS is provided by a variety of sources: EHRs, imaging laboratories, clinical studies and wearable devices. These are not easily generalized and reproducible models as different formats, imaging protocols and standards of recording are involved. Poor or unbalanced information may produce a false forecast and expose patients to danger. Thus, standardization of data capture, labeling and reporting is critical to sound AI in all clinical environments.

11.9.2. *Testing, interpretation and usability*

A great number of AI models, particularly DL networks, are black-box models. Clinicians must be able to know the way in which a model makes its recommendations. In the absence of interpretability, trust is lost, adoption is slowed and legal or ethical concerns are brought up – especially when high-stakes treatments are being controlled by decisions. The creation of understandable AI systems that present the logic behind the prediction is essential to the clinical utilization of AI, which can be considered safe.

11.9.3. *Ethical and privacy concerns*

The AI in MS processes sensitive data: wearable behavior, scans and genetics. The security of data and privacy are of primary importance. Ethical issues also exist, concerning consent and ownership of data, as well as the misuse of predictions. Patients should be aware of how their information is gathered, stored and used, and there should be a regulation that demands stern protection against unauthorized exploration or prejudice.

11.9.4. *Implementation clinically and into workflow*

It is possible that even the correct AI implementations will not work until they are integrated into regular clinical procedures. The miscellaneous factors involve a lack of technical infrastructure, poor interoperability with the existing EHRs and the insufficient training of clinicians. Models should also be tested in a wide variety of populations to do equally well. These practical issues need to be addressed using deployment plans so that their use in real MS care is safe and effective.

11.9.5. *Limitations of current AI models*

The existing MS AI is limited in a number of aspects. Small retrospective datasets are used in many of the models, and this is detrimental to generalization. We run the risk of overfitting – being predictive on training data, but not with new patients. This is technically difficult to integrate clinical, imaging and omics data and would need a powerful computing platform and architecture. Such gaps will require continuous methodology research and powerful future testing.

11.10. Future directions and clinical translation

11.10.1. *integration of real-world data*

Although this is a powerful source of information on AI, real-world data, including records related to electronic health systems, patient registries and wearables, serves as a valuable data source. The AI models of the future will be based on longer-term real-life information to comprehend the entire spectrum of MS variability. Using this data, predictive tools will be able to take into account comorbidity, lifestyle habits and adherence to treatment plans observed among the patients. The outcome is a less generalized risk evaluation and treatment recommendation. This patient-centered and data-driven method will allow treatments to change with time in real-life contexts.

11.10.2. *Multisensory modeling and multidimensional modeling*

The next generation of AI will incorporate numerous types of data and generate one predictive model of the brain images, genetics, proteins, metabolic and clinical history. The tools of DL, such as graph neural networks and transformer models, will aid in the capture of complex links that are present at all of these levels. The models will also be able to predict the progression of the disease, as well as uncover the mechanisms of the disease, indicating new biomarkers and drug targets to be used to customize treatment.

11.10.3. *AI-assisted clinical trials*

AI will be able to change MS clinical trials by improving the selection of participants, forecasting results and enhancing efficiency. Models are able to identify high-risk groups of patients, who are more likely to progress or respond to therapy, hence resulting in enrolling into shorter trials and more directed enrollment. Adaptive, AI-based designs will allow the change of treatment arms during the flow of the patients, allowing therapies to be introduced to patients earlier, resulting in faster trials.

11.10.4. *Personalized digital therapeutics and telemedicine*

The integration of AI with mobile health (mHealth) platforms, telemedicine and wearable sensors will enable personalized digital therapeutics for MS. Patients can receive individualized exercise programs, cognitive rehabilitation or fatigue management strategies guided by AI algorithms that continuously adapt to their condition.

Real-time monitoring and feedback loops will support patient engagement, adherence and early intervention, reducing the reliance on in-person visits and enhancing accessibility to care, particularly in remote or underserved areas.

11.10.5. *Ethical and regulatory considerations for future integration*

As AI becomes more integral to personalized MS care, ethical and regulatory frameworks must evolve to ensure patient safety, privacy and equitable access. Explainable AI, transparent model validation and standardized reporting protocols will be essential for clinician trust and regulatory approval. Policymakers and healthcare institutions will need to balance innovation with oversight, establishing clear guidelines for the deployment, monitoring and continuous evaluation of AI-driven interventions.

11.11. Conclusion

With the help of AI and sophisticated analytics integration, personalized medicine in MS develops rather rapidly. AI delivers advantages at all stages of MS treatment: early and precise diagnostics, predictive analytics, choice of customized treatment, combination of multi-omics, neuro-imaging analysis and constant monitoring of the patient. The tools enable clinicians to provide individualized treatment based on the biology, clinical profile and lifestyle of the patient, rather than using a population strategy. However, it is difficult to use AI in individual MS treatment. Data heterogeneity, the inability to interpret algorithms, ethical issues, privacy and the necessity to incorporate AI tools into the current clinical workflow are major challenges. Addressing these challenges will require cooperation between the clinicians, data scientists, ethicists and policymakers, and the development of AI models that are robust, transparent and clinically verified. The integration of AI, multi-omics and digital health, as well as real-world evidence in the future, will afford a completely tailored form of care and treatment to MS. Predictive, preemptive and precision strategies will offer clinicians an opportunity to anticipate disease activity, refine treatment and engage patients in self-management activities. Since AI systems continuously learn based on various data, they will change with the existing patient population, making personalized medicine an effective, scalable and dynamic evidence-based solution.

11.12. References

Afzal, H.R., Luo, S., Ramadan, S., Lechner-Scott, J. (2022). The emerging role of artificial intelligence in multiple sclerosis imaging. *Multiple Sclerosis Journal*, 28(6), 849–858.

Ali, S.G., Zhang, C., Guan, Z., Chen, T., Wu, Q., Li, P., Yang, P., Ghazanfar, Z., Jung, Y., Chen, Y. et al. (2024). AI-enhanced digital technologies for myopia management: Advancements, challenges, and future prospects. *The Visual Computer*, 40(6), 3871–3887.

Amin, M., Martínez-Heras, E., Ontaneda, D., Prados Carrasco, F. (2024). Artificial intelligence and multiple sclerosis. *Current Neurology and Neuroscience Reports*, 24(8), 233–243.

Antar, A.D., Kratz, A., Banovic, N. (2023). Behavior modeling approach for forecasting physical functioning of people with multiple sclerosis. *Proceedings of the ACM on Interactive, Mobile, Wearable and Ubiquitous Technologies*, 7(1), 1–29.

Aslam, N., Khan, I.U., Bashamakh, A., Alghool, F.A., Aboulnour, M., Alsuwayan, N.M., Alturaif, R.A., Brahimi, S., Aljameel, S.S., Al Ghamdi, K. (2022). Multiple sclerosis diagnosis using machine learning and deep learning: Challenges and opportunities. *Sensors*, 22(20), 7856.

Chen, O.Y., Lipsmeier, F., Phan, H., Dondelinger, F., Creagh, A., Gossens, C., Lindemann, M., De Vos, M. (2023). Personalized longitudinal assessment of multiple sclerosis using smartphones. *IEEE Journal of Biomedical and Health Informatics*, 27(7), 3633–3644.

Chen, Y.M., Hsiao, T.H., Lin, C.H., Fann, Y.C. (2025). Unlocking precision medicine: Clinical applications of integrating health records, genetics, and immunology through artificial intelligence. *Journal of Biomedical Science*, 32(1), 16.

Creagh, A.P., Dondelinger, F., Lipsmeier, F., Lindemann, M., De Vos, M. (2022). Longitudinal trend monitoring of multiple sclerosis ambulation using smartphones. *IEEE Open Journal of Engineering in Medicine and Biology*, 3, 202–210.

Dara, M., Dianatpour, M., Azarpira, N., Tanideh, N. (2025). The transformative role of artificial intelligence in genomics: Opportunities and challenges. *Gene Reports*, 41, 102314.

Ganjgahi, H., Häring, D.A., Aarden, P., Graham, G., Sun, Y., Gardiner, S., Su, W., Berge, C., Bischof, A., Fisher, E. et al. (2025). AI-driven reclassification of multiple sclerosis progression. *Nature Medicine*, 31, 3414–3424.

Gashi, S., Oldrati, P., Moebus, M., Hilty, M., Barrios, L., Ozdemir, F., PHRT Consortium, Kana, V., Lutterotti, A., Rätsch, G. et al. (2024). Modeling multiple sclerosis using mobile and wearable sensor data. *npj Digital Medicine*, 7(1), 64.

Guo, K., Wu, M., Soo, Z., Yang, Y., Zhang, Y., Zhang, Q., Lin, H., Grosser, M., Venter, D., Zhang, G. et al. (2023). Artificial intelligence-driven biomedical genomics. *Knowledge-Based Systems*, 279, 110937.

Gupta, S., Gupta, U., Sharma, M., Malik, K. (eds) (2025). *Generative Intelligence in Healthcare: Transforming Patient Care with AI Creativity*. CRC Press, Boca Raton.

Jayasinghe, Y.A. (2024). Developments and future prospects of personalized medicine in head and neck squamous cell carcinoma diagnoses and treatments. *Wiley-Cancer Reports*, 7(3), e2045.

Johnson, K.B., Wei, W.Q., Weeraratne, D., Frisse, M.E., Misulis, K., Rhee, K., Zhao, J., Snowdon, J.L. (2021). Precision medicine, AI, and the future of personalized healthcare. *Clinical and Translational Science*, 14(1), 86–93.

Jonna, S.T. and Natarajan, K. (2025). EEG signal processing in neurological conditions using machine learning and deep learning methods: A comprehensive review. *The European Physical Journal Special Topics*, 234, 3981–3999.

Mottaghi-Dastjerdi, N. and Soltany-Rezaee-Rad, M. (2024). Advancements and applications of artificial intelligence in pharmaceutical sciences: A comprehensive review. *Iranian Journal of Pharmaceutical Research: IJPR*, 23(1), e150510.

Mouazen, B., Bendaouia, A., De Marco, G. (2025). Machine learning and clinical EEG data for multiple sclerosis: A systematic review. *Artificial Intelligence in Medicine*, 166, 103116.

Nabizadeh, F., Ramezannezhad, E., Kargar, A., Sharafi, A.M., Ghaderi, A. (2023). Diagnostic performance of artificial intelligence in multiple sclerosis: A systematic review and meta-analysis. *Neurological Sciences*, 44(2), 499–517.

Naji, Y., Mahdaoui, M., Klevor, R., Kissani, N., Raymond, K. (2023). Artificial intelligence and multiple sclerosis: Up-to-date review. *Cureus*, 15(9), e45412.

Naskar, S., Sharma, S., Kuotsu, K., Halder, S., Pal, G., Saha, S., Mondal, S., Biswas, U.K., Jana, M., Bhattacharjee, S. (2025). The biomedical applications of artificial intelligence: An overview of decades of research. *Journal of Drug Targeting*, 33(5), 717–748.

Patil, M.S., Lin, L.Y., Ford, R.K., James, E.J., Morton, S., Marsh-Wakefield, F., Hawke, S., Grau, G.E. (2025). Harnessing artificial intelligence for the diagnosis, treatment and research of multiple sclerosis. *Sclerosis*, 3(2), 15.

Praet, J., Anderhalten, L., Comi, G., Horakova, D., Ziemssen, T., Vermersch, P., Lukas, C., Van Leemput, K., Steppe, M., Aguilera, C. et al. (2024). A future of AI-driven personalized care for people with multiple sclerosis. *Frontiers in Immunology*, 15, 1446748.

Ramezanian, M., Benis, D.S., Nikakhtar, R., Gorjizadeh, N., Asadi, F., Bagherianlemraski, M., Rad, N.K., Sarikhani, P., Rezvanimehr, A., Asghari, S.F. et al. (2025). Artificial intelligence in genomic medicine: Improving diagnostic accuracy and treatment outcomes. *Kindle*, 5(1), 1–215.

Uddin, M.R., Sovon, M.S., Mondal, S., Ahmed, S., Al-Mizan, M.A., Aktar, F., Amran, M.S. (2025). Artificial intelligence and machine learning in pharmaceutical sciences: Unpacking regulatory guidance, opportunities, and challenges for safe and effective drug development. *International Journal of Medical Informatics*. doi: 10.2139/ssrn.5505018.

Villar-Delfino, P.H., Pereira Christo, P., Volpe, C.M. (2025). Drug repurposing and artificial intelligence in multiple sclerosis: Emerging strategies for precision therapy. *Sclerosis*, 3(3), 28.

Voigt, I., Inojosa, H., Dillenseger, A., Haase, R., Akgün, K., Ziemssen, T. (2021). Digital twins for multiple sclerosis. *Frontiers in Immunology*, 12, 669811.

Wang, Z. and Tang, H. (2025). *A Comprehensive Survey of AI Models in Precision Medicine*. Authorea Preprints.

Yousef, H., Malagurski Tortei, B., Castiglione, F. (2024). Predicting multiple sclerosis disease progression and outcomes with machine learning and MRI-based biomarkers: A review. *Journal of Neurology*, 271(10), 6543–6572.

12

Artificial Intelligence Applications in Sleep Medicine and Neurological Disorders

Artificial intelligence (AI) is changing the face of modern medicine by introducing new instruments to the diagnostic process and personal care, as well as predictive modeling. AI can bring about changes in clinical workflow, making diagnoses more accurate and allowing clinicians to track complicated brain processes in real time in the field of sleep medicine and neurological care. Sleep disorders include insomnia, sleep apnea and narcolepsy, among others. These disorders are frequently undiagnosed due to the limitations of the normal polysomnography and subjective reporting. Machine learning and deep learning-enabled AI systems are capable of independently identifying sleep stages and identifying irregular patterns, as well as forecasting the progression of the disease with a high degree of accuracy. Similarly, AI enhances neuroimaging readings, synthetic biomarkers and prognostic models in epileptiform diseases, Alzheimer's disease, Parkinson's disease and multiple sclerosis. Such developments are able to detect problems in the initial stages, customize treatment plans and monitor the progress of the disease over time. A combination of various types of data, such as electroencephalography (EEG), magnetic resonance imaging (MRI), wearable sensors and electronic health records, provides a full view of the health of a patient and aids in precision medicine in the field of neurology and sleep science. Nevertheless, there are still issues related to the standardization of data, understanding algorithms and dealing with the ethical issues of the application of AI in clinical practice. This chapter focuses on the current progress in AI in sleep and neurological disorders, the achievements of recent progress, the existence of integration opportunities and the necessary barriers that have to be addressed to implement AI safely, effectively and, above all, fairly in healthcare.

Chapter written by Swati JAGTAP and Sharifnawaj Y. INAMDAR.

12.1. Introduction

Artificial intelligence (AI) is no longer a research instrument and is now a major force for innovation in healthcare. Through the latest innovations in machine learning (ML), deep learning (DL) and data science, AI is able to analyze complex and high-dimensional data automatically. It is also capable of detecting latent relationships that are not always apparent in traditional statistics and can be very helpful, particularly in problem domains that depend on large longitudinal and multimodal datasets, including sleep medicine and neurology (Bajwa et al. 2021).

Neurological diseases, along with sleep disorders, put a tremendous burden on the world. Sleep disorders such as insomnia, obstructive sleep apnea (OSA), narcolepsy and restless leg syndrome occur in as many as one-third of adults in the world. They are associated with heart disease, diabetes, poor diet, depression and poor quality of life (Naik et al. 2024). Among the leading causes of disability and death in the world, neurological disorders include ailments such as epilepsy, Alzheimer's disease (AD), Parkinson's disease (PD), multiple sclerosis (MS) and stroke. They can require a lifetime of assistance, lead to high healthcare costs and burden patients, caregivers and health systems (Wang et al. 2023). These areas have received lower priority in AI research, despite the urgent need for more effective diagnostic and monitoring solutions.

Conventional diagnostic procedures are accurate but also have major shortcomings. A polysomnography (PSG), an overnight laboratory test with a manual scoring of electroencephalography (EEG), electromyography (EMG) and electrooculography (EOG), is the gold standard of sleep medicine. This is both expensive and time-consuming, and can lack consistency among scorers. In neurology, magnetic resonance imaging (MRI), EEG, positron emission tomography (PET) and neuropsychological examination are the main means of testing, all of which are labor-intensive and require specialist interpretation. Subjective reports from patients, such as sleepiness in the daytime or memory issues, introduce a variability that slows down diagnosis and updates on the progress of the disease (Chari 2024).

A large portion of these challenges can be solved through AI. It is possible to have algorithms that automatically analyze raw EEGs to label sleep stages, identify microarousals or identify apnea events without human intervention. This intelligence could be used in the field of neurology, where we can use large imaging datasets to detect structural and functional abnormalities and negative biomarkers of neurodegeneration, or even to forecast the risk of seizures. Such tools minimize the workload of clinicians, enhance reproducibility and increase access to care on a large scale. The latest trends in AI technologies include the integration of wearables and mobile health devices, which will facilitate continuous data collection and remote monitoring outside of clinical settings for chronic conditions, in which follow-ups must be provided over an extended period.

Although there has been an improvement, AI usage in sleep medicine and neurology has barriers to use. The heterogeneity of the data, inconsistency of the protocols and limitation of large annotated datasets obstruct the training of models and generalization. Several DL models are black boxes, and this can make predictions unclear, resulting in less trust in clinicians. Before AI can be safely introduced into routine care, ethical concerns such as patient privacy, bias and equitable access should also be addressed (Bajwa et al. 2021; Chari 2024).

This chapter studies the existing AI in the fields of neurology and sleep medicine. It discusses the use of AI in automated sleeping phases, sleep-disorder diagnostics, wearable tracking, seizure tracking, neuroimaging diagnostics and disease-progression simulation. It also talks about multimodal data integration, predictive analytics, ethical concerns and future trends. This chapter will provide clinicians, researchers and policymakers with a current perspective of the ways AI is changing these areas, and what impediments stand in the way of safe and effective clinical translation.

12.2. AI in sleep medicine

12.2.1. *Sleep stage classification*

A proper determination of the sleep stages is essential in the diagnosis of sleep disorders and sleep physiology. The gold standard is currently a PSG, which monitors several aspects of physiological signals during the night, including EEG, EOG or EMG. However, the scoring of the process by sleep technicians is lengthy and the outcome may differ depending on who does it. AI offers an alternative that is also quite powerful, relying on the automation of sleep stage classification, enhancing the efficiency and consistency of the results (Yang et al. 2024).

The initial developments of ML were based on handcrafted features of EEG and other PSG signals. Although these models were better than manual scoring, they were still not as precise as human experts. The latest DL is now able to process raw signals in an end-to-end manner, without the need for handcrafted features. Convolutional neural networks (CNNs) preserve both the spatial and temporal features of EEG, whereas recurrent networks such as recurrent neural networks (RNNs) and long short-term memories (LSTMs) are used to learn the long-term relationship in the relationship between sleep sessions. Such DL models are able to learn the task with accuracy comparable to or even better than human experts when trained using big annotated datasets (Morokuma et al. 2023; Somaskandhan et al. 2023).

12.2.2. *Sleep disorder diagnosis*

In addition to the staging, AI is currently able to identify certain problems in sleep with high accuracy. The most common issue is OSA, which used to be traditionally diagnosed through the collection of an apnea–hypopnea index using PSG. The current AI systems automatically detect apnea events based on the EEG, airflow, oximetry and heart-rate measurements with good sensitivity and specificity. The problems of insomnia and narcolepsy, which are not commonly diagnosed due to the subjective symptoms described by patients, are also currently assessed using AI models trained on physiological and behavioral levels (Miller et al. 2022).

Recent research has focused on multimodal AI, which combines PSG signals with wearables and actigraphy. Using this holistic system, more information on sleep disorders is obtained, which can be identified both in the laboratory and at home. As an example, the combination of EEG, heart-rate variability and movement patterns leads to a better detection of apneic events and minor sleep disturbances that traditional measures cannot detect (Lee et al. 2023).

12.2.3. *Wearables and home-based monitoring*

Wearables have expanded the use of AI in the field of sleep medicine. Wristbands, headbands and other sensor-enabled devices constantly monitor physiological indicators such as heart rate, movement and skin temperature. These streams are processed by AI algorithms to approximate the length of sleep, its efficiency and sleep development in real time. This daily or weekly monitoring is more revelatory of habitual sleep patterns than a single PSG (Birrer et al. 2024).

Home-based monitoring is especially implemented in areas with low resources, where access to sleep laboratories is limited. Artificially intelligent platforms allow patients to monitor quality of sleep over time, identify sleep disorders early and promote individualized interventions. An evaluation of validation demonstrates that

AI-powered wearables can be used in the same way as a PSG to classify sleep stages and detect apnea, which allows an expansion of clinical use (Svensson et al. 2024).

12.3. AI in neurological disorders

12.3.1. *Epilepsy*

Epilepsy is a persistent neurological disorder, which is the cause of recurrent seizures. More than 50 million individuals are affected by this disorder throughout the world. Good care must include the timely identification of the problem and an accurate observation of any seizures. Conventional EEG and video-EEG research is expensive to conduct in terms of human resources and seizures can often be missed, making it difficult for clinicians to determine the frequency and type of seizures. These challenges can be overcome with the help of AI.

ML detectors identify seizures by observing the indications of EEG signals. The earliest systems used handcrafted capabilities, such as spectral power, amplitude and rhythmicity, to divide the ictal and interictal periods. In recent work within modern settings, raw EEG data is directly analyzed using deep learning models, effectively bypassing the traditional hand-crafted feature extraction stage (Kerr et al. 2024). They are able to capture delicate pre-ictal events and provide real-time seizure forecasting and warnings. There is limited clinical evidence on AI-driven seizure-detecting devices (worn on a headband or embedded EEG sensors), but these devices have significantly higher recognition compared to traditional detection methods (Bai et al. 2025).

AI is also useful in searching for areas of seizure onset, which are critical to patients with drug-resistant epilepsy who may require surgery. The EEG is used together with neuroimaging such as MRI and functional magnetic resonance imaging (fMRI) to identify epileptogenic regions accurately using advanced algorithms. The methods can reduce the need for invasive surgery and contribute to the customization of surgery plans (Jiang et al. 2022).

12.3.2. *AD and dementia*

AD and other forms of dementia are progressive diseases that are debilitating in terms of impaired cognitive ability and a reduction in quality of life. In preclinical or mild cognitive impairment (MCI), an early diagnosis is essential since medicine is more effective at these levels. The old methods (cognitive tests and MRI) tend to overlook symptoms at an early stage, which slows down the process.

Neuroimaging, genetics and behavioral information are used by AI to enhance early diagnosis. ML models that have been trained using structural MRI, PET scans and cerebrospinal fluid markers are capable of detecting AD, following the slightest brain changes that can indicate AD years before symptoms manifest (Fei et al. 2025). Naturally, non-invasive biomarkers are provided by natural language processing (NLP) on speech and writing. Vocabulary, syntax and coherence changes are predictors of cognitive issues and are monitored over time (Hajjar et al. 2023).

AI can also assist with precise prognosis and treatment. Predictive models determine the rate of decline, response to medication or the appropriateness of a patient to participate in a clinical trial. Multimodal data incorporations into AI schemes lead to accuracy in prescribing medication for treating dementia (Ding et al. 2024).

12.3.3. *PD*

PD has motor (tremor, slowed movement, stiffness, balance problems) and non-motor (cognitive impairment, sleep challenges and autonomic malfunction) symptoms. The conventional tests are based on physical examinations and anecdotal patient history.

AI uses wearable sensors and smartphone apps for objective and continuous monitoring. The motor activity is recorded by accelerometers, gyroscopes and pressure sensors, and processed by ML algorithms that measure the severity of tremor, gait and bradykinesia. The systems are used to identify initial motor alterations and monitor disease progression over time (Sotirakis et al. 2023).

AI aids PD diagnosis by using imaging. MRI or dopamine transporter (DAT) models are also able to distinguish between PD and atypical syndromes of parkinsonism. The use of voice and speech analysis powered by AI can identify early vocal symptoms preceding motor symptoms, which are used as prodromal physical signs (Sigcha et al. 2023). These multimodal AI tools offer end-to-end clinical and research evaluation.

12.3.4. *MS and other neurological arguments*

MS is a demyelinating condition that has no uniform symptoms or rates of progression. It is essential that the lesion loads and disease progression are tracked in order to make treatment decisions. The application of AI to a brain MRI makes the detection, segmentation and measurement of lesions automated, eliminating observer variability and enhancing longitudinal tracking (Spagnolo et al. 2023). Serial imaging predictive models can predict relapses and progression and treatment responses, assisting in personalized care.

Other conditions, such as amyotrophic lateral sclerosis (ALS), stroke and trauma, are also the focus of AI. ML models are applied in ALS to predict the progression and functional deterioration of the disease based on digital biomarkers such as voice records and information on fine-motor tasks. In stroke care, AI integrates imaging technologies with laboratory and clinical data to predict patient outcomes, guide rehabilitation and improve acute care management (Kamraoui et al. 2022).

12.4. Multimodal data integration and predictive analytics

12.4.1. *Rationale for multimodal approaches*

Sleep medicine and neurology are complicated disciplines. Single-modality data do tend to ignore critical signals. Sleep dysfunctions involve neural functioning, the respiratory system, the heartbeat and behavior. Neurological illnesses involve structural, functional and molecular deviations throughout the central nervous system. Conventional measurements tend to be based on a single modality (EEG sleep-staging or MRI neurodegeneration), and this has the potential to be incomplete. AI can integrate diverse data sources – including onboard imaging, electrophysiology, wearables and clinical records – into predictive modeling systems that improve diagnostic accuracy and forecasting capability (Albarrati et al. 2025).

12.4.2. *Integration of neuroimaging, physiological and behavioral data*

Contemporary research illustrates that the connection of various sources of data enhances our knowledge concerning illness. AI models based on structural MRI, PET scans and speech-based digital biomarkers detect cognitive deterioration sooner than those of the single-modality approach in AD (Wang et al. 2025). Models that combine EEG, heart rate variability and breathing patterns with actigraphy are found to be more effective in the detection of OSA and subtle sleep issues that go unnoticed with just the PSG approach in sleep medicine. Wearables and mobile health-related devices provide continuous behavior and physiological information on movement, heart rate, oxygen saturation and sleep. Integrated with lab-based measurements, AI models can track the disease development, detect initial deviations and predict flare-ups. As an example, wearable activity data that is connected to a PSG to predict nightly sleep efficiency can be predicted using an AI model. When combined with EEG data, wearable accelerometers can accurately predict epileptic seizure events, even outside clinical settings.

12.4.3. *Disease progression predictive models*

A potential clinical contribution of AI, and one of the most promising, is predictive analytics. Training AI on longitudinal and multimodal data will allow the prediction of disease progression, course and outcome, which can be used to prevent disease. The predictive models used in PD use imaging, wearable sensors and clinical tests to predict motor deterioration and risk of falling, and provide individualized treatments. By analogy, in MS, the repeated MRI images and clinical measures generate models predicting lesion expansion and later disability to assist clinicians in tailoring their treatment (Tariq 2025). Predictive models may be innovated in sleep medicine to identify patients with potential cardiovascular or metabolic issues related to untreated sleep apnea so that the problem can be addressed prior to occurrence. ML algorithms compare trends from long-term PSG, wearables and clinical data to emphasize personal risk scores, which help to determine patient-focused opportunities in counseling and tailor treatment to patients.

12.4.4. *Predictive modeling for disease progression*

Multimodal integration is not without its challenges, though. The heterogeneity of the data makes it difficult to train data because of the varied sampling rate, signal quality and format among devices and centers. A lack of data, the quality of variable annotation and a discrepancy of measurements performed at home and in the lab can also compromise reliability. To ensure consistency in performance, AI models should therefore have effective preprocessing, normalization and missing-data processing. In addition, a large number of modalities can increase model complexity, increasing risks of overfitting, interpretability problems and computing time.

12.4.5. *Future perspectives*

The future of multimodal AI in sleep medicine and neurology lies in the development of scalable, interpretable and clinically deployable frameworks. Federated learning approaches can train models across multiple centers without sharing raw patient data, addressing privacy concerns while improving generalizability. Explainable AI (XAI) techniques, including attention mechanisms, feature importance analyses and visualization tools, can help clinicians understand which modalities or features drive predictions, fostering trust and adoption. The integration of genomics, metabolomics and other "omics" data alongside neuroimaging, electrophysiology and behavioral data represents the next frontier for comprehensive, personalized disease modeling (Albarrati et al. 2025; Wang et al. 2025; Tariq 2025). Table 12.1 lists the applications of AI in sleep and neurological disorders.

Clinical area	AI technique/model	Data source/modality	Objective/application	Outcome/impact
Sleep stage classification	Deep learning (CNN, LSTM)	EEG, EOG, EMG, PSG signals	Automatic scoring of sleep stages	Accuracy comparable to human experts; reduced scoring time
Sleep apnea detection	ML and DL models	PSG, airflow, oximetry, heart rate signals	Automated detection of apnea and hypopnea events	High sensitivity and specificity; non-invasive home diagnosis
Wearable-based sleep monitoring	Embedded AI algorithms	Wristbands, headbands, actigraphy, HR sensors	Continuous real-time sleep tracking and disorder screening	Enables at-home, long-term monitoring; PSG-level validation
Epilepsy	CNN, RNN-based EEG models	EEG, video-EEG	Seizure detection and prediction	Real-time forecasting; localization of seizure onset zones
Alzheimer's and dementia	Multimodal ML and NLP	MRI, PET, speech, CSF biomarkers	Early diagnosis, cognitive decline prediction	Detects preclinical AD; digital biomarkers via speech
Parkinson's disease	Wearable sensor ML models	Accelerometer, gyroscope, voice data	Motor and speech symptom monitoring	Early detection, progression tracking, digital biomarker creation
Multiple sclerosis	Deep learning for MRI segmentation	MRI (T1, T2, FLAIR)	Lesion detection, progression prediction	Automated tracking of disease activity; personalized care
Multimodal predictive analytics	Ensemble and federated models	EEG, MRI, wearables, clinical data	Disease progression modeling and risk prediction	Enables precision medicine and early intervention

Table 12.1. *Applications of artificial intelligence in sleep and neurological disorders*

12.5. Ethical, legal and clinical challenges

12.5.1. *Data quality, bias and generalizability*

To work effectively, AI systems require high-quality representative data. Sleep medicine and neurology have a plethora of small datasets, often based on a single institution or biased towards specific groups. Such biases may result in AI models not functioning well among underrepresented people, which may bring up the issues of fairness and reliability (Georgin et al. 2025). Indicatively, a seizure-detecting model that was largely trained using adult patients may be unable to detect seizures in children, and a sleep-staging algorithm that has been trained on a healthy volunteer population may erroneously categorize signals in patients with other illnesses. To mitigate these limitations, multi-center collaborations, larger and more demographically diverse datasets, and rigorous external validation are essential to ensure model generalizability across patient populations.

12.5.2. *Explainability and clinician trust*

Numerous successful AI systems, in particular DL models, are black-box predictors, producing predictions with no apparent explanation of how they do so. In medical practice, it is crucial to know the reason an AI makes a decision in order to trust the clinician, for patient safety, and follow regulations. Attention maps, feature-importance rankings and counterfactual reasoning are XAI methods that indicate what inputs support the predictions (De Oliveira et al. 2025). As an example, when it comes to seizure detection, to ensure that the AI output is correct, neurologists can highlight the parts of the EEG that are the most likely to signal an ictal seizure. XAI approaches are currently in development. An incorrect understanding of an explanation may result in clinical errors, and thus, the methods need to be thoroughly incorporated in clinical practices.

12.5.3. *Privacy, data governance and federated learning*

Sleep and neurological data contain extremely sensitive personal data, such as EEG and MRI data, as well as behavioral and mobile health data. Ensuring patient privacy while preserving it alongside ongoing AI innovation represents a critical ethical and legal challenge. It would be useful to train AI models in multiple institutions using federated learning, which does not require moving raw data and thus minimizes privacy risks and enables the usage of more extensive datasets. Nevertheless, federated approaches are not without their own problems, including data heterogeneity, disproportionate data quality and technical complexity when consolidating models (De Oliveira et al. 2025; Georgin et al. 2025; Singh et al. 2025).

12.5.4. *Regulatory and liability considerations*

The regulation of AI-powered medical appliances is changing. Developers will have to adhere to the Good Machine Learning Practice (GMLP), show clinical performance, implement comprehensive monitoring and update plans. Who is responsible is also not clear: in the event of a misdiagnosis or a negative outcome of an AI algorithm, no one can determine who is to blame: the manufacturer, the healthcare provider or the institution (Singh et al. 2025).

12.5.5. *Equity of access and health system integration*

AI has the potential to provide increased access to sleep and neurological services through remote tracking and automatic analysis. Nevertheless, it could also increase existing inequalities. Individuals without wearable devices, smartphones and a stable internet connection will probably be excluded from the interventions driven by AI. Health systems have to implement AI fairly with a consideration of the infrastructures, cost, culture and education at each design and implementation phase. Close follow-up on real-life results is necessary to ensure that AI really enhances care and does not cause any unintended harm (De Oliveira et al. 2025; Georgin et al. 2025).

12.6. Future directions

12.6.1. *Federated, multicenter and open data initiatives*

The field of sleep medicine, as well as neurology, will be improved by AI, mostly on large and eclectic datasets developed via federated, multi-center partnerships. Federated learning ensures that models can learn from numerous institutions without transferring patient data, and thus, privacy is ensured and learning is increased. Reproducibility, comparisons and faster innovation are facilitated by open and pending projects, clear labeling standards and shared benchmarks.

As an illustration, multisite datasets of EEG, MRI, PSG and wearable data contribute to the construction of algorithms that are effective across different ages, devices and clinical contexts (Shen et al. 2025).

12.6.2. *Hybrid human–AI workflows*

AI is best used in combination with the knowledge of clinicians instead of as a substitute for it. Hybrid workflows – where AI provides preliminary suggestions or flags high-priority and critical events, such as candidate seizure segments, suspected apneas, or early signs of cognitive decline – enable clinicians to make the final and most effective decisions. This model is called human-in-the-loop, where a human maintains responsibility and provides clinical supervision, and can be adopted into regular practice. Future studies should be directed towards the maximization of these workflows based on user-intended design, electronic health record integration and feedback systems that boost the performance of AI and/or its acceptance by clinicians (Shen et al. 2025).

12.6.3. *Multimodal foundation models and transfer learning*

Clinical AI is being redefined to involve large-scale multimodal foundation models. These models are a combination of imaging, electrophysiology, behavior and long-term clinical data. They acquire these representations, which can then be generalized to numerous tasks. As an illustration, a base model that was trained on EEG and MRI data from several institutions can be refined to meet the small task of early-onset Alzheimer's diagnosis, sleep-stage classification or seizure prediction, and can thus be deployed quickly across hospitals and populations (He et al. 2024).

12.6.4. *Continuous learning with safe update mechanisms*

The information provided in healthcare is continuously evolving, and AI applications implemented in clinics have to adapt to new equipment, target patients or communication regimes. Ongoing performance checks, periodic reviews of these models by a clinician and ongoing deployment of continuous learning pipelines in conjunction with stated change-control rules support the accuracy of these models in the long term. Safety in updating and tracking the evolution is crucial to prevent the model diminishing, save lives and comply with laws. Research in the future must establish frameworks that are flexible, accountable, repeatable and contain risk management (He et al. 2024).

12.7. Conclusion

AI will revolutionize sleep medicine and neuroscience, with correct diagnosis, timely and ongoing evaluation, and tailored care. Within sleep medicine, AI recognizes the stages of sleep automatically, identifies sleep disorders, such as sleep apnea and narcolepsy, and operates with devices measuring sleep in patients that can be performed anywhere, not necessarily in a lab. These are available in low-resource and non-high-resource areas, offer more diagnostic accuracy and minimize the workload associated with the use of labor-intensive PSG. In neurology, AI can be used to identify and forecast seizures, and assist in early recognition and the monitoring of Alzheimer's and other dementias, as well as motor and non-motor symptoms of Parkinson's disease. ML and DL process neuroimaging, electrophysiology, behavior and wearable data and provide definitive, quantitative information that can be used to supplement routine clinical examination. Predictive models allow preventive medical care, improved disease treatment and intelligent patient selection to undergo clinical trials by enhancing precision medicine. Even with such advantages, the implementation of AI in everyday routine care should be approached cautiously, considering the ethical, legal and practical challenges. The most significant problems are data quality, bias, privacy, explanations of decisions by the AI, regulatory regulations and equitable access. These variables determine the extent to which AI tools will be reliable, safe and acceptable. Future advancements will rely on cross-site collaboration, multimodal data integration, synergistic human–AI workflows, continuous learning platforms, and the development of digital patient biomarkers. With a well-constructed and properly tested AI, the future of diagnosing, monitoring and treating sleep and neurological issues could change. AI can enhance the results of care, increase its efficiency and assist in proactive and personalized care, supporting the expertise of clinicians with data-driven insights.

12.8. References

Abd-Alrazaq, A., Aslam, H., AlSaad, R., Alsahli, M., Ahmed, A., Damseh, R., Aziz, S., Sheikh, J. (2024). Detection of sleep apnea using wearable AI: Systematic review and meta-analysis. *Journal of Medical Internet Research*, 26, e58187.

Albarrati, A.M., Abdelwahab, S.I., Nazer, R.I. (2025). A comprehensive bibliometric analysis of disability research in Saudi Arabia: Trends, gaps, and future directions. *Journal of Disability Research*, 4(2), 20250003.

Bai, L., Litscher, G., Li, X. (2025). Epileptic seizure detection using machine learning: A systematic review and meta-analysis. *Brain Sciences*, 15(6), 634.

Bajwa, J., Munir, U., Nori, A., Williams, B. (2021). Artificial intelligence in healthcare: Transforming the practice of medicine. *Future Healthcare Journal*, 8(2), e188–e194.

Birrer, V., Elgendi, M., Lambercy, O., Menon, C. (2024). Evaluating reliability in wearable devices for sleep staging. *NPJ Digital Medicine*, 7(1), 74.

Chari, P.V. (2024). On computational imaging in the era of neural sensing: The sensor, the data and the algorithm. Thesis, University of California, Los Angeles.

De Oliveira, A.C., Azevedo, J.P., Ruback, L., Moreira, R., Teixeira, S.S., Teles, A.S. (2025). Effect of explainable artificial intelligence on trust of mental health professionals in an AI-based system for suicide prevention. *IEEE Access*, 13, 60987–61005.

Ding, K., Chetty, M., Noori Hoshyar, A., Bhattacharya, T., Klein, B. (2024). Speech based detection of Alzheimer's disease: A survey of AI techniques, datasets and challenges. *Artificial Intelligence Review*, 57(12), 325.

Fei, Z.H., Li, Z., Liang, L., Ru, G.W., Yi, H.L., Zhen, W. (2025). Network meta-analysis based on the improvement of motor ability. In *Advances in Parkinson's Disease Research: Exploring Biomarkers and Therapeutic Strategies for Halting Disease Progression*, Bougea, A. and Degirmenci, Y. (eds). Frontiers Media SA, Lausanne.

Georgin, J., Ramos, C.G., de Oliveira, J.S., Dehmani, Y., El Messaoudi, N., Meili, L., Franco, D.S. (2025). A critical review of the advances and current status of the application of adsorption in the remediation of micropollutants and dyes through the use of emerging bio-based nanocomposites. *Sustainability*, 17(5), 2012.

Hajjar, I., Okafor, M., Choi, J.D., Moore, E., Abrol, A., Calhoun, V.D., Goldstein, F.C. (2023). Development of digital voice biomarkers and associations with cognition, cerebrospinal biomarkers, and neural representation in early Alzheimer's disease. *Alzheimer's & Dementia: Diagnosis, Assessment & Disease Monitoring*, 15(1), e12393.

He, Y., Huang, F., Jiang, X., Nie, Y., Wang, M., Wang, J., Chen, H. (2024). Foundation model for advancing healthcare: Challenges, opportunities and future directions. *IEEE Reviews in Biomedical Engineering*, 18, 172–191. doi: 10.1109/RBME.2024.3496744.

Jiang, R., Zhang, L., Wei, H.-L., Crookes, D., Chazot, P. (2022). *Recent Advances in AI-enabled Automated Medical Diagnosis*. CRC Press, Boca Raton, FL.

Kamraoui, R.A., Mansencal, B., Manjon, J.V., Coupé, P. (2022). Longitudinal detection of new MS lesions using deep learning. *Frontiers in Neuroimaging*, 1, 948235.

Kerr, W.T., McFarlane, K.N., Figueiredo Pucci, G. (2024). The present and future of seizure detection, prediction, and forecasting with machine learning, including the future impact on clinical trials. *Frontiers in Neurology*, 15, 1425490.

Lee, T., Cho, Y., Cha, K.S., Jung, J., Cho, J., Kim, H., Kim, D., Hong, J., Lee, D., Keum, M. et al. (2023). Accuracy of 11 wearable, nearable, and airable consumer sleep trackers: Prospective multicenter validation study. *JMIR mHealth and uHealth*, 11(1), e50983.

Miller, D.J., Sargent, C., Roach, G.D. (2022). A validation of six wearable devices for estimating sleep, heart rate and heart rate variability in healthy adults. *Sensors*, 22(16), 6317.

Morokuma, S., Hayashi, T., Kanegae, M., Mizukami, Y., Asano, S., Kimura, I., Tateizumi, Y., Ueno, H., Ikeda, S., Niizeki, K. (2023). Deep learning-based sleep stage classification with cardiorespiratory and body movement activities in individuals with suspected sleep disorders. *Scientific Reports*, 13(1), 17730.

Naik, K., Goyal, R.K., Foschini, L., Chak, C.W., Thielscher, C., Zhu, H., Lu, J., Lehár, J., Pacanoswki, M.A., Terranova, N. et al. (2024). Current status and future directions: The application of artificial intelligence/machine learning for precision medicine. *Clinical Pharmacology & Therapeutics*, 115(4), 673–686.

Shen, Y., Yu, J., Zhou, J., Hu, G. (2025). Twenty-five years of evolution and hurdles in electronic health records and interoperability in medical research: Comprehensive review. *Journal of Medical Internet Research*, 27, e59024.

Sigcha, L., Borzì, L., Amato, F., Rechichi, I., Ramos-Romero, C., Cárdenas, A., Gascó, L., Olmo, G. (2023). Deep learning and wearable sensors for the diagnosis and monitoring of Parkinson's disease: A systematic review. *Expert Systems with Applications*, 229, 120541.

Singh, V., Cheng, S., Kwan, A.C., Ebinger, J. (2025). United States Food and Drug Administration regulation of clinical software in the era of artificial intelligence and machine learning. *Mayo Clinic Proceedings: Digital Health*, 3(3), 100231.

Somaskandhan, P., Leppänen, T., Terrill, P.I., Sigurdardottir, S., Arnardottir, E.S., Ólafsdóttir, K.A., Serwatko, M., Sigurðardóttir, S.Þ., Clausen, M., Töyräs, J. et al. (2023). Deep learning-based algorithm accurately classifies sleep stages in preadolescent children with sleep-disordered breathing symptoms and age-matched controls. *Frontiers in Neurology*, 14, 1162998.

Sotirakis, C., Su, Z., Brzezicki, M.A., Conway, N., Tarassenko, L., FitzGerald, J.J., Antoniades, C.A. (2023). Identification of motor progression in Parkinson's disease using wearable sensors and machine learning. *npj Parkinson's Disease*, 9(1), 142.

Spagnolo, F., Depeursinge, A., Schädelin, S., Akbulut, A., Müller, H., Barakovic, M., Melie-Garcia, L., Cuadra, M.B., Granziera, C. (2023). How far MS lesion detection and segmentation are integrated into the clinical workflow? A systematic review. *NeuroImage: Clinical*, 39, 103491.

Svensson, T., Madhawa, K., Chung, U.I., Svensson, A.K. (2024). Validity and reliability of the Oura Ring Generation 3 (Gen3) with Oura sleep staging algorithm 2.0 (OSSA 2.0) when compared to multi-night ambulatory polysomnography: A validation study of 96 participants and 421,045 epochs. *Sleep Medicine*, 115, 251–263.

Tariq, R. (2025) Machine learning methods for personalized treatment response characterization using clinical care brain MRI and non-imaging data in multiple sclerosis. Master's Thesis, University of Calgary, Calgary.

Wang, N.N., Zhu, B., Li, X.L., Liu, S., Shi, J.Y., Cao, D.S. (2023). Comprehensive review of drug–drug interaction prediction based on machine learning: Current status, challenges, and opportunities. *Journal of Chemical Information and Modeling*, 64(1), 96–109.

Wang, R., Peng, S., Zhu, J., Xu, Y., Wang, M., Zhang, L., Qiu, Y., Hou, D., Wang, Q., Liu, R. (2025). Innovations in Alzheimer's disease diagnostic technologies: Clinical prospects of novel biomarkers, multimodal integration, and non-invasive detection. *Frontiers in Neurology*, 16, 1651708.

Yang, L., Ding, Z., Zhou, J., Zhang, S., Wang, Q., Zheng, K., Wang, X., Chen, L. (2024). Algorithmic detection of sleep-disordered breathing using respiratory signals: A systematic review. *Physiological Measurement*, 45(3), 03TR02.

13

Virtual and Augmented Reality Coupled with AI for Cognitive Rehabilitation

Cognitive rehabilitation is now part of contemporary neurorehabilitation since it meets shortcomings in memory, attention, executive functioning and problem-solving. These impairments usually occur due to the neurologic disorders involving strokes, traumatic brain injuries and neurodegenerative disorders. Conventional treatment procedures are therapeutically useful. They are, however, not always engaged, do not adapt to the needs of individual patients and have difficulty providing consistent long-term care. New technologies such as virtual reality (VR) and augmented reality (AR) have made some initial steps in revolutionizing this area by providing immersive, interactive and personalized experiences with rehabilitation. These technologies, when integrated with artificial intelligence (AI), extend beyond passive exercises to enable data-driven and adaptive cognitive training environments. AI facilitates real-time performance monitoring, dynamically adjusts task difficulty, and leverages predictive analytics to personalize and optimize therapy based on the unique cognitive profile of each patient. Remote rehabilitation and telehealth provision are also more easily accessed and administered with the help of VR and AR platforms timed by AI, which eliminates discrepancies in access and care delivery. The latest developments show that combining VR, AR and AI does not only make patients more motivated but will also contribute to higher neuroplasticity through involvement in engaging, repetitive and meaningful tasks. Multimodal sensing technologies with AI algorithms allow the evaluation of minor behavioral and physiological signs, which contributes to the accuracy of cognitive rehabilitation.

This chapter will discuss the integration of VR and AR with AI in the sphere of cognitive rehabilitation, its clinical possibilities, the principle of its work, technology development, limitations and prospects. This chapter highlights the promise of AI-based VR/AR interventions to influence the future of the next generation of personalized neurorehabilitation policies by summarizing the existing knowledge base.

Chapter written by Omkar KULKARNI and Amruta B. KALE.

13.1. Introduction

Cognitive impairments are usually due to neurological conditions such as strokes, traumatic brain injuries (TBIs), Alzheimer's, Parkinson's and other neurodegenerative disorders. They are able to influence attention, memory, executive function, problem-solving and processing the speed that significantly limits everyday functioning and quality of life (Zhang et al. 2025). Conventional forms of rehabilitation, such as exercises led by the therapist, paper-and-pencil, and memory, have been effective. Nevertheless, they tend to not be relevant to real-life settings, become monotonous and are not able to adapt to the specific needs of each patient, which may reduce the engagement and adherence in the long term (Al-Rajab et al. 2025).

Cognitive rehabilitation has been altered by the emergence of digital technology. Virtual reality (VR) and augmented reality (AR) offer simulative environments, which engage and simulate real-life activities within a risk-free and controlled setting. VR immerses patients in entirely computer-generated environments, where therapists can vary cognitive and motor demands in precise manners. AR introduces digital data to the physical world, which allows patients to rehearse their skills in natural environments. Such technologies make exercises more relatable and relevant, as well as having a higher degree of ecological validity, which aids patients in clinically applying their skills to everyday living (Maggio et al. 2025).

A combination of VR and AR with artificial intelligence (AI) moves the rehabilitation to the next level. Machine learning (ML) and reinforcement learning (RL) are AI algorithms that monitor performance of patients in real time, as well as analyze behaviors and regulate the difficulty, sequence and feedback of the tasks involuntarily. It makes the therapy challenging and personal enough, promotes neuroplasticity and accelerates recovery (Maggio et al. 2025).

VR and AR prove to be effective in cognitive rehabilitation, which is gradually supported in clinical research. Research indicates an enhancement of attention, memory and executive functioning, as well as spatial navigation among diverse groups of patients. AI platforms are also able to track progress in the long run, predict recovery routes and support remote treatment, which is a benefit for resource-lacking or remote areas. Collectively, these technologies have the potential to shift care beyond the ordinary procedures to evidence-based, patient-centered care rehabilitation (Al-Rajab et al. 2025; Zhang et al. 2025).

In addition to cognitive benefits, VR/AR-AI systems increase patient engagement and motivation. Incorporating games, simulations, and immediate feedback makes treatment more engaging, which is essential for long-term adherence and retention. It is also possible to have clinicians develop programs that focus on multiple skills simultaneously, such as memory drills, combined with attention training, or motor and cognitive tasks. Such multi-domain interventions are a representation of the daily life complexities, and more extensive rehabilitation results are achieved with them (Al-Rajab et al. 2025).

VR, AR and AI are also useful in research and public health. They produce fine-pointed data that can be used to investigate the cognitive aging, neuroplasticity and recovery pathways. Analyzing trends of a large number of users, the researchers can identify predictors of successful therapy, take protocols to the next level and develop new treatment models. Telerehabilitation and remote monitoring services can increase access to care, continuity and the reduction of disparities in care provision (Maggio et al. 2025).

Even though VR, AR and AI have tremendous potential, there are still challenges. They are expensive, technically intricate and require extensive clinical validation. The ethical concerns such as data privacy, transparency of the algorithms used and fair access should be addressed. Nevertheless, combining immersive technology and AI is a significant breakthrough in cognitive rehabilitation that provides individualized, interactive and effective interventions, which could help a large number of neurological patients.

13.2. Foundations of cognitive rehabilitation

Cognitive rehabilitation is a reflective therapeutic model based on evidence aimed at enhancing brain memory, attention, problem-solving and executive disrupted functions due to neurological processes. It is mainly aimed at compensating or restoring the same deficits so that such people can become more independent and enhance their daily functioning (Al-Rajab et al. 2025).

There are two prevailing approaches: restorative and compensatory. Restorative interventions involve repetitive training that in turn activates neural pathways as well as promoting restoration of impaired cognition. Compensatory interventions are aimed at instructing strategies and applying outside assistance, including scheduled programs, reminders or computer applications to avoid deficits and optimize functional performance (Rajkumar 2025).

Cognitive rehabilitation depends on the nature of neuroplasticity as a capacity of the brain to organize itself and create new connections during the process of learning and experience. Repetitive, task-relevant and increasingly challenging therapeutic exercises are important to activate and strengthen these neuroplastic processes and are therefore full-fledged cognitive recovery agents (MindMaze n.d.). Nevertheless, standard rehabilitation procedures may be significantly unable to maintain patient attention as well as tailor the interventions in response to personal progress.

Such an absence has provided the opportunity for new technologies such as VR and AR, which can present ecologically valid, motivating and immersive tasks. When paired with AI, these technologies provide real-time customization, whereby the level of task and therapeutic strategies is modified to be in close alignment with the neurobiological principles that govern effective rehabilitation.

13.3. VR in cognitive rehabilitation

Donning VR has become one of the most promising mechanisms of cognitive rehabilitation due to its capability to provide immersive, controlled and engaging therapeutic activities. In contrast to traditional interventions, which are based on abstract exercises, VR offers simulated environments, which are reminiscent of the real-life situations. This allows patients to train on functional activities in safe rehearsing conditions (Georgiev et al. 2021). As an example, VR applications can replicate real-life tasks (shopping, navigation, cooking, etc.), and the people with cognitive disabilities can practice the skills that are directly related to the further increase of their independence.

The ecological validity is one of the primary outcomes of VR. Challenges that are represented in VR environments resemble real-life challenges more closely than the traditional exercises and such cognitive tasks enhance the relationships between therapy and everyday living. The literature shows that patients tend to feel that VR-based rehabilitation is fun and encouraging, and therefore, patients are more likely to adhere and practice more often than due to paper-based or therapist-led rehabilitation (Ding et al. 2025). This is an economically important motivational element because long-term engagement is the vital feature in fostering neuroplasticity and long-term cognitive rehabilitation.

It is also possible to track and evaluate patient performance using VR. All of the interactions in the virtual environment are loggable and analyzable, which leads to the objective data of reaction time, error rate, task completion and other figures. These datasets provide clinicians with detailed information on the development of cognitive skills, which can be used in a more informed way during the therapeutic decisions. Also, VR enables real-time feedback – an aspect that enables the patient to figure out their mistake and modify their performance during the task in real time, and this aspect further promotes learning.

The second strength of VR is that it has the possibility of a progressive increase in complexity. Environments may also be modified to gradually challenge the patient. Examples of this are to include distractions and raise task demands or multitasking. This is flexible enough and enables rehabilitation to follow the rate of recovery of the patient. Furthermore, VR machines are being modified to use remote or home-based rehabilitation, which eliminates the necessity to frequently visit the hospital and increases the writers of underserved populations (Hao et al. 2024).

Although these are the advantages, VR in cognitive rehabilitation also has its weaknesses. Immersive systems based on high quality can be rather costly in terms of hardware, which is a reason to doubt their scalability and availability. Also, pregnancy among patients may cause cybersickness upon extended use and, therefore, the design of therapeutic sessions must be done carefully. Finally, VR-based rehabilitation cannot be considered as substitution for therapist-led treatment but as an augmentation tool to be part and parcel of more comprehensive treatment options.

Altogether, VR is a huge step toward the concept of cognitive rehabilitation, as it provides immersive, exciting and quantifiable therapeutic possibilities that are not only consistent with the principles of neuroplasticity but are also based on the needs of patients.

13.4. AR in cognitive rehabilitation

AR is a new technology that promises to be highly useful in cognitive rehabilitation. In contrast to VR, which makes users plunge into a fully computer-generated space, AR places digital objects in the real world, i.e. images, sounds or interactive hints. This combination allows patients to experience virtual and real stimuli in parallel, which provides a therapeutic experience that can be considered immersive and contextual (Navarro-Ramos et al. 2025).

The key benefit of AR is its context-sensitive interventions. Cognitive activities can also be woven into an ordinary environment of a patient and increase ecological validity and the narrowing of the boundary between therapy and life. An example is that in AR, reminders, cues or instructions can be projected onto objects in the household, so that those with memory lapses can cope with the everyday world of cooking, dressing or taking medication (Piszcz et al. 2024). With the integration of training within a real-life scenario, AR assists in stimulating generalization of the skills, which is frequently ignored by rehabilitation methods.

The other important advantage is a reduced adoption barrier. In comparison to VR, it usually requires having expensive head-mounted displays and a strong computer. In contrast, AR can work on mobile phones or even lightweight smart glasses. This portability enables AR interventions to be made available and usable at home or in the community rehabilitation, as well as in low-resource clinical settings. Patients are able to exercise within normal settings with no special tools and complicated systems.

AR provides interactive responses, as well as real-time adjustment. AR systems can also change the challenge of tasks dynamically by monitoring how people use them and analyzing the patterns with the help of AI. One example in memory training involves adapting prompts by providing additional cues when a patient struggles to recall information and gradually removing them as recall performance improves. This system of adaptation perpetuates involvement and maximizes treatment value (Ding et al. 2025).

In addition, AR enhances communal interaction and community rehabilitation. Applications may include the use of a caregiver, family member or even the therapists, who may be able to achieve or join in exercises with the patient. Such a feature does not only enhance adherence, but it also promotes social connectedness , which is essential toward cognitive and emotional well-being.

The AR platforms should characteristically have an appropriate calibration and tracking to prevent disorientation, particularly in patients with neurological defects. Privacy and security also play a significant role since the AR systems can gather sensitive behavioral and health-related information. Clinical trials over the long run are required to test the efficiency of AR-based interventions relative to the conventional rehabilitative techniques.

13.5. AI for adaptive therapy

AI is changing the cognitive rehabilitation process to introduce data-driven, personalized and adaptive therapies. Conventional techniques in many cases do not correspond to the changing abilities of a patient with rising tasks. AI works to provide real-time performance monitoring, prediction of recovery curves and real-time adjustment of therapy, thus enhancing performance (Wong et al. 2025).

ML algorithms that receive large datasets created in the course of therapy are the core of AI-based rehabilitation. All interactions with a patient, including the correctness of the responses, reaction speed and the errors occurring in them, leave traces of data that are processed by ML models to recognize the progress, stagnation or deterioration. These understandings enable the therapy systems to customize the interventions to the needs of individuals (Makmee and Wongupparaj 2025). Indicatively, a supervised ML can be used to classify the severity of cognitive impairment, whereas an unsupervised grouping can be used to find patient subgroups that react similarly to specific treatment.

The field of deep learning (DL) has opened up even more possibilities of AI. Convolutional neural networks (CNNs) and recurrent neural networks (RNNs) are able to provide the processing of multimodal data such as speech, eye-tracking or movement information recorded in VR and AR in sessions. These models identify minute cognitive variations that the clinician may overlook and can offer an opportunity to intervene sooner and better plan therapy. The natural language processing is also facilitated by DL, which provides the opportunity to speak to patients when they are doing rehabilitation tasks, provided that the conversational agent or a virtual coach is involved.

Another effective method is RL, which is a type of learning through trial and error using algorithms to maximize therapeutic gain. Cognitive rehabilitation RL has the ability to identify the best sequence and intensity of tasks with a particular patient. A reinforcement learning-based system can gradually increase task complexity as performance consistently improves, or introduce supportive aids when performance declines. This makes treatment difficult, but not impossible, eliminating frustration and apathy (Alshami et al. 2025).

In addition to adaptation, AI can be used to provide predictive analytics, which forecast recovery curves and patients with a high risk of unfavorable outcomes. These predictions aid in clinical decision-making and resource mobilization as well as provide patients and families with realistic expectations. Remote monitoring through AI-driven platforms also helps make telerehabilitation a possibility, hence continuity of care in other clinical settings.

Regardless of these benefits, there are still problems in holding AI models transparent and credible. Most ML and DL systems are black boxes and give predictions without any clear explanations that may hamper clinical adoption. Ethics, including cases of data privacy as well as bias in the algorithms, should also be prioritized to make AI widely applicable in the healthcare field.

13.6. Synergistic role of VR/AR coupled with AI

Although all three components, VR, AR and AI, can be beneficial to cognitive therapy, they may form a synergistic ecosystem, which is more than the aggregate of their individual powers. VR and AR have interactive and immersive settings and model real-life tasks. AI is also used to add diversity to the therapy, making it personalized, conducting predictive analytics and giving adaptive feedback. The two combine to create an intelligent rehabilitation model that personalizes treatment according to the cognitive profile of every person (Jiao 2025).

An ecosystem would be depicted by a conceptual diagram that would describe three layers:

– *An immersive layer (VR/AR environments):* in this layer, the patients are subjected to virtual supermarkets, a navigational task or a memory test.

– *A data layer (sensors and monitoring)*: this is where eye-tracking, motion capture, voice input and physiological data (i.e. heart rate variation) are registered during the therapy session.

– *An AI layer (analytics and adaptation)*: ML and RL algorithms process incoming data and modify the difficulty of a task, as well as predict future advancements.

This feedback loop is created through this integration. To illustrate, when a patient is unable to memorize the items on a VR shopping experience, the AI system can automatically decrease the items to improve confidence and slowly increase complications as the patient makes progress. In the same way, during an AR medication-management task, the AI can track the lag of responses and provide prompt real-time responses, guaranteeing constant activity and success in practice (Zhu et al. 2023).

Precision rehabilitation can also be achieved during the joint action of these technologies. Through multimodal data stream analysis, AI is able to identify the subtle cognitive shifts and modify therapy prior to it being reflected in functional decline. This forward-looking practice is differentiated from traditional rehabilitation, which in many cases is subjective to observations made by clinicians. Also, AI-powered VR/AR platforms facilitate longitudinal care, which enables clinicians to monitor progress throughout the weeks or months and adjust their care plans accordingly.

The other important benefit to this synergy is that remote and scalable therapy is facilitated. AR-based training is available to the patients at home through mobile phones, and VR training can be implemented in lightweight headsets.

The information of such sessions is sent safely to AI-based systems, and clinicians are provided with data on progress reports. The model makes it less reliant on face-to-face meetings and increases the reach of patients in rural or resource-constrained settings (Xie et al. 2024).

Nonetheless, integration is also problematic. The large computational requirements, incompatibility between devices and the necessity to have powerful data-security models may pose an impediment to large-scale adoption. Besides, it is also vital to balance automation and human control. Even though the use of AI is flexible regarding the workload, therapists are crucial in result interpretation and responding to the psychological requirements.

13.7. Clinical applications and case studies

There has been a significant promise of the use of VR, AR and AI in the area of cognitive rehabilitation with regard to a variety of neurological conditions. Some of the case studies and clinical trials that prove the effectiveness of these technologies are listed in the following sections.

13.7.1. *Stroke rehabilitation*

One study examined the VR-based interventions as a means to promote cognitive and motor abilities in patients who have suffered a stroke. The subjects were involved in a VR simulation of an immersive environment, as well as one created to activate cognitive processes during motor activities. It was shown that both cognitive performance and motor skills have significantly improved, which means that VR can be a good post-stroke rehabilitation instrument (Banikova et al. 2025).

Likewise, one more study investigated the joint impact of VR and AI on the patients suffering with chronic strokes. The AI system customized exercises of the rehabilitation process dynamically and changed the level of difficulty according to the performance. This method caused an increase in interactions and better recovery results that indicate the potential synergies between VR and AI in stroke recovery (Sarkar and Alqasemi 2025).

13.7.2. *TBI*

A randomized controlled trial was used in the TBI rehabilitation protocol to investigate the use of VR-based cognitive stimulation exercises among older adults with a cognitive impairment. Those who experienced VR training also showed better outcomes with respect to memory, attention and cognitive performance, which would have been otherwise poor under regular therapy, making VR a necessity in improving cognitive performance following TBI (Wen et al. 2021).

13.7.3. *Dementia and Alzheimer's disease*

AI-enhanced VR technologies have also been applied in dementia care. In one study, a VR–AI system with adaptive therapy and interactive interaction with patients with Alzheimer's disease was introduced. It provided individuals with customized cognitive procedures, which led to a higher cognitive engagement and emotional well-being. The findings presented demonstrate how AI-based VR interventions can help in solving cognitive and affective interventions in the management of dementia (Wen et al. 2021).

In addition, meta-analyses of VR interventions in patients with a Mild Cognitive Impairment (MCI) indicate that they have a significant beneficial effect on global cognition, attention and quality of life, especially when semi-immersive VR environments are used in several sessions weekly (Wen et al. 2021).

13.8. Technological innovations and tools

Over recent years, significant technological changes have transformed VR, AR and AI into technologies being used in cognitive rehabilitation. Such innovations can be new hardware, software or AI platforms. They facilitate individualized, comprehensive and evidence-based therapy (Naqvi et al. 2024).

13.8.1. *VR and AR hardware*

Full immersion devices, including the Oculus Quest3 and the HTC VivePro, are high-fidelity VR devices. Patients have the opportunity to communicate in simulated situations. The gadgets are motion tracked, have hand controllers and are haptic. This enables clinicians to track movements and interactions at a fine level. Lightweight smart glasses such as Microsoft HoloLens 3 and Magic Leap are used in AR to project digital data on actual objects. Patients complete mental activities that are in sync with the natural environment. Hardware VR and AR are now smaller and easier to carry, so home-based and community-based programs are viable (Naqvi et al. 2024).

13.8.2. *Software platforms*

Computerized cognitive rehabilitation is provided through new software platforms. Some examples include NeuroRehab VR, MindMaze and COGNISPACE. They offer immersive modules that address memory, attention and executive function.

These are platforms that typically apply gamification, provide live feedback and measure performance, enhancing motivation and compliance. AR applications (AR-MemoryTrainer and Rehago) allow therapists to overlay interactive cues onto real tasks. They provide adaptive cues toward everyday living. Each patient can be treated with therapies that can be tailored to them, making the work hard but not impossible (Piszcz et al. 2024).

13.8.3. *AI implementation and analytics software and applications*

VR and AR systems are now supported by AI to enable adaptive therapy. Rewards and penalties are handled by ML and RL models based on performance outcomes. They also vary and modify the difficulty of tasks and the sequence. AI is able to identify critical mistakes, predict ways of recovery and propose changes in therapy. The analytics are provided by the Cloud so that remote monitoring and long-term tracking become possible. Clinicians receive relevant feedback without having to be monitored all of the time in person (Ding et al. 2025).

The current rehab systems take multimodal sensors to gather richer data. Physiological analyzers and motion sensors, as well as eye-tracking cameras, document detailed behaviors and body language. Based on these data, AI algorithms identify insidious changes in cognition. The full-color feedback contributes to the precision of the process of rehabilitation and planning further sessions.

13.9. Challenges and ethical considerations

Despite the promising advancements of VR, AR and AI in cognitive rehabilitation, several technical and ethical challenges must be addressed to ensure safe, effective and equitable implementation.

13.9.1. *Technical challenges*

Cost and accessibility are huge technical challenges. VR headsets with high fidelity, smart glasses and AI-enabled platforms may depend on massive financial investment. This reduces their accessibility to low-resource or rural environment (Zhichao and Yu 2025). Although portability and ease of use are improving, the complexity of the system remains a hindrance in the older patients or in patients with severe cognitive impairment.

Interoperability and integration are other challenges. Integrating VR/AR devices with AI analytics and multimodal sensors requires standard instructions and untouchable exchange of data. Poor calibration or unsuitable compatibility between software can decrease therapy quality, monitoring accuracy and adverse patient outcome.

There is also concern relating to data reliability and robustness. The software uses quality and long-term data to accurately predict and modify interventions so that AI can use the new data. The presence of noise or missing data or faulty sensors may harm the performance of the model further, resulting in inappropriate or suboptimal therapeutic alterations. Moreover, cybersickness, fatigue or sensory fatigue caused by VR may reduce patient involvement, as well as the length of the session.

13.9.2. *Ethical and privacy concerns*

AI-focused VR/AR technologies accumulate vast behavioral and physiological data, which provoke concerns regarding privacy, security and informed consent (Maggio et al. 2025). Sensitive health data should be well-kept, shared and analyzed. Data ownership, sharing and retention should be clearly outlined to safeguard patients' rights.

Ethical issues concern equity and accessibility. Advanced technologies can boost healthcare disparities without any purposeful design and distribution policies, benefiting patients in urban settings with strong resources and disadvantaging marginalized groups.

The additional ethical issues are transparency and interpretability of AI systems. Most ML algorithms are black boxes, where they do not provide a rational justification as to how they arrived at a particular answer. Such an inability to interpret may undermine clinicians and restrain patient acceptance. There must be established guidelines on clinician supervision and human-in-the-loop decision-making to be responsible in deployment (Rabin et al. 2015).

Last, but not least, are the psychological effects of immersive therapy. Long-term exposure to VR/AR may lead to stress or feelings of disorientation in some patients, particularly those with severe cognitive impairments. The implementation of ethical practice should be performed with moderate immersion under the name of patient comfort and safety.

13.10. Future directions and research opportunities

The amalgamation of immersive technologies, AI and models of the next generation of biofeedback is how the future of cognitive rehabilitation is going to be viewed. The new trends are directed toward VR and AR, which, together with the high-level AI and wearable technologies, generate exceptionally personalized, flexible and multi-sensory rehabilitation experiences (Ziyi 2018).

One of the most promising directions is the use of brain–computer interfaces (BCIs), along with the VR/AR systems. BCIs can be used to monitor the neural activity in real time, and the system can change cognitive tasks based on the neural activity of the patient. In the case of fatigue or attentional lapses, the system will be able to change the task difficulty or provide assistance. This would be an implementation of neurofeedback to speed up neuroplasticity and perform better than traditional mechanisms.

Another radical trend is wearable sensors. Motion tracking, gaze, heart-rate variation and galvanic skin response devices offer extensive multimodal information to an AI. The information allows specific tracking of cognitive activity, emotional state and biological reactions, and the therapy can become dynamic. Remote rehabilitation with the help of wearables is also possible, and continuous at-home treatment is supported by controls of a therapist.

VR/AR rehabilitation is becoming more and more multi-sensory by including auditory, tactile and haptic feedback. These systems increase learning, memory retention and task generalization because they are involved in combination with several senses. AI will streamline how often, how strong and how various stimuli are presented to each patient to create a genuinely personalized environment.

Longitudinal data analytics and predictive model are emerging fields of research. By combining performance data on groups of patients, AI is capable of determining trends that would predict the course of recovery, the likelihood of recurrence or indicate how patients respond to particular treatment. These pieces of information guide the design of therapy, allocation of resources and the planning of care for the individual, thus introducing accuracy to the field of cognitive rehabilitation.

The scalability, accessibility and inclusiveness must be addressed in future studies. The most important issues to be considered in order to reach diverse patient groups are the reduction of costs of hardware, simplification of user interfaces and the design of culturally and linguistically adaptive content. The ethical issues, such as privacy of data, transparency in algorithms and human supervision, will still be observed in responsible deployment (Corrigan et al. 2014; Geerts and Spiros 2020).

13.11. Conclusion

VR, AR and AI are altering the cognitive rehabilitation approach. They provide comprehensive, engaging and flexible treatment, which allows therapy to overcome typical issues of standard approaches: patients usually become demotivated, care is not always personalized, and it is not always easy to deliver real-world or consistent training. As soon as AI is integrated with VR and AR, a task can vary in time, recovery routes can be forecasted, and care can be monitored. This will make certain that each patient receives therapy that is tailored to their cognitive profile. Research on TBI patients and patients who have suffered a stroke demonstrates that the interventions enhance cognitive functioning and raise the level of functional independence, as well as quality of life. The prospective advancements, such as BCIs, wearable sensors and multi-sensory stimulation, should allow the increasing of accuracy, improving the outcomes and expanding access to rehabilitation programs. Simultaneously, we should manage technical impediments and ethical aspects, as well as equitable deployment in a careful manner, to gain the maximum benefits without compromising on safety, privacy and inclusivity. On balance, the fusion of VR, AR and AI is one of the steps in the transformation of personalized, data-oriented and immersive cognitive rehabilitation. Continued research, technology and clinical trials will help convert these tools from experiments to standard neurorehabilitation. This provides optimism on the improved results of innumerable patients.

13.12. References

Al-Rajab, M., Lu, J., Amawi, S., Elmehalawy, N., Babillie, B., Alasmi, Y., Ibrahim, H.S., Ellahham, S., Sawsaa, A., Al Zraiqat, S. (2025). A smart secure virtual reality immersive application for Alzheimer's and dementia patients. *Scientific Reports*, 15(1), 30584.

Alshami, A., Nashwan, A., AlDardour, A., Qusini, A. (2025). Artificial intelligence in rehabilitation: A narrative review on advancing patient care. *Rehabilitación*, 59(2), 100911.

Banikova, S., Najsrova, A., Szegedi, I., Vitová, K., Fiedorova, I., Trda, J., Volny, O. (2025). Patient satisfaction and tolerance of virtual reality rehabilitation in subacute ischemic stroke: A pilot study. *Frontiers in Rehabilitation Sciences*, 6, 1660766.

Corrigan, B., Ito, K., Rogers, J., Polhamus, D., Stephenson, D., Romero, K. (2014). Clinical trial simulation in Alzheimer's disease. In *Applied Pharmacometrics,* Schmidt, S. and Derendorf, H. (eds). Springer, New York, 451–476.

Ding, K., Ma, Y., Zhang, L., Gu, Y., Pan, H., Gu, Z.E., Zhang, H. (2025). Patient-centered insights into virtual reality rehabilitation for stroke: A systematic review and qualitative meta-synthesis. *Journal of Neuroengineering and Rehabilitation*, 22(1), 124.

Geerts, H. and Spiros, A. (2020). Simulating the effects of common comedications and genotypes on Alzheimer's cognitive trajectory using a quantitative systems pharmacology approach. *Journal of Alzheimer's Disease*, 78(1), 413–424.

Georgiev, D.D., Georgieva, I., Gong, Z., Nanjappan, V., Georgiev, G.V. (2021). Virtual reality for neurorehabilitation and cognitive enhancement. *Brain Sciences*, 11(2), 221.

Hao, J., Crum, G., Siu, K.C. (2024). Effects of virtual reality on stroke rehabilitation: An umbrella review of systematic reviews. *Health Science Reports*, 7(9), e70082.

Jiao, D. (2025). AI-enhanced digital therapeutics for cognitive impairment: Integrating mobile applications, virtual reality, and wearable devices. *Discover Artificial Intelligence*, 5(1), 69.

Maggio, M.G., Maione, R., Cotelli, M., Bonasera, P., Corallo, F., Pistorino, G., Luca, A., Marra, A., Quartarone, A., Nicoletti, A. et al. (2025). Cognitive rehabilitation using virtual reality in subjective cognitive decline and mild cognitive impairment: A systematic review. *Frontiers in Psychology*, 16, 1641693.

Makmee, P. and Wongupparaj, P. (2025). VR cognitive-based intervention for enhancing cognitive functions and well-being in older adults with mild cognitive impairment: Behavioral and EEG evidence. *Psychosocial Intervention*, 34(1), 37–51.

MindMaze (n.d.). MindMotion: Neurorehabilitation across the continuum of care [Online]. Available from: https://mindmaze.com/digital-therapies-for-neurorehabilitation/.

Naqvi, W.M., Naqvi, I.W., Mishra, G.V., Vardhan, V.D. (2024). The future of telerehabilitation: Embracing virtual reality and augmented reality innovations. *Pan African Medical Journal*, 47(1), 157.

Navarro-Ramos, C.D., Murataya-Gutiérrez, J., Acosta-Quiroz, C.O., García-Flores, R., Echeverría-Castro, S.B. (2025). Effects of cognitive training with virtual reality in older adults: A systematic review. *Brain Sciences*, 15(9), 910.

Piszcz, A., Rojek, I., Mikołajewski, D. (2024). Impact of virtual reality on brain–computer interface performance in IoT control: Review of current state of knowledge. *Applied Sciences*, 14(22), 10541.

Rabin, L.A., Smart, C.M., Crane, P.K., Amariglio, R.E., Berman, L.M., Boada, M., Buckley, R.F., Chételat, G., Dubois, B., Ellis, K.A. et al. (2015). Subjective cognitive decline in older adults: An overview of self-report measures used across 19 international research studies. *Journal of Alzheimer's Disease*, 48(s1), S63–S86.

Rajkumar, M. (2025). Transformative learning. In *AI Applications and Pedagogical Innovation*, Wang, V. (ed.). IGI Global Scientific Publishing, Hershey, PA.

Sarkar, S. and Alqasemi, R. (2025). Neural interfaces for robotics and prosthetics: Current trends. *Journal of Sensor and Actuator Networks*, 14(6), 105.

Wen, D., Fan, Y., Hsu, S.H., Xu, J., Zhou, Y., Tao, J., Lan, X., Li, F. (2021). Combining brain–computer interface and virtual reality for rehabilitation in neurological diseases: A narrative review. *Annals of Physical and Rehabilitation Medicine*, 64(1), 101404.

Wong, W.W., Wong, G.H., Choy, J.C., Pui Li, D.S., Lo, Y.L. (2025). Utilization of immersive virtual reality in cognitive stimulation therapy (IVR-CST) for elderly with mild cognitive impairment: A randomized controlled pilot study protocol. *PLoS One*, 20(8), e0330686.

Xie, X., Shi, R., Yu, H., Wan, X., Liu, T., Duan, D., Li, D., Wen, D. (2024). Executive function rehabilitation and evaluation based on brain–computer interface and virtual reality: Our opinion. *Frontiers in Neuroscience*, 18, 1377097.

Zhang, J., Liu, M., Yue, J., Yang, J., Xiao, Y., Yang, J., Cai, E. (2025). Effects of virtual reality with different modalities on upper limb recovery: A systematic review and network meta-analysis on optimizing stroke rehabilitation. *Frontiers in Neurology*, 16, 1544135.

Zhichao, Z. and Yu, L. (2025). AI and stroke rehabilitation: The past, present and future. *Regenesis Repair Rehabilitation*, 1(4), 6–11.

Zhu, Y., Wang, C., Li, J., Zeng, L., Zhang, P. (2023). Effect of different modalities of artificial intelligence rehabilitation techniques on patients with upper limb dysfunction after stroke: A network meta-analysis of randomized controlled trials. *Frontiers in Neurology*, 14, 1125172.

Ziyi, L. (2018). Development of a high-sensitivity method for the measurement of human nasal $A\beta_{42}$, tau, and phosphorylated tau. Thesis, Shiga University of Medical Science.

14

AI-Driven Drug Discovery Pipelines for Neurological and Mental Health Therapies

Neurological and mental illnesses are some of the most pressing health concerns worldwide, and their increasing number, limited number of treatment options and socioeconomic burden are rapidly increasing. The classic pipelines of drug-making to treat these diseases have been very tedious, costly and prone to high chances of failure, given that it may take more than a decade and cost billions of dollars before a single drug sees the light of the day. The recent innovations in artificial intelligence (AI) are altering the sphere, with the implementation of computational speed, improved prediction and data-driven insights at all stages of drug discovery. Machine learning, deep learning, and natural language processing are among the AI approaches used to analyze biomedical literature, predict molecular interactions, and design novel compounds targeting complex brain processes. Additionally, the integration of multi-omics data with neuroimaging and electronic health records enables more comprehensive and precise modeling. Reproductive AI models and reinforcement learning assist in making more absorbent, distributive, metabolic, excreted and safe drug-like molecules. AI provides effective representation of phenotypic screening, drug repurposing and customization of therapy plans in mental health care. Nonetheless, barriers to usage like variability in the data, inability to interpret it, and ethical and regulatory barriers continue to restrict widespread implementation. This chapter provides a comprehensive background on the findings of AI in neurological and psychiatric drug discovery, along with concepts, technologies, case studies, limitations and opinions. Finally, the advancement of AI can result in accelerated drug development, reduced clinical failure rates and more tailored therapy for complicated brain disorders.

14.1. Introduction

One of the largest health issues on a global scale is neurological and mental health disorders. Alzheimer's disease, Parkinson's disease, epilepsy, depression, schizophrenia and bipolar disease are significant burdens causing reduced quality of

Chapter written by Sharad KSHIRSAGAR and Ashish N. PATIL.

life and a lot of disability-adjusted life years (DALYs) across the world (Carroll 2019). Decades later, there is still a very low success rate in drug development for diseases of the central nervous system (CNS). CNS drug discovery has a higher rate of failure, longer development period and is more expensive than other areas of medicine (DiMasi et al. 2016).

The classic drug deployment process is a linear process, whereby the target is discovered, the hit is discovered, the lead is optimized, preclinical studies are conducted and clinical trials are undertaken. Every step consumes numerous resources and may even come to a stop. The complexity of the brain and variability in patients complicate the translation of the brain in neurological and psychiatric research (Paul et al. 2010). Alzheimer's trials have had numerous promising pre-clinical trials fail in the late stages and psychiatric trials usually fail to proceed as there are many symptoms and responses that are not similar among patients.

A transformative factor is artificial intelligence (AI), which has the potential to alter this route. Machine learning (ML), deep learning (DL), reinforcement learning and generative models allow AI to provide speed, predictability and efficiency to drug development processes (Vamathevan et al. 2019). In contrast to other types of bioinformatics applications, AI can combine large diverse data sets, including genomics, proteomics, neuroimaging and electronic health records (EHRs), in order to identify patterns that would otherwise be neglected by standard statistics.

AI provides particular advantages in the neurological and mental health treatment process. It is also useful in finding new molecular drug targets using integrated biomarker analytics, synthesizing drug-like molecules using generative algorithms, accelerating virtual screening and drug repurposing, and enabling precision psychiatry in personalized treatment of patients. Another area where AI is applied is the simulation of drug–brain interaction, side effect prediction, and refinement of the choice of candidates prior to costly clinical tests.

Nevertheless, AI application in this field is problematic. The heterogeneity in data, low interpretability of the model and regulatory challenges impede general use (Chen et al. 2018). The presence of ethical concerns such as algorithmic bias, patient privacy and accountability also makes the use of AI more problematic in sensitive specialist fields (neurology and psychiatry).

This chapter will provide an in-depth overview of AI-powered drug-discovery pipelines of neurological and mental health treatments. It also provides the fundamental principles of AI in drug development, applications at all pipeline phases, case studies and success stories, limitations and future directions. This chapter indicates that AI has the potential to transform the manner in which therapies for some of the most complicated brain-related ailments are conceived, validated and delivered by using current evidence and new technologies.

14.2. Principles of AI in drug discovery

The use of AI in drug discovery has emerged as a fundamental part of contemporary drug discovery and how scientists tackle the complexities of biology, projecting molecular interactions and building new molecules. In contrast to traditional methods of computation, AI systems are trained on large datasets and do not reach independence in their performance at once, and thus they are able to discover relationships that are unnoticed by humans (Jumper et al. 2021). The underlying principles of the applications of AI in drug discovery can be classified into various major paradigms: ML, DL, natural language processing (NLP), generative modeling and reinforcement learning.

14.2.1. *Predictive modeling via ML*

ML is the use of algorithms to enhance performance, based on learning (data) instead of a priori factors. ML models are a common technology applied in drug discovery to predict compound bioactivity, pharmacokinetics and toxicity profiles. The techniques of supervised learning are trained using known ligand-target binding affinities to predict the activity of new molecules. Unsupervised learning, on the contrary, works by clustering unmarked data to demonstrate latent or concealed atypical patterns, and this can be especially applicable in determining subtypes of neurological disorders that may react differently to treatment (Ching et al. 2018). Random forests and gradient boosting are examples of ensemble approaches, which additionally contribute to predictive accuracy by making use of a number of models.

14.2.2. *DL and neural networks*

DL, a subdivision of ML, is based on multilayered neural networks that approximate hierarchical representations of data. DL has transformed the discovery of drugs due to the ability to handle high-dimensional and multimodal data. As an example, convolutional neural networks (CNNs) are better at analyzing neuroimaging, whereas recurrent neural networks (RNNs) are better applied to sequential data, such as health records. Graph neural networks (GNNs) have more recently become effective in drug discovery, using the chemistry of molecular representations as a graph, with atoms as nodes and bonding between atoms as edges. By doing so, molecular properties and binding affinities can be predicted accurately, which is important in the creation of drugs targeting the neurological pathways (Tian et al. 2025).

14.2.3. *NLP as a knowledge extraction*

Frequently, the discovery of drugs involves the search for large masses of biomedical literature, patents and clinical trial data. NLP allows AI to automatically learn valuable information about unstructured text, determine possible drug–disease relationships and propose repurposing ideas (Ghosh et al. 2011). As an example, NLP can be applied to mental health studies to find patterns of drug reaction among groups of people, namely EHRs and clinical notes. This has been greatly improved by the use of transformer-based models like BERT and GPT to facilitate contextual interpretation of complex biomedical language.

14.3. AI in target identification and biomarker discovery

The initial step in drug development is target identification and biomarker discovery. They establish the biological pathways and mechanisms that the therapies will be targeting. This is particularly difficult in cases of neurology and mental problems, as the brain is very complicated and scientists are unaware of the disease processes. Due to this uncertainty, it is challenging to select trustworthy targets. Also, a great number of varying symptoms are demonstrated by patients, further complicating the search for valid biomarkers (Vieira et al. 2017). AI could be of use. Through a large number of data sources, AI is able to identify hidden patterns and rank the possible targets and biomarkers in a systematic manner.

14.3.1. *Multi-omics integration to discover novel targets*

Alzheimer's, Parkinson's, and multiple sclerosis are examples of neurological diseases that have numerous interacting molecules in genomics, transcriptomics, proteomics and metabolomics. Single-omics research can only provide a few details. When AI techniques are used to combine these data layers, we are provided with the entire picture of the illness. Support-vector machines and random forests are ML algorithms that have been used to identify genes and pathways that monitor disease progression. Interaction maps can be drawn to new therapeutic targets using deep learning models, and particularly, GNNs (Dwyer et al. 2018).

In the case of psychiatric disorders such as depression and schizophrenia, the hereditability is very strong and the underlying mechanisms are not clearly understood. Transcriptomic AI, which connects genome-wide association studies

(GWASs) to AI, has identified novel pathways. Such discoveries aid in the identification of druggable proteins and the subdivision of patients into biologically unique groups, a direction towards precision psychiatry.

14.3.2. *Biomarkers of neuroimaging and AI*

Brain disorders can only be studied through neuroimaging. Magnetic resonance imaging (MRI), functional magnetic resonance imaging (fMRI), positron emission tomography (PET) and electroencephalography (EEG) generate massive datasets exhibiting structural and functional issues. Deep neural networks have performed quite well when analyzing these high-dimensional images. Seeing the tiny details that are associated with disease development or progression, AI can identify biomarkers in imaging that can be used in diagnosis and treatment.

Indicatively, AI applications developed on the basis of MRI can identify, with certainty and many years in advance, that an individual with a mild impaired cognitive disorder will develop Alzheimer's. However, resting-state fMRI ML of major depressive disorder has identified patterns in the brain networks that indicate whether the patients will react to therapy (Beam and Kohane 2018). These findings exemplify the role imaging biomarkers play in influencing drug development and also the selection of patients for clinical trials.

14.3.3. *EHR and phenotypic data*

Another resource that can be rich but is usually untapped when finding targets and biomarkers is EHRs. NLP has the potential to extract useful information from clinical notes, patient history and diagnostic records. AI processing of EHR data can also show drug exposure, clinical outcomes and disease pathways, which facilitate biomarker selection (Rifaioglu et al. 2019). Among psychiatric diseases with limited objective biological characteristics, EHR mining has demonstrated novel relationships between lifestyle and comorbidity variables and treatment outcomes. These lessons indicate potential disease risk and disease progression biomarkers.

14.4. AI in hit discovery and lead optimization

The process of drug discovery requires hit discovery and lead optimization, which play significant roles in drug discovery that help to identify potential molecules, optimize them and validate their therapeutic development. These steps are especially difficult in the neurological and psychiatric case of drug discovery, as they need to penetrate the blood–brain barrier (BBB), reduce off-target effects and maneuver neurochemical pathways that are usually quite complex (Bilbrey et al. 2021). These phases are changing with AI, making screening processes virtual, producing other compounds and refining the pharmacological properties with prediction modeling.

14.4.1. *Virtual screening and high-throughput prediction*

Conventional approaches of high-throughput screening (HTS) use experimental systems to test compound libraries for interest in activity against a specific target. Effective but costly, labor-intensive and constrained by the size of existing libraries, HTS is expensive. This process can be greatly improved by using AI-based virtual screening to support a computational assessment of millions of compounds in silico. Intense ML models based on available bioactivity data are capable of predicting binding affinities between ligands and targets (Merk et al. 2018). Deep-, graph- and interaction-based convolutional networks (GCNs) are the frameworks of DL representing molecules as regular graphs, allowing fine-scale prediction of binding interactions.

In the context of CNS drug discovery, lipophilicity and molecular weight can be used as constraints to ensure that AI-based virtual screening chooses compounds more likely to be BBB permeable. Such dual filtering, namely activity prediction and neuropharmacokinetic modeling, makes it faster to identify targets that have realistic therapeutic potential.

14.4.2. *Generative AI in de novo molecule design*

In addition to screening known molecules, AI can also create novel drug-like molecules that are specific to the neurological target. Variational autoencoders, generative adversarial networks and diffusion models are examples of generative models that can explore extensive chemical space and produce new molecular scaffolds that will have desirable characteristics. These molecules can also be further refined through reinforcement learning, thus they are considered selective, safe and BBB-penetrating through reward functions.

As a case in point, AI-based platforms have already suggested candidate molecules against conditions including Alzheimer's and amyotrophic lateral sclerosis (ALS), with structures that have anticipated nanomolar affinities and positive pharmacokinetics. This feature finds an application especially in psychiatric drug discovery, where the majority of the current drugs are based on repurposed drugs and not on rationally designed agents (Segler et al. 2018).

14.4.3. *Optimizing a lead using multi-parameter modeling*

After identification, the promising hits have to be optimized into leads of increased potency, selectivity and safety. The process sometimes takes a lot of medicinal chemistry and consists of cycles of synthesis and testing. Multi-parameter optimization (MPO) can be achieved with the help of AI when multiple models are being used to assess several drug-like properties at once (Pushpakom et al. 2019).

The key components of this stage are the predictive models of absorption, distribution, metabolism, excretion and toxicity (ADMET). In the case of neurotherapeutics, ADMET modeling will also need to include the parameters that are specific to CNS drugs, like passive diffusion across the BBB, efflux pump interactions and risks of toxicity that are specific to CNSs. The combination of these limitations allows AI to direct chemists towards structural modifications that enhance drug-like properties in general and CNS viability.

14.5. AI in drug repurposing for neurological and mental health disorders

Drug repurposing (also repositioning) is the approach to exploiting new therapeutic uses of known medications. It is particularly useful in neuroscience and psychiatric studies, in which the traditional drug development process is slow, expensive and hazardous. The fact that the repurposed drugs have known safety profiles allows them to be developed into trials faster (Himmelstein et al. 2017). This approach relies on AI because this method generates diverse data and can identify previously unknown drug–disease relationships and predict new benefits.

14.5.1. *Data-driven repurposing strategies*

AI can use extensive biomedical datasets, such as genomics, transcriptomics, proteomics, neuroimaging and clinical records to identify new capable opportunities of known compounds. ML models project drug-gene-disease networks, pointing out the candidates of complex diseases like Alzheimer's or schizophrenia. As an illustration, transcriptomic data can be clustered to indicate drug-reversing disease-mimicking gene signatures (Brown and Patel 2017).

Phenotypic screening is another field where AI is applied to psychiatric studies, where drugs are tested both on cell cultures or on patient-made models. Compounds that induce desirable changes in phenotype by a mechanism that is not well understood are detected using algorithms. This is most applicable for mental health conditions whose biology is yet to be discovered.

14.5.2. *Literature mining NLP*

The amount of biomedical literature and clinical trial data is overwhelming, making it challenging to identify promising lines of evidence without a need to sift through it. NLP is an AI technology that allows unstructured text such as research articles, patents, trial reports and others to be analyzed to yield structured knowledge, through mapping co-occurrences of drugs, diseases and targets. Many therapeutic opportunities that were overlooked in previous studies have been revealed by NLP tools, including the unexpected interactions between anti-inflammatory agents and enhanced cognition and thus interest in repurposing these compounds in neurodegenerative disease arises (Morselli Gysi et al. 2021). Likewise, when considering psychiatric case reports, NLP has also demonstrated mood-stabilizing effects on drugs that were not specifically designed to be used psychiatrically.

14.5.3. *Actual data and EHRs*

Repurposing has copious real-world evidence available in EHRs and pharmacovigilance databases. The utilization of AI models on EHRs may identify the trends of off-label prescribing that relate to improved outcomes in neurological and psychiatric patients. As an example, it can be observed that patients who are treated with some antihypertensives have been observed to have fewer cases of dementia, and this can indicate new treatment paths. The use of AI in detecting adverse events in signal processing can also identify drug-based unintended positive outcomes (Zarin et al. 2019). In psychiatry, where the empirical reactions hold significance, EHR mining contributes to the sorting of patients who would probably have a positive impact on repurposed medication.

14.6. AI in preclinical and clinical trial design for neurological and mental health therapies

It is particularly hard to develop drugs treating neurological and psychiatric disease. Clinical trials fail more often than not, disease mechanisms are complex and patients are highly heterogeneous. These challenges cannot be well captured in traditional trial designs. They are ineffective and costly. AI is an innovative technique (Sudlow et al. 2015). It will be able to reconsider preclinical and clinical approaches, enhance patient selection, optimize endpoints, make predictions and become more efficient.

14.6.1. *AI in preclinical research*

The preclinical phases normally depend on animal models and in vivo systems. Such models are not always able to replicate human illness. AI assists in closing the gap by combining the preclinical data with human-derived data. Indicatively, the use of DL in induced pluripotent stem cell (iPSC) models to induce neurodegeneration can be more effective in translational efficacy prediction. Neuropathology analysis of animal models is also better evaluated by AI-driven image analysis, which increases the reliability of the preclinical experiments (Rodrigues 2017).

One more important area is silico modeling. AI is used to simulate drug–target and drug–disease interactions prior to the expensive wet-lab studies. This minimizes the use of less predictive studies in animals and puts emphasis on compelling compounds to be tested.

14.6.2. *Patient stratification in clinical trials*

The heterogeneity of patients is one of the greatest reasons why trials fail in psychiatry and neurology. The AI-based stratification involves using genomic, neuroimaging and clinical data to place patients into subgroups that have a higher chance of responding to the treatment (Coravos et al. 2019). For instance, MRI scans can be used to identify the neuroanatomical subtypes of depression using the clustering algorithms that thus tend to respond to antidepressants differently.

In the trials for Alzheimer's, ML picks potential patients who have developed dementia during the study. This increases the sample size and trial power. AI produces more accurate results by diversifying cohorts with accelerating progressors to increase the variability and the probability of finding treatment effects.

14.6.3. *Endpoints and biomarkers optimization*

Conventional clinical outcomes, such as psychiatric scale or cognitive test scores, are usually subjective and changeable. AI identifies wearable sensors, smartphones and speech patterns, which are considered digital biomarkers. These are more sensitive and continuous measures of response. An example is NLP, which monitors minor speech variations, which are indicators of early psychosis or cognitive impairment.

Surrogate endpoint validation is also enhanced by ML. As a result of longitudinal data analysis, AI determines changes in which biomarkers, including amyloid PET signal, EEG signatures, metabolic markers, etc., are predictive of long-term outcomes. This enables shorter and more efficient trials (Tjoa and Guan 2020).

14.6.4. *Predictive modeling of good trial results*

Predictive analytics based on AI allows sponsors to have trial simulations and then implement them. AI identifies designs that can be used to achieve maximum success by simulating different recruitment strategies, dosing regimens and endpoints. Reinforcement learning models are capable of learning protocols as new data is known in real-time, and it is an increasing practice in adaptive clinical trials. In mental trials with elevated placebo effects, AI simulates the placebo reaction curve and modifies the examination strategies. This reduces the chances of false negatives due to the variability of placebos (U.S. Food and Drug Administration 2021). Table 14.1 shows the applications of artificial intelligence across the drug discovery pipeline for neurological and mental health therapies.

14.7. Ethical, regulatory, and societal implications of AI in neurological and psychiatric drug discovery

14.7.1. *Ethical considerations*

Data privacy is one of the largest ethical issues in AI-based discoveries. Neurological and psychiatric studies are increasingly turning to sensitive neuroimaging, genetic profiles and EHRs as a source of information. The use or violation of this information without the consent of the patient may result in a lack of confidentiality and heighten the stigma of mental illness (Floridi et al. 2021). To reduce such risks, AI systems should hence use privacy-preserving tricks, such as federated learning and differential privacy.

The other ethical concern is bias in AI models. When the training data does not represent all demographics worldwide, it is possible that alternative populations will not be predicted as accurately, thus increasing or deepening healthcare disparities that already exist. For example, the neuroimaging datasets, for the most part, predominantly include western participants, which may give AI models false classifications or cause crucial features to be missed that are of importance to non-western governments. To deal with this issue, we will have to make a conscious effort to diversify training data and use fairness-conscious algorithms.

Stage of drug discovery	AI techniques used	Applications/outcomes	Examples in neurological and mental health disorders
Target identification and biomarker discovery	Machine learning, deep learning, graph neural networks	Integration of multi-omics data; identification of disease-related genes and pathways; neuroimaging biomarker analysis	AI models predicting Alzheimer's progression using MRI and fMRI data; GWAS-linked transcriptomics in schizophrenia
Hit discovery and lead optimization	Virtual screening, generative AI, reinforcement learning	In silico prediction of ligand–target binding affinities; de novo molecule generation; ADMET property optimization	Graph convolutional networks generating CNS-penetrant drug candidates; AI-driven screening for anti-Parkinson agents
Drug repurposing	Natural language processing (NLP), knowledge graphs, machine learning	Literature mining for hidden drug–disease links; analysis of EHR data for off-label effects	NLP-identifying antidepressant potential of anti-inflammatory drugs; EHR-based dementia risk reduction from antihypertensives
Preclinical research	Deep learning, image recognition, predictive modeling	In silico modeling of drug–target interaction; automated analysis of animal model pathology	AI analysis of iPSC-derived neuronal degeneration; preclinical toxicity prediction for ALS drugs
Clinical trial design and optimization	Reinforcement learning, clustering algorithms, digital biomarkers	Patient stratification; adaptive trial simulations; endpoint optimization	AI-based clustering for depression subtypes; speech and motion analysis for early psychosis detection
Ethical and regulatory oversight	Explainable AI (XAI), federated learning, differential privacy	Model transparency, data protection, bias mitigation	Use of privacy-preserving algorithms for psychiatric data; fairness-based validation frameworks

Table 14.1. *Applications of artificial intelligence across the drug discovery pipeline for neurological and mental health therapies*

14.7.2. *Regulatory challenges*

Regulatory bodies around the globe are grappling with the process of assessing and regulating AI-based tools in drug discovery and clinical trials. One of the major issues is that there are no standardized validation models for AI models. As opposed to standard biomarkers, or statistical approaches, AI algorithms may develop and adapt dynamically according to the newer information, a feature that makes them more difficult to approve, as most traditional methods rely on unchanging validation.

Other organizations, including the United States Food and Drug Administration (FDA) and the European Medicines Agency (EMA), have begun to publish guidelines concerning digital health and AI-based medical technologies. Nonetheless, there are not yet clear avenues for AI in drug discovery. There are still questions regarding the measurement of the concept of algorithmic transparency, reproducibility and interpretability (Niazi 2025). The most concerned regulators are the ones where AI output is involved in high-stakes decisions, for example, including patients in the trial or given drug candidates a priority.

14.7.3. *Societal implications*

Regulatory and technical issues are not the only problems that have a social implication on AI in the discovery of neurological and psychiatric drugs. The trust that people place in AI applications is a key factor, particularly in the field of psychiatry, since patients may not have much trust in medical facilities. To create acceptance, it is crucial to clearly communicate that AI supplements and does not diminish the knowledge and experience possessed by humans.

Another issue is equal access. Changes in AI technologies and AI-enabled drug pipelines are known to be concentrated in per capita-intensive pharmaceutical enterprises and academic firms, making potential so-called therapeutic solutions inaccessible to low-resource locations (Stokes et al. 2020). Therapeutic AI innovations need to be applied to patient groups that are diverse and, therefore, policymakers have to examine mechanisms that may be used to achieve this goal, including open-access data sharing and the existence of partnership between the government and the commercial sector.

14.7.4. *Pathways forward*

A number of measures are gradually arising to solve these dilemmas. To begin with, explainable AI (XAI) methods seek to more readily interpret the outputs of algorithms so that clinicians and regulators can comprehend the predictions they are based on. Second, collaborative models of governance, uniting regulators, industry and patient advocacy organizations are also being designed in order to develop collective standards of AI validation (Schneider 2018). Third, incorporating ethics-by-design moral ideas into AI creation may prove to be a way of making sure that privacy, fairness and accountability are not introduced as an afterthought but instead as a key aspect of AI creation.

14.8. Future directions and emerging trends in AI-driven drug discovery for neurological and mental health therapies

14.8.1. *Integration of multi-modal data*

Future AI pipelines will increasingly integrate multi-modal datasets, combining genomics, transcriptomics, proteomics, metabolomics, neuroimaging, EHRs and digital phenotyping data. Multi-modal integration allows models to capture complex relationships between molecular, cellular, structural and behavioral levels of brain function, enabling more accurate identification of therapeutic targets and patient subgroups (Tian et al. 2025). For example, integrating genetic risk scores with longitudinal neuroimaging and wearable sensor data may facilitate highly personalized interventions in psychiatric disorders.

14.8.2. *Generative AI and automated molecular design*

Generative AI is likely to play an even more central role in future drug design. Advances in diffusion models, transformer-based architectures and reinforcement learning will enable the generation of molecules with increasingly complex and tailored properties. Coupled with automated synthesis platforms, these AI-generated compounds could be rapidly produced and screened, creating closed-loop discovery pipelines that significantly shorten development timelines (Brown and Patel 2017). Such platforms hold particular promise for neurotherapeutics, where balancing blood–brain barrier permeability, receptor selectivity and safety are critical.

14.8.3. *Digital biomarkers and remote monitoring*

The adoption of digital biomarkers is expected to expand, leveraging smartphones, wearables and passive environmental sensors. Continuous monitoring of sleep patterns, cognitive function, mood and behavior provides high-resolution phenotypic data, which AI models can analyze to predict disease progression, assess drug efficacy and optimize dosing regimens. This trend will enable more agile, real-world-informed clinical trials, reducing reliance on intermittent in-clinic assessments and enhancing patient-centric care (Paul et al. 2010).

14.8.4. *Personalized and adaptive therapeutics*

AI-driven personalization of therapy is likely to become the norm. ML models that predict individual drug response, adverse event susceptibility and optimal dosing strategies will guide precision interventions in neurological and psychiatric disorders. Furthermore, adaptive clinical trial designs, powered by AI simulations and real-time data analysis, will allow dynamic modification of study parameters based on interim outcomes, enhancing efficiency and reducing failure rates.

14.9. Conclusion

AI stands out as a potential game changer in the discovery of drugs used in neurological and mental treatments to address the issues of complexity, heterogeneity and the high attrition rates that have challenged the disease over time. ML combined with DL, generative modeling and NLP is useful because, in this way, AI provides the complete workflow, including the identification of targets, the discovery of biomarkers, the creation of hits, the optimization of leads, drug repurposing and the design of clinical trials. The technologies enhance the predictive accuracy, speed of decision-making and, in prospect, the ability for more personalized interventions, applicable to Alzheimer's, Parkinson's, depression and schizophrenia. AI is particularly useful in neurological and psychiatric conditions, where traditional approaches can easily be complicated with biological, structural and behavioral factors that are complex. Multimodal information (genomics and proteomics, neuroimaging and digital phenotyping) can be incorporated into the system to target new therapeutic targets, as well as specific patient subpopulations that were previously inaccessible. In addition, AI-based repurposing (with predictive models) is capable of reducing the durations and expenses of development, whereas the adaptive clinical trial design can increase the likelihood of success. However, there are obstacles to the implementation of AI, such as the heterogeneity of data, its interpretability, ethical issues and lack of regulatory certainty. It will require the cooperation of researchers, clinicians, regulators and patients, as well as the implementation of understandable, explicable and fair AI endeavors to overcome these concerns.

14.10. References

Beam, A.L. and Kohane, I.S. (2018). Big data and machine learning in health care. *JAMA*, 319(13), 1317–1318.

Bilbrey, J., Ward, L., Choudhury, S., Kumar, N., Sivaraman, G. (2021). Evening the SCORE: Targeting SARS-CoV-2 protease inhibition in graph generative models for therapeutic candidates. arXiv preprint, arXiv:2105.10489, 7 May.

Brown, A.S. and Patel, C.J. (2017). A standard database for drug repositioning. *Scientific Data*, 4(1), 1–7.

Carroll, W.M. (2019). The global burden of neurological disorders. *The Lancet Neurology*, 18(5), 418–419.

Chen, H., Engkvist, O., Wang, Y., Olivecrona, M., Blaschke, T. (2018). The rise of deep learning in drug discovery. *Drug Discovery Today*, 23(6), 1241–1250.

Ching, T., Himmelstein, D.S., Beaulieu-Jones, B.K., Kalinin, A.A., Do, B.T., Way, G.P., Ferrero, E., Agapow, P.M., Zietz, M., Hoffman, M.M. et al. (2018). Opportunities and obstacles for deep learning in biology and medicine. *Journal of the Royal Society Interface*, 15(141), 20170387.

Coravos, A., Khozin, S., Mandl, K.D. (2019). Developing and adopting safe and effective digital biomarkers to improve patient outcomes. *NPJ Digital Medicine*, 2(1), 14.

DiMasi, J.A., Grabowski, H.G., Hansen, R.W. (2016). Innovation in the pharmaceutical industry: New estimates of R&D costs. *Journal of Health Economics*, 47, 20–33.

Dwyer, D.B., Falkai, P., Koutsouleris, N. (2018). Machine learning approaches for clinical psychology and psychiatry. *Annual Review of Clinical Psychology*, 14, 91–118.

Floridi, L., Cowls, J., King, T.C., Taddeo, M. (2021). How to design AI for social good: Seven essential factors. In *Ethics, Governance, and Policies in Artificial Intelligence*, Floridi, L. (ed.). Springer, Cham, 125–151.

Ghosh, S., Matsuoka, Y., Asai, Y., Hsin, K.Y., Kitano, H. (2011). Software for systems biology: From tools to integrated platforms. *Nature Reviews Genetics*, 12(12), 821–832.

Himmelstein, D.S., Lizee, A., Hessler, C., Brueggeman, L., Chen, S.L., Hadley, D., Green, A., Khankhanian, P., Baranzini, S.E. (2017). Systematic integration of biomedical knowledge prioritizes drugs for repurposing. *eLife*, 6, e26726.

Jumper, J., Evans, R., Pritzel, A., Green, T., Figurnov, M., Ronneberger, O., Tunyasuvunakool, K., Bates, R., Žídek, A., Potapenko, A. et al. (2021). Highly accurate protein structure prediction with AlphaFold. *Nature*, 596(7873), 583–589.

Merk, D., Friedrich, L., Grisoni, F., Schneider, G. (2018). De novo design of bioactive small molecules by artificial intelligence. *Molecular Informatics*, 37(1–2), 1700153.

Morselli Gysi, D., Do Valle, Í., Zitnik, M., Ameli, A., Gan, X., Varol, O., Ghiassian, S.D., Patten, J.J., Davey, R.A., Loscalzo, J. et al. (2021). Network medicine framework for identifying drug-repurposing opportunities for COVID-19. *Proceedings of the National Academy of Sciences*, 118(19), e2025581118.

Niazi, S.K. (2025). Artificial intelligence in small-molecule drug discovery: A critical review of methods, applications, and real-world outcomes. *Pharmaceuticals*, 18(9), 1271.

Paul, S.M., Mytelka, D.S., Dunwiddie, C.T., Persinger, C.C., Munos, B.H., Lindborg, S.R., Schacht, A.L. (2010). How to improve R&D productivity: The pharmaceutical industry's grand challenge. *Nature Reviews Drug Discovery*, 9(3), 203–214.

Pushpakom, S., Iorio, F., Eyers, P.A., Escott, K.J., Hopper, S., Wells, A., Doig, A., Guilliams, T., Latimer, J., McNamee, C. et al. (2019). Drug repurposing: Progress, challenges and recommendations. *Nature Reviews Drug Discovery*, 18(1), 41–58.

Rifaioglu, A.S., Atas, H., Martin, M.J., Cetin-Atalay, R., Atalay, V., Doğan, T. (2019). Recent applications of deep learning and machine intelligence on in silico drug discovery: Methods, tools and databases. *Briefings in Bioinformatics*, 20(5), 1878–1912.

Rodrigues, T.C. (2017). A socio-technical multicriteria approach for the construction of indices in the presence of value interactions among indicators: Application to population health in Portugal. PhD Thesis, Universidade de Lisboa, Lisbon.

Schneider, G. (2018). Automating drug discovery. *Nature Reviews Drug Discovery*, 17(2), 97–113.

Segler, M.H., Kogej, T., Tyrchan, C., Waller, M.P. (2018). Generating focused molecule libraries for drug discovery with recurrent neural networks. *ACS Central Science*, 4(1), 120–131.

Stokes, J.M., Yang, K., Swanson, K., Jin, W., Cubillos-Ruiz, A., Donghia, N.M., MacNair, C.R., French, S., Carfrae, L.A., Bloom-Ackermann, Z. et al. (2020). A deep learning approach to antibiotic discovery. *Cell*, 180(4), 688–702.

Sudlow, C., Gallacher, J., Allen, N., Beral, V., Burton, P., Danesh, J., Downey, P., Elliott, P., Green, J., Landray, M. et al. (2015). UK biobank: An open access resource for identifying the causes of a wide range of complex diseases of middle and old age. *PLoS Medicine*, 12(3), e1001779.

Tian, C., Hao, Y., Fu, H., Shao, X., Cai, W. (2025). From AI-driven sequence generation to molecular simulation: A comprehensive framework for antimicrobial peptide discovery. *Journal of Chemical Information and Modeling*, 65(18), 9566–9575.

Tjoa, E. and Guan, C. (2020). A survey on explainable artificial intelligence (XAI): Toward medical XAI. *IEEE Transactions on Neural Networks and Learning Systems*, 32(11), 4793–4813.

U.S. Food and Drug Administration (2021). Artificial intelligence/machine learning (AI/ML)-based software as a medical device action plan. Report, FDA, Silver Spring, MD.

Vamathevan, J., Clark, D., Czodrowski, P., Dunham, I., Ferran, E., Lee, G., Li, B., Madabhushi, A., Shah, P., Spitzer, M. et al. (2019). Applications of machine learning in drug discovery and development. *Nature Reviews Drug Discovery*, 18(6), 463–477.

Vieira, S., Pinaya, W.H., Mechelli, A. (2017). Using deep learning to investigate the neuroimaging correlates of psychiatric and neurological disorders: Methods and applications. *Neuroscience & Biobehavioral Reviews*, 74, 58–75.

Zarin, D.A., Goodman, S.N., Kimmelman, J. (2019). Harms from uninformative clinical trials. *JAMA*, 322(9), 813–814.

15

Ethical, Legal and Societal Implications of AI in Neurology and Medicine

Artificial intelligence (AI) has established an influential force in neurology and medicine. It has spurred the progress of diagnosis, treatment planning and management of patients. Predictive analytics, machine-learning algorithms and natural language processing have become a part of clinical practice. These technologies provide superior medical results, increase operational efficiency, as well as personal care. However, there are grave ethical, legal and sociocultural issues with these advances. Some ethical issues in this area include patient privacy, bias in algorithms, transparency and accountability of clinical decisions. The legal problems are regarding liability, intellectual property and compliance with regulations. In society, these are the questions that we should ask ourselves: Is it fair to have access to AI? How will the labor market evolve? Do we trust the robots? And what will be the influence of AI on the relationship between patients and physicians? At the social level, there become issues regarding equal access to AI-facilitated care. A disruptive workforce is a visible problem. There has to be reliance on the automated systems. And the long-term impact of patient–physician relations is not known. AI finds application in neurology in the prediction of seizures, analysis of neuroimages and support of decision-making regarding neurodegenerative diseases. The issues are particularly acute since data about the nervous system are delicate, and the consequences of decisions made by the clinician are significant. This chapter looks at the moral, legal and social AI-related topics in neurology and medicine. It focuses on the potential and the threats. It compiles relevant literature, providing an overall picture of the AI changes in healthcare. This chapter also emphasizes the importance of powerful systems, which should balance responsibility and innovativeness. These issues need to be discussed so that AI can positively affect the care conditions of patients, promote medical ethics and contribute to the society.

Chapter written by Dipali JANKAR and Anil SAHU.

15.1. Introduction

AI has been a groundbreaking technology in the contemporary medical field, helping in promoting new clinical decision-making, patient diagnosis, managing treatments and patients. In the last 10 years, computing power, machine learning, deep learning and natural language processing have helped make AI systems analyze large and intricate datasets to produce actionable insights, which previously would have demanded different methods (Voigtlaender et al. 2024). This is necessary in neurology, where symptoms are subtle and often overlapping and therefore critical. AI has demonstrated itself in the neuroimaging field, predicting seizures, management of neurodegenerative conditions or diseases and rehabilitation to help clinicians in decision-making and bettering its outcomes (Ratti et al. 2025).

AI delivers much more personalized care, which has the ability to streamline treatments and predict disease progression. Algorithms are used in neurology to learn the early signs of Alzheimer's, Parkinson's, multiple sclerosis and epilepsy without any human eye contact by identifying patterns. Such predictive skills are important since it is possible to modify the course of disease and the quality of life when treated in a preliminary manner (Kundu and Bardhan 2025).

Nevertheless, the introduction of AI into the clinical practice is associated with ethical, legal and societal concerns. Ethically, there are concerns regarding autonomy of patients, informed consent, transparency, accountability and bias of algorithms. Training data can include many biases that can be reinforced by AI models and therefore result in disproportionate performance between populations. Also, most models are opaque, and on this basis, clinicians and patients fail to make informed consent, as it is difficult to know the logic underpinning predictions (Pham 2025).

Regulations are yet to keep up with technology, as far as laws are concerned. A problem of liability occurs in the case of AI misuse of patient's information. It is complicated to define who is responsible: developers, institutions or clinicians (Salles and Farisco 2024). The legal environment also becomes complicated with intellectual property (IP) rights on AI-generated diagnostics or biomarkers, which describes why clear harmonized rules are necessary.

Access to specialized care can be enhanced through AI with the use of telemedicine and remote monitoring, but differences in technology and digital literacy and affordability can increase existing disparities in society. There is also a risk of altered trust dynamics in the field of AI because patients will feel they are not managed by a human. The acceptance is conditional on transparency, explainability and safety, which are proven, which means that patient engagement and education should be emphasized.

The sphere of neurology is a high-stakes area. The neurological disorders may have a devastating impact on the brain and motor performance, and the wrong diagnosis may lead to irreversible damage. Neuroimaging, electrophysiology and genetics all hold sensitive information that raises the issue of privacy and security (Willem et al. 2024). Thus, it is important to be aware of the ethical, legal and social consequences of AI in the field of neurology and minimize the risks as well as make sure that AI brings more benefits than harm to patients.

This chapter provides a complete overview of the ethical, legal and social concerns regarding AI in neurology and medicine. It also tries to guide clinicians, researchers, policymakers and technology developers through challenges and potential opportunities. These points are crucial for responsible AI implementation, which would bring benefit and uphold the rights of patients, provide equity and keep the population trustful.

15.2. AI in neurology and medicine: an overview

AI will provide healthcare with one of the most important elements of innovation: in the industries that use imaging and electrophysiology in unconventional ways and in fields that avert longer patient data. The best example is in the field of neurology, where the accuracy of diagnosis and prompt treatment heavily affects patient outcome. In contrast to conventional techniques that primarily depend on human judgment, AI is able to analyze large and multimodal datasets, identify any subtle patterns and deliver real-time insights (Singh et al. 2025). AI applications in neurology and medicine have been used primarily in the fields of diagnostics, treatment and prognosis, research and drug discovery, as well as clinical workflow integration.

15.2.1. *AI in diagnostics*

Diagnosis in neurology should be accurately performed, since a lot of diseases such as epilepsy, multiple sclerosis and dementia possess comparable symptoms. AI has developed this area by analyzing neuroimaging and electrophysiology. Convolutional neural networks (CNNs) and other deep-learning models are reasonably accurate at detecting brain tumors, ischemic stroke lesions and the initial stages of neurodegeneration (Dankwa-Mullan 2024). An example is that AI used in magnetic resonance imaging (MRI) establishes the presence of structural abnormalities more than some radiologists, and this will assist in the timely identification of Alzheimer's and Parkinson's diseases (Saeidnia et al. 2024).

In epilepsy, AI algorithms, which are trained on the electroencephalography (EEG) data, can anticipate the seizures several minutes before they occur and provide patients and clinicians with an opportunity to prevent them in a timely manner (Chustecki 2024). Similarly, automatic image-analysis devices can now differentiate ischemic strokes and hemorrhagic strokes in emergency rooms and accelerate the decision-making processes by reducing the response that can be made within a relative treatment timeframe (Khan et al. 2025).

15.2.2. *AI in the treatment and prognosis*

In addition to diagnosis, AI helps individual treatment regimen and forecasts prognosis. Machine-learning algorithms are able to group patients based on their response to drugs, and this is able to reduce trial-and-error in the case of epilepsy and Parkinson's disease (Gómez-González et al. 2020). Predictive algorithms have been used in stroke care, to ascertain patients who can qualify under reperfusion treatments, including thrombolysis and thrombectomy, and deliver the correct treatment to them promptly (BenJaMins and Salazar García 2019).

AI is also useful in improving rehabilitation, especially among patients who have suffered a stroke or brain trauma. Smart sensors and AI applications used in conjunction with wearables monitor this progress and provide personalized exercise plans, which therapists can alter on a case-by-case basis (Lekadir et al. 2025). Such innovations will result in faster recoveries, and the strain on the healthcare systems will be diminished.

15.2.3. *AI in research and drug discovery*

AI accelerates the overall neurological research through identification of novel therapeutic targets as well as expediting the drug-development pipeline. AI models accelerate the time and cost of new drugs by modeling protein–ligand interactions (Mondal and Mondal 2024). Once applied to pathological issues (such as Alzheimer's), AI proposes numerous digital biomarkers that indicate minor cognitive and motor changes much earlier before they manifest themselves (Karimian et al. 2022).

Massive data assembly makes it possible to find genetic and molecular associations to neurological diseases. By integrating clinical records with genomic information, AI can pinpoint patient subgroups that could have a therapy that benefits them, therefore innovating precision medicine in neurology (Lund et al. 2025).

15.2.4. *Integration into clinical practice*

The success of AI in medicine depends not only on technological performance but also on its integration into existing clinical workflows. Many AI tools are designed as decision-support systems rather than replacements for clinicians, augmenting human expertise rather than supplanting it (Kawamleh 2023). For example, AI-enabled platforms can flag abnormal neuroimaging findings, allowing radiologists to prioritize urgent cases without removing their oversight role.

Telemedicine and mobile health applications are increasingly incorporating AI features to support remote monitoring of neurological patients. For instance, smartphone-based AI applications can assess gait abnormalities in Parkinson's patients or track speech changes in individuals with dementia, providing valuable longitudinal data to clinicians.

15.2.5. *Opportunities and risks*

There are still a lot of possibilities for AI in medicine and neurology. AI medicine is still in its early stages. The risks of its use are also starting to show. The quality of AI outputs is a product of the quality of the training data. Inaccurate outcomes could entail serious clinical risks due to biased and incomplete datasets (Kawamleh 2023). The trustworthiness of AI systems could also be undermined due to the "black box" phenomena, in which rationales for AI's decisions cannot be explained to the clinician or the patient. These risks must be addressed and are the focus of the following sections.

15.3. Ethical implications

AI application in neurology and medicine is fraught with numerous ethical issues. These obstacles are due to the fact that there is a dynamic between clinical care, patient rights and some new technology. In spite of the fact that AI holds great potential to enhance performance, it also entails the question of autonomy, consent, data use, algorithmic fairness and accountability (Li et al. 2022). These concerns need to be addressed to ensure AI does not disrupt the fundamental principles of medical ethics of beneficence, non-maleficence, autonomy and justice.

15.3.1. *Patient autonomy and informed consent*

Clinical practice must respect the autonomy of patients. Informed consent implies that patients should know what the treatment is and the benefits and risks of it. AI makes this difficult due to the fact that its decision-making process is frequently opaque and inscrutable to non-experts (Chandio et al. 2024). In the field of neurology, such as stroke treatment recommendations or certain stroke prognosis, AI can recommend treatments and patients will not easily understand how these recommendations are made. Such doubt in informed consent and the question of whether patients can make informed choices when they have access to black-box results are pertinent (Burger 2020).

This is done by developing explainable AI (XAI) models that provide the reasons behind their decisions in a clear language to enhance informed consent. Clinicians assist in closing the technical gap by making AI results applicable to an existing body of medical knowledge (Hirani et al. 2024).

15.3.2. *Data privacy and confidentiality*

Neurological information is one of the most vulnerable medical data. It is demonstrated through brain scans, EEGs and genetic data exposing the reasons for disease and also human cognition and behavior. The training of AI with this information increases the possibility of invasion and abuse (Kaufman 2024). Indicatively, in some cases, re-identification attacks have the potential of restoring identities of individual patients when the data presented is anonymized, therefore undermining confidentiality.

To use AI ethically, it is vital to meet such data-protection regulations as the General Data Protection Regulation (GDPR) in the European Union (EU) and the Health Insurance Portability and Accountability Act (HIPAA) in the USA. Secure storage, powerful encryption and constant identification of cybersecurity risks should also be developed in healthcare organizations to prevent unauthorized access (Upadhyay et al. 2023).

15.3.3. *Algorithmic bias and fairness*

The causes of AI bias are non-representative training data and poor models. In neurology, minority groups can have diagnosis or under-treatment problems, resulting in increased health inequalities (Nizamullah et al. 2024). As an illustration, when an AI model is primarily trained with Western data, it might obtain poor results on patients of a different region, giving victims unfair results.

It is necessary to reach fairness by having various, representative data, extensive validation of all demographic groups and audit biases frequently to identify and eliminate them. The need to provide fairness is both an ethical and a social requirement that safeguards vulnerable individuals and helps in sustaining justice during healthcare (Čartolovni et al. 2022).

15.3.4. *Transparency and explainability*

OpenAI systems are essential when it comes to clinical trust and ethical application. Neurological choices may have the strongest impact on patients, including the use of aggressive treatment or prognosis of diseases. Unless clinicians understand the way AI comes to its conclusion, they might be skeptical of using it – or even have a tendency of over relying on it without proper evaluation (Krook et al. 2025).

Explainable AI approaches attempt to address this issue by highlighting which features influenced predictions, such as brain regions in MRI scans or waveform patterns in EEGs.

15.3.5. *Accountability in ethical use*

There is also no clarity on who can be blamed when AI commits an error. As an example, who takes the blame when a brain tumor is misdiagnosed by an AI model? Is it the software developer, the hospital that implemented the technology, or is it the clinician who believed in the output of the technology? The vast majority of ethical innovations require collective responsibility and insist that AI is designed to assist and not substitute human judgment (Krook et al. 2025).

The designers also have a moral responsibility to come up with safe, long-lasting and bias-free systems. The clinicians have to interpret the AI recommendations in the entire clinical context. AI deployment requires sufficient supervision, education and regulation of the hospitals. AI integration into neurology and medicine can be ethical only with the help of shared responsibility.

15.4. Legal implications

The accelerating nature of the introduction of AI into the field of neurology and medicine has far outpaced the development of detailed legal frameworks. Although AI-powered systems are likely to be more accurate and efficient in clinical care, their implementation raises the important legal issue of liability, IP, regulating authorities and meeting the current standard. The absence of definite law standards will pose a threat to accountability and patient safety (Xu and Shuttleworth 2024).

15.4.1. *Liability and accountability for errors*

One of the most urgent legal issues is deciding on the liability in cases where AI systems aid in medical mistakes. Such an AI tool would have serious ramifications in neurology and miss diagnosing a stroke or possibly detecting damage in the early stages of dementia. It is also unclear whether the algorithm developer, the healthcare provider who used the tool or the institution that implemented the tool is liable (Karimian et al. 2022).

Other legal scholars would include a shared liability model, which would share the responsibility among the parties involved so that no single party would be considered too responsible. Other individuals suggest new types of legal liability, including the idea of the so-called algorithmic liability, to take care of the damage done by similar AI-based recommendations. Until a real law is put in place, clinicians are still left as the decision-makers and legal uncertainty prevails due to the ambiguity.

15.4.2. *IP rights*

AI systems are based on proprietary algorithms, edited datasets and calculation models. The idea of IP gains particular importance in the context of AI-related or assisted breakthrough in the field of diagnostics or the development of new treatment methods in neurology (Shabankareh et al. 2025). To take the example of an AI platform that finds a new biomarker of Parkinson's disease, should we not know who owns the discovery, the developer of the software, the healthcare institution or the researchers who collected the information?

Laws should balance national security in safeguarding commercial innovation with the similar requirement to ensure open accessibility of national information and tools to promote national health. Over-protective legislation of IP can become an obstacle to cooperation, and a lack of protection can decrease innovation incentives.

15.4.3. *Regulatory frameworks for AI in healthcare*

Regulatory oversight is essential for ensuring that AI tools in medicine meet standards of safety, efficacy and reliability. Agencies such as the US Food and Drug

Administration (FDA) and the European Medicines Agency (EMA) have begun to establish pathways for approving AI-based medical devices. However, most regulations were designed for static technologies, whereas AI systems evolve over time through continuous learning (Xu and Shuttleworth 2024).

15.4.4. *Compliance with medical and data standards*

The use of AI in the field of neurology is also subject to adherence to set medical rules on medical data protection. The healthcare entities implementing AI should aim at compliance with the provisions of such frameworks as the GDPR in Europe, the HIPAA in the United States or other laws in the countries with regulations of data concerning patients (Karimian et al. 2022). Lack of compliance might subject institutions to legal fines and loss of patient confidence.

15.5. Societal implications

Neurology and medicine are at the heart of the AI revolution. Its impacts extend way beyond treating patients. AI has many impacts regarding care access, the structure of the workforce, patient–physician relationship and the social approach to medical questions. Whereas AI has the potential to enhance care delivery and patient outcomes, it brings concerns of equity, mistrust and utilization of this technology. To be sure that AI can help all people and will not make current inequalities even worse, we need to cognize and resolve these social issues.

15.5.1. *Fairness and fairness to access AI-enhanced care*

AI has the potential to enhance health equity through the diagnostic and treatment assistance in underserved regions. One such area is AI-managed telemedicine, allowing low-resource or rural areas to get special neurological guidance at a distance, eliminating distance and lack of infrastructure. The distribution of resources, the prioritization of patients based on urgency and a reduction of wait times on urgent cases such as stroke or epilepsy are also improved with the aid of AI, since it is essential when it comes to time (Xu and Shuttleworth 2024).

Nevertheless, digital inequity may be constrained by inequality in the technological infrastructure, finances and digital skills. Expensive AI technology and the requirement to have fast Internet access or sophisticated imageries mainly serve urban and wealthy populations, excluding rural or poor populations. Also, AI algorithms primarily trained on the data of developed countries may be insufficiently effective on a population with different genetics, environment or socioeconomic status, which will reinforce health inequalities without purpose. Such issues can be resolved only with the help of conscious policies: subsidizing the purchase of AI in the low-resource regions, investing in digital infrastructure and creating AI models that are more representative of cultural and demographic diversity.

15.5.2. *Workforce transformation in medicine*

AI changes the roles and functions of healthcare workers. Simple and routine measures such as image analysis, record entry and initial diagnostics can be automated now, and this may decrease the workload of clinicians and enable their attention towards complex decision-making and interaction with patients.

In the field of neurology, AI is applied to allow radiologists to identify minor abnormalities on MRI images and to allow neurologists to track the progression of neurodegenerative conditions over time through streams of continuous data (Karimian et al. 2022).

Simultaneously, the transformation in the workforce can alter the characteristics of work and clinicians will need to acquire AI literacy and computational skills. Positions can change or be eliminated, and a new possibility of collaboration between clinicians, data scientists and engineers emerges. Continuing education and training programs are necessary to give healthcare professionals the knowledge and skills they require to operate well with the AI systems.

15.5.3. *Patient–physician relationship in the AI era*

The adoption of AI may fundamentally alter the patient–physician relationship. While AI can provide clinicians with precise, data-driven recommendations, there is a risk that patients may perceive a reduction in personalized care if human judgment appears secondary to algorithmic outputs. Trust, empathy and communication remain central to medical care, and AI integration must preserve these relational aspects (Shabankareh et al. 2025).

Dimension	Key issue	Description/example	Impact on neurology and medicine	Proposed mitigation strategies
Ethical	**Patient autonomy and informed consent**	AI decision-making opacity complicates patient understanding of treatment choices	Reduces patient participation in clinical decisions; weakens informed consent	Promote explainable AI (XAI); clinician mediation in decision-making
Ethical	**Data privacy and confidentiality**	Neurological data (EEG, MRI and genetic) highly sensitive and vulnerable to re-identification	Threatens trust and violates data protection norms	Apply GDPR/HIPAA compliance, encryption and data anonymization
Ethical	**Algorithmic bias and fairness**	Training data underrepresents minorities or certain demographics	Diagnostic inaccuracies and unequal treatment outcomes	Use diverse datasets; perform demographic audits and fairness testing
Ethical	**Transparency and explainability**	"Black-box" models hinder clinician understanding and accountability	Decreased clinical trust and misinterpretation risks	Use model interpretability tools and transparency reporting frameworks
Legal	**Liability and accountability**	Ambiguity about who is responsible for AI-driven errors	Legal uncertainty in malpractice or misdiagnosis cases	Develop shared or algorithmic liability frameworks
Legal	**Intellectual property (IP) rights**	Ownership ambiguity in AI-generated discoveries (e.g. new biomarkers)	Limits innovation sharing and hinders clinical translation	Define IP-sharing models between developers, clinicians and institutions
Legal	**Regulatory compliance**	Evolving legal oversight lags behind adaptive AI models	Challenges for approval, auditing and safety validation	Establish adaptive regulatory pathways and post-market surveillance

Societal	**Equitable access to AI care**	Rural or low-income populations lack access to AI tools	Reinforces healthcare disparities	Subsidize AI implementation; invest in digital infrastructure
Societal	**Workforce transformation**	Automation alters clinical roles and skill requirements	Clinicians may need AI literacy to maintain relevance	Continuous AI training and interdisciplinary education
Societal	**Patient–physician relationship**	Overreliance on AI may erode human empathy in care	Decreases patient trust and satisfaction	Implement hybrid human–AI decision-making frameworks

Table 15.1. *Ethical, legal and societal dimensions of AI in neurology and medicine*

15.6. Challenges and future perspectives

Even though AI has the ability to revolutionize neurology and medicine, it is not possible to provide safe and widespread application of AI due to numerous obstacles. Such barriers are technical, ethical, legal, as well as social in nature. Addressing them is critical so that AI can gain the most benefits (and minimum risks) to make patient care, efficiency and fairness better.

15.6.1. *Technical challenges*

AI relies on high-quality and various training information. The presence of variations, a lack of records and a small number of instances of rare cases in the neurology domain lower the reliability and generalizability of a model. The existence of biases in the data may result in poor performance among the various groups of demographics, further exacerbating the current healthcare disparity (Xu and Shuttleworth 2024).

The other major technical problem is interpretability. Deep-learning models are black boxes that provide unprocessed results, without explaining their creation. It is unlikely that doctors can trust or rely on AI advice unless it is made clear to them that it is especially in cases of stroke, seizure or staging of neurodegenerative diseases. The essential approaches to address these issues include the creation of XAI techniques, estimating uncertainty and combining AI outcomes with the opinion of clinicians.

Viable obstacles are also provided by interoperability and workflow integration. AI should be integrated with the electronic health records (EHRs), imaging equipment and monitoring tools without requiring any additional effort (Karimian et al. 2022). The requirement of compatibility with most platforms and settings implies general rules, comprehensive testing and constant updating.

15.6.2. *Harmonization of ethics and legal alignment*

AI raises ethical and legal problems that are closely connected. The safeguarding of patient choice, informed consent, privacy and fairness implies that laws must be updated to match the latest technology. The current rules usually lag behind AI advancement, and gaps in liability, accountability and intellectual-property protection arise (Shabankareh et al. 2025).

The solutions of the future should contain teams comprising doctors, ethicists, lawyers and AI makers to create pliable regulations to keep patients safe, just and transparent. Ethical and legal compliance skills require continual monitoring and audits of AI throughout the process. The novel legislation might establish adaptive approval paths of AI appliances, after-market inspections and responsibility models of algorithms.

15.6.3. *Social preparedness and inequality in the world*

The success of AI will not be achieved unless society is prepared, rather than technology, since differences in digital tools, funding and patient knowledge may create uneven usage, creating disparities across regions between the rich and poor. To provide an example, intelligent neuroimaging can be urban but not rural, therefore disadvantaging equity.

The attitude of people towards AI is also important. Honesty about the capabilities and limitations of AI, being truthful about it, and openness create credibility. Engaging patients in the design, educating and speaking fluently contribute to people accepting AI. Educating physicians and patients regarding digital skills will allow them to work safely on AI and eliminate any misunderstandings and usage abuse.

15.6.4. *Pathways for responsible AI deployment*

Solving these issues requires a number of steps. To begin with, robust data governance ensures various, quality data with privacy. Second, predictable AI is clear, and therefore, it is trusted by doctors and patients. Third, the regulating flexibility should continuously verify AI security. Fourth, ethics requires responsibility and fairness, transparency and equity inbuilt into AI.

It is essential to educate physicians, scientists and patients to use AI. Providing equal access to AI worldwide prevents the development of disparities in health globally. Collaborating with legislators, hospitals, developers and patient organizations assists in the creation of standard regulations that will achieve optimal outcomes without posing a threat.

15.7. Conclusion

Neurology and medicine are changing as a result of AI. It provides new methods of enhancing diagnostics, individualizing treatment and increasing patient outcomes. From the initial diagnosis of neurological conditions to adaptive rehabilitation and targeted therapies, AI can help to make care more precise and individualized. However, the advantages of these technologies are complex ethically, legally and socially and they have to be tackled. The essential ethical issues are autonomy of patients, informed consent, privacy of data, and fairness and accountability of algorithms. To tackle these issues, the AI systems should be transparent and human-oriented. There are also legal concerns such as legal liabilities, IP and compliance with the regulations. A clear structure is required to safeguard the patients and health professionals. It needs to have solid legal protection to protect AI usage. On a wider social scale, there are other consequences that need to be taken into account. To accept AI, there must be balanced access to the tools, workplace change, patient–physician relationship differences and trust in the technology. These aspects demonstrate the broader effect of AI on society. To overcome the obstacles, there is a need to have interdisciplinary cooperation, good governance and forward-looking policymakers. AI has the potential to augment, rather than substitute, clinical judgment by fostering transparency, equity and accountability. The outcome of such an approach is an ethical, effective and patient-centered healthcare environment.

15.8. References

BenJaMins, V.R. and Salazar García, I. (2019). Towards a framework for understanding societal and ethical implications of artificial intelligence. In *Vulnerabilidad y cultura digital: riesgos y oportunidades de la sociedad hiperconectada*, Alfonso, I.B., Fernández-Martínez, L.M., Suarez-Alvarez, R. (eds). Dykinson, Madrid.

Burger, M. (2020). The risk to population health equity posed by automated decision systems: A narrative review. *arXiv*.

Čartolovni, A., Tomičić, A., Mosler, E.L. (2022). Ethical, legal, and social considerations of AI-based medical decision-support tools: A scoping review. *International Journal of Medical Informatics*, 161, 104738.

Chandio, S.A., Rehman, A.U., Bano, S., Hammed, A., Hussain, A. (2024). Enhancing trust in healthcare: The role of AI explainability and professional familiarity. *The Asian Bulletin of Big Data Management*, 4(1).

Chustecki, M. (2024). Benefits and risks of AI in health care: Narrative review. *Interactive Journal of Medical Research*, 13(1), e53616.

Dankwa-Mullan, I. (2024). Health equity and ethical considerations in using artificial intelligence in public health and medicine. *Preventing Chronic Disease*, 21, E64.

Gómez-González, E., Gomez, E., Márquez-Rivas, J., Guerrero-Claro, M., Fernández-Lizaranzu, I., Relimpio-López, M.I., Dorado, M.E., Mayorga-Buiza, M.J., Izquierdo-Ayuso, G., Capitán-Morales, L. (2020). Artificial intelligence in medicine and healthcare: A review and classification of current and near-future applications and their ethical and social Impact. arXiv preprint, arXiv:2001.09778, 22 January.

Hirani, R., Noruzi, K., Khuram, H., Hussaini, A.S., Aifuwa, E.I., Ely, K.E., Lewis, J.M., Gabr, A.E., Smiley, A., Tiwari, R.K. et al. (2024). Artificial intelligence and healthcare: A journey through history, present innovations, and future possibilities. *Life*, 14(5), 557.

Karimian, G., Petelos, E., Evers, S.M. (2022). The ethical issues of the application of artificial intelligence in healthcare: A systematic scoping review. *AI and Ethics*, 2(4), 539–551.

Kaufman, D. (2024). Logic and foundations of artificial intelligence and society's reactions to maximize benefits and mitigate harm. *Filosofia Unisinos*, 25, e25110.

Kawamleh, S. (2023). Against explainability requirements for ethical artificial intelligence in health care. *AI and Ethics*, 3(3), 901–916.

Khan, M.M., Scalia, G., Shah, N., Umana, G.E., Chavda, V., Chaurasia, B. (2025). Ethical concerns of AI in neurosurgery: A systematic review. *Brain and Behavior*, 15(2), e70333.

Krook, J., Winter, P., Downer, J., Blockx, J. (2025). A systematic literature review of artificial intelligence (AI) transparency laws in the European Union (EU) and United Kingdom (UK): A socio-legal approach to AI transparency governance. *AI and Ethics*, 5, 4069–4090.

Kundu, T. and Bardhan, M. (2025). Artificial intelligence in neurology, ethics, recent guideline, and law – an Indian perspective. *Frontiers in Neurology*, 16, 1515041.

Lekadir, K., Frangi, A.F., Porras, A.R., Glocker, B., Cintas, C., Langlotz, C.P., Weicken, E., Asselbergs, F.W., Prior, F., Collins, G.S. et al. (2025). FUTURE-AI: International consensus guideline for trustworthy and deployable artificial intelligence in healthcare. *BMJ*, 388, e081554.

Li, F., Ruijs, N., Lu, Y. (2022). Ethics & AI: A systematic review on ethical concerns and related strategies for designing with AI in healthcare. *AI*, 4(1), 28–53.

Lund, B., Orhan, Z., Mannuru, N.R., Bevara, R.V., Porter, B., Vinaih, M.K., Bhaskara, P. (2025). Standards, frameworks, and legislation for artificial intelligence (AI) transparency. *AI and Ethics*, 5, 3639–3655.

Mondal, H. and Mondal, S. (2024). Ethical and social issues related to AI in healthcare. In *Artificial Intelligence in Microbiology: Scope and Challenges, Volume 1,* Srivastava, A. and Mishra, V. (eds). Academic Press, London, 247–281.

Nizamullah, F., Fahad, M., Abbasi, N., Qayyum, M.U., Zeb, S. (2024). Ethical and legal challenges in AI-driven healthcare: Patient privacy, data security, legal framework, and compliance. *International Journal of Innovative Research in Science, Engineering and Technology*, 13, 15216–15223.

Pham, T. (2025). Ethical and legal considerations in healthcare AI: Innovation and policy for safe and fair use. *Royal Society Open Science*, 12(5), 241873.

Ratti, E., Morrison, M., Jakab, I. (2025). Ethical and social considerations of applying artificial intelligence in healthcare—a two-pronged scoping review. *BMC Medical Ethics*, 26(1), 68.

Saeidnia, H.R., Hashemi Fotami, S.G., Lund, B., Ghiasi, N. (2024). Ethical considerations in artificial intelligence interventions for mental health and well-being: Ensuring responsible implementation and impact. *Social Sciences*, 13(7), 381.

Salles, A. and Farisco, M. (2024). Neuroethics and AI ethics: A proposal for collaboration. *BMC Neuroscience*, 25(1), 41.

Shabankareh, M., Khamoushi Sahne, S.S., Nazarian, A., Foroudi, P. (2025). The impact of AI perceived transparency on trust in AI recommendations in healthcare applications. *Asia-Pacific Journal of Business Administration*. doi: 10.1108/APJBA-12-2024-0690.

Singh, M.P., Keche, Y.N., Keche, Y. (2025). Ethical integration of artificial intelligence in healthcare: Narrative review of global challenges and strategic solutions. *Cureus*, 17(5), e84804.

Upadhyay, U., Gradisek, A., Iqbal, U., Dhar, E., Li, Y.C., Syed-Abdul, S. (2023). Call for the responsible artificial intelligence in the healthcare. *BMJ Health & Care Informatics*, 30(1), e100920.

Voigtlaender, S., Pawelczyk, J., Geiger, M., Vaios, E.J., Karschnia, P., Cudkowicz, M., Dietrich, J., Haraldsen, I.R., Feigin, V., Owolabi, M. et al. (2024). Artificial intelligence in neurology: Opportunities, challenges, and policy implications. *Journal of Neurology*, 271(5), 2258–2273.

Willem, T., Fritzsche, M.C., Zimmermann, B.M., Sierawska, A., Breuer, S., Braun, M., Ruess, A.K., Bak, M., Schönweitz, F.B., Meier, L.J. et al. (2024). Embedded ethics in practice: A toolbox for integrating the analysis of ethical and social issues into healthcare AI research. *Science and Engineering Ethics*, 31(1), 3.

Xu, H. and Shuttleworth, K.M. (2024). Medical artificial intelligence and the black box problem: A view based on the ethical principle of "do no harm". *Intelligent Medicine*, 4(1), 52–57.

16

Federated Learning and Collaborative AI Models in Neuroscience Research

Current research is transforming the field of neuroscience with the approach of federation learning (FL) and collaborative artificial intelligence (AI), addressing the following issues: data privacy, heterogeneity and scalability. Conventional centralized machine-learning systems store sensitive patient or research data in one or several repositories, and this system has ethical, regulatory and logistical concerns. Conversely, FL trains models at the local level on data maintained on each institution or device and communicates only model changes and not raw data. The privacy of the data is ensured by this decentralized method of integrating various sources of clinical and experimental data. Federated functional learning (FFL) is a principle applied in neuroscience, neuroimaging and electrophysiological signal processing, in predicting neurodegenerative diseases using cognitive models. Collaborative AI is based on this premise, to allow institutions to collaborate to produce models that use multimodal data, such as magnetic resonance imaging, electroencephalography, genomic data and digital biomarkers. Such frameworks generate high-fidelity models that reveal subtle neurobiological patterns and comply with strict data governance regulations such as the General Data Protection Regulation (GDPR) and the Health Insurance Portability and Accountability Act (HIPAA). AI and FL have enormous potential in making breakthroughs in the field of precision diagnostics, the predictive modeling of brain disorders and real-time adaptive neuro-technologies. Nonetheless, there are still issues of standardization, interoperability, efficiency of communication and minimization of bias in distributed data sets. This chapter presents the latest developments, examines the applications to the field of neuroscience, outlines the existing drawbacks and considers future research directions to harness FL and collaborative neural networks to transform neuroscience.

16.1. Introduction

Research in the field of neuroscience is evolving at a very fast pace since artificial intelligence (AI) and machine learning (ML) are considered to be the

---

Chapter written by Dipali JANKAR and Sanjay L. BADJATE.

primary means of investigating brain operation, cognition and neurodegenerative conditions. Conventional computational approaches have involved collecting large amounts of neuroimaging, electrophysiological and behavioral data in a centralized location where it can be trained. Although it can result in strong predictions, this method is associated with significant issues: threat to the privacy of the data, organizational isolation, issues getting the consent of the patient and difficulties with fulfilling regulatory rules. Decentralized training is a new solution to federated learning (FL) and collaborative AI that is aimed at replacing the centralized model (Sheller et al. 2020).

FL is a collaborative learning system that allows a large number of institutions or devices to train AI models in concert without including the raw data. Rather than transmitting real data, the participants share model parameters or gradients, keeping the sensitive information safely in its initial location. Such an approach is important in neuroscience, where medical imaging, electrophysiological measurements and genomic data may carry very recognizable and personal information (Li et al. 2020). FL provides an ethical and technically robust method to carry out neuroscience studies by balancing privacy against the statistical power of a big dataset.

The technical aspects of FL are not the only aspects of collaborative AI. It also incorporates inter-institutional, inter-disciplinary and inter-project collaboration in the creation of AI models. The field of neuroscience uses many different types of data. Functional magnetic resonance imaging (fMRI) studies differ in terms of scanners, protocols and populations (Warnat-Herresthal et al. 2021). Similarly, there is high inter-subject variation in electroencephalography (EEG) or magnetoencephalography (MEG) recordings, and therefore, cross-site cooperation is required. Such heterogeneous data streams are combined with collaborative AI models to facilitate the development of generalized models that can be used in clinical, research and translational settings.

These innovations are arriving at a particularly timely moment. The data that is being produced by neuroscience is beyond anything that has ever been produced before. Neuroimaging, high-density neural recording equipment and digital behavioral tracking advances generate terabyte-sized information. Centralizing such vast volumes of data is not practically feasible and would risk excluding underrepresented institutions that lack the necessary computational infrastructure (Kaissis et al. 2020). FL and collaborative models will democratize AI-based neuroscience, whereby distributed contributors have a chance to manipulate a shared model without relocating their data.

These strategies, in addition to logistical advantages, are in line with the increasing needs of ethical and legal conformity. Strict rules such as the General Data Protection Regulation (GDPR) of the European Union and the Health

Insurance Portability and Accountability Act (HIPAA) of the United States strictly restrict data flow and utilization. FL automatically complies with these requirements since the data on patients is stored in a safe local environment. Collaborative AI also advances the transparency and responsibility of the stakeholders, which resolves the skepticism around bias, equity and inclusivity in neuroscientific discovery (Dayan et al. 2021). In this chapter, we investigate the way FL and collaborative AI are incorporated in neuroscience studies. We present recent developments in methodology, practice, issues and their perspectives.

16.2. Fundamentals of FL in neuroscience

16.2.1. *Principles of FL*

FL as a paradigm is an ML paradigm that is decentralized at its core. A global model is constructed by amalgamating local computed updates by a number of clients. Rather than transmitting raw data to a central server, individual participants, for example, a hospital, a research institute or a device, train on their own data and only share model parameters, for example, weight updates or gradients. These are in turn incorporated, typically using a Federated Averaging (FedAvg) algorithm, to generate a better global model. This communication cycle is repeated over numerous rounds of communication until the model converges.

This is how the primary issue of privacy in neuroscience will be addressed. fMRI, structural MRI, diffusion tensor imaging (DTI) or EEG images can all contain identifying information about the patient. Ethical and legal regulations often bar sharing such data across institutions or even borders. FL has the advantage of storing the data locally, which means the reduction of the need to violate privacy regulations and the possibility of sharing intelligence (Basnin et al. 2025).

16.2.2. *FL architectures in applications*

There are a number of FL architectures, varying in their impact on neuroscience research:

– *Cross-silo FL*: applicable where not many companies, but those with large precisely structured datasets, work together. This is best suited to multi-center neuroimaging processes.

– *Cross-device FL*: encompasses a large number of clients including mobile telephones, wearable devices or implanted brain–computer interface (BCI) devices. In neuroscience, it is able to learn from a vast amount of people through digitized biomarkers gathered through smartphones or wearable EEG.

– *Hybrid structures*: these combine both styles, allowing the institutions and individual components to play their part at the same time. This is being applied increasingly to digital neuroscience, in which institutional image data can be merged with real-world behavioral data from consumer electronics (Xu et al. 2021).

16.2.3. *Privacy-preserving mechanisms*

While FL reduces the need for direct data sharing, it is not immune to privacy threats. Malicious actors could infer sensitive information from shared gradients or updates. To counter this, privacy-preserving mechanisms are commonly integrated into FL frameworks:

– *Differential privacy*: adds statistical noise to local updates before transmission, reducing the risk of reconstructing original data.

– *Secure multiparty computation (SMPC)*: ensures that updates are aggregated without being individually visible to the central server.

– *Homomorphic encryption*: allows computations on encrypted updates, providing mathematical guarantees of privacy (Dou et al. 2021).

16.2.4. *Challenges in implementing FL in neuroscience*

Despite its potential, FL also introduces new challenges:

– *Non-IID data*: neuroscience datasets across institutions often follow non-identical and non-independent distributions (e.g. age, ethnicity, scanning protocol variations). This reduces model convergence and generalizability (Ghader et al. 2023).

– *Communication overhead*: iterative updates require stable and high-bandwidth connections, which may be difficult in large-scale collaborations.

– *Model interpretability*: FL models, such as many deep learning frameworks, are often considered "black boxes", raising concerns in clinical neuroscience where explainability is crucial.

– *Infrastructure disparities*: smaller institutions may lack the computational power to perform local training on high-dimensional datasets such as fMRI.

Addressing these challenges requires innovative solutions such as personalized FL, adaptive aggregation techniques and resource-aware optimization methods (Cheplygina et al. 2019; Torre et al. 2023).

16.3. Collaborative AI models in neuroscience

FL establishes a privatized technical base. Collaborative AI builds on that base but extends the paradigm to a broader system that bridges institutions, disciplines and computational systems. Cross-disciplinary integration, which involves the integration of biology, psychology, medicine and engineering, is necessary in neuroscience. The technical challenge associated with distributed data can be overcome with the help of collaborative AI models in order to provide environments wherein knowledge, expertise and computational resources can be shared and used in unison. This section discusses the main ideas, design principles and those based on the neuroscience of collaborative AI.

16.3.1. *Conceptual foundations of collaborative AI*

Collaborative AI implies that within a scientific or clinical objective, distributed AI systems, humans and institutional resources are brought together to achieve a shared outcome. In contrast to the typical generally centralized AI pipelines, collaborative models operate through the input of a large number of parties, including research laboratories, hospitals or computational agents, and each one contributes to the value, using specialized information, specialized algorithms or encoded area knowledge (Stripelis et al. 2021).

Cooperation in neuroscience, by and large, has been confined to data-sharing projects, such as the Human Connectome Project or the Alzheimer's Disease Neuroimaging Initiative (ADNI). Collaborative AI is more than just a data exchange: it also allows various institutions to co-train models, jointly optimize algorithms and merge multimodal data without data motion. The resultant effect is the outcome of a more efficient learning system that is difficult to break and more representative of real populations.

16.3.2. *Multi-institutional AI collaborations*

Among the most notable benefits of collaborative AI, the opportunity to form multi-institutional projects within which research organizations mutually engage in training models, is also possible. Indicatively, neuroimaging datasets acquired in various hospitals will likely differ because of scanner types, acquisition procedures and the demographics of the population. Poor generalizability will be experienced when a single AI model is trained on a single dataset. Through collaborative AI designs, models will be able to learn the entire heterogeneity of distributed data, which will result in better diagnostic and predictive results (Perera et al. 2016).

Collaborative AI

In addition to neuroimaging, collaboration on a large-scale study of electrophysiology, EEG or MEG records acquired under different conditions can be combined. In the case of clinical neuroscience, multi-site partnerships are likely to help find digital biomarkers of diseases such as epilepsy, Parkinson's disease and multiple sclerosis (MS) much faster. It is also noteworthy that smaller institutions with limited data can also take part in collaborative models in which the contributions toward state-of-the-art neuroscience are democratized.

16.3.3. *Human–AI collaboration in neuroscience research*

Collaborative AI is not only about machines working with one another but also the interaction of humans and AI processes. Neuroscience frequently involves intricate theories that require professional decoding. Shared AI systems offer the concept of human-in-the-loop systems, whereby neuroscientists and clinicians are able to enhance AI systems iteratively. As an example of this, in the case of brain tumor segmentation, radiologists have the option to edit AI-generated boundaries and the corrections can be sent back to the system to further enhance the system, and thus, the process recurs (Munaweera and Yapa 2024).

The synergy that exists between human expertise and machine intelligence is of particular interest to the activities that require interpretability.

Cognitive neuroscience

Cognitive neuroscience has been suggested to use collaborative AI to design experiments by identifying unforeseen correlations in behavioral or neural data. These findings can then be confirmed by experts. Human–AI co-learning models are created to develop trust and efficiency.

16.3.4. *Multi-modal collaborative AI in neuroscience*

Multi-modal data or the collection of imaging, electrophysiology, genetics and behavioral measures are becoming more important for neuroscience research. Shared AI systems perform especially well in the integration of these heterogeneous streams of data. To cite one example, researchers take structural connectivity methods by using MRI and EEG-based functional connectivity to construct more elaborate brain network models. These types of collaborative models enable dedicated institutions to add their expertise without centralizing raw data, leaving the data decentralized (Jiang et al. 2025).

In neurodegenerative diseases, multimodal collaborative AI models can be used to combine clinical records, biomarkers in imaging and genetic risk factors to promote early identification. More generally, collaborative models in psychiatric neuroscience, where symptoms tend to be heterogeneous and diffuse, yield integrative models, which better capture the pathophysiology (Baghersalimi et al. 2021; Wen et al. 2023).

16.4. Applications of FL and collaborative AI in neuroscience

16.4.1. *Neuroimaging applications*

One of the most promising areas of FL use is neuroimaging since it entails large volumes of sensitive patient images and different scan protocols across different institutions. Disease (e.g. Alzheimer's, MS, brain tumor, etc.) diagnostic models require big, heterogeneous data, to be effective inter-site. The privacy regulations of strict privacy rules often make it difficult to pool data centrally. However, FL can construct strong models using local model updates across hospitals and imaging centers without direct sharing of the raw images (Dentamaro et al. 2024).

As a case in point, federated brain-tumor segmentation projects demonstrated that models trained in multiple institutions are superior to those developed using a single dataset. The distributed training takes into consideration variations in hardware and settings of the scanner, enhancing the precision and dependability in clinical practice.

Other uses of FL include automated cortical-thickness estimation, white-matter integrity mapping and functional connectivity analysis in addition to tumor detection. These are reproducible neurodegenerative and psychiatric disorder biomarkers using such methods (Rai and Avila-Quezada 2024).

Image harmonizing is also part of collaborative AI. Performing structural MRI, diffusion tensor imaging (DTI) and positron emission tomography (PET) images across different locations, federated frameworks construct multimodal works that are more complex. This integrability is vital in diseases such as Alzheimer's disease, in which structural, metabolic and functional alterations occur in a coordinated fashion.

16.4.2. *Neural signal analysis and electrophysiology*

The data provided by electrophysiological recordings (EEG, MEG, invasive local-field potentials, etc.) are of high dimensionality, but take a lot of time, thus challenging to share due to their bulk, as well as sensitivity. FL provides an alternative to training models with distributed electrophysiological data to identify and forecast neurological occurrences.

A major use would be in seizure detection in epilepsy studies. Federated methods help hospitals on the other side of the world to donate to shared models, and they do not have to transfer sensitive recordings of EEGs (electroencephalograms). These models, trained with varied electrode setups, surroundings of noise and different patient groups, extrapolate more and result in dependable seizure prediction systems (Wang et al. 2022).

FL is also used in the advancement of studies into Parkinson's that combine the patterns of neural activities of deep brain stimulation (DBS) electrodes. Overall, collaborative models that are trained using distributed datasets assist in optimizing the parameters of DBS, preconditioning the development of personalized treatment. Federated EEG analysis is used in non-invasive settings, as it assists the brain–BCI development of generalization between users, devices and experimental conditions, by leveraging distributed learning.

16.4.3. *Digital biomarkers and remote monitoring*

Mhealth technologies are also creating new avenues in neuroscience studies that can be performed outside of the laboratory. This behavioral and physiological data can be registered continuously by smartphones, wearable EEGs and motion sensors. These recordings will form digital biomarkers that can assist in detecting cognitive deterioration, psychiatric symptoms, and motor impairments.

Through the data processed by machines, researchers can get to know about entire populations without violating the privacy of individual users through the training of AI models.

Demonstrating the shift of the voice through the analysis of digital speech is one such example before Alzheimer's disease presents itself in other ways. An FL model enables devices in smartphones to record speech in numerous distinct countries and the information can be used to create a common model. The scheme retains the original audio files in the phone of the user, and therefore, no confidential audio is transferred to a central storage.

The other example is suitable with gait and tremor data collected by wearable accelerators. The gadgets capture the manner in which individuals walk and shake. Through an amalgamation of the information of numerous users, scientists would be able to enhance the early diagnosis of Parkinson's disease and track the advancement of the disease over time (Yang et al. 2021).

Such applications are particularly valuable in low-resource settings where traditional neuroimaging infrastructure may be unavailable. By enabling decentralized contributions, FL and collaborative AI democratize access to precision neuroscience tools globally.

16.4.4. *Cognitive and behavioral neuroscience*

Reconfigurable AI models have been applied to simple cognition and behavior research. The sharing of big data in psychology and cognitive science would enable the effort to jointly analyze the data and discover similar trends among the population in the learning, memory and decision-making process.

Experimental neuroscience is usually deficient in reproducibility. Collaborative AI also allows researchers to verify findings made in several labs without the dissemination of raw data. As one of the examples, neural cognition signatures can be observed both in a universal and culturally unique manner when FL models are distributed with training on working memory tasks in various groups (Dubey et al. 2025).

Adaptive experiments can be done in real time with collaborative AI. Distributed behavioral data can be used to modify the parameters of the tasks dynamically through reinforcement-learning models running across institutions. This accelerates the testing of hypotheses in fields such as attention, executive functioning and emotional control.

16.4.5. *Neurodegenerative and psychiatric disorders*

Perhaps the most impactful applications of FL and collaborative AI lie in clinical neuroscience, where decentralized models offer new avenues for disease detection, prognosis and treatment personalization:

– *Alzheimer's disease*: collaborative AI has been used to train predictive models on multimodal data (MRI, PET, genetics and cognitive assessments), improving early diagnosis before clinical symptoms fully manifest.

– *MS*: distributed learning enables the integration of MRI lesion load, spinal cord imaging and functional measures across institutions to develop models for disease progression and treatment response.

– *Psychiatric disorders*: FL has been applied to harmonize data across heterogeneous cohorts in depression and schizophrenia research, where differences in symptom presentation and comorbidities complicate model generalization (Huang et al. 2023).

16.4.6. *BCIs and neurotechnology*

BCIs and neurotechnologies represent a new frontier for FL and collaborative AI. Due to the difficult centralization of neural recordings, large datasets are needed for the training and decoding of BCI neural algorithms. Federated models allow for privacy protective continuous learning for end-users from disparate and separate BCI devices, while user privacy is preserved.

Application domain	Data modality	Objective/outcome	Collaborative/ federated approach	Key benefits
Neuroimaging	MRI, fMRI, PET, DTI	Disease diagnosis, cortical thickness mapping, tumor segmentation	Multi-institutional federated model aggregation across hospitals	Improves generalizability and privacy-preserving analysis
Neural signal analysis (EEG/MEG)	Electrophysiological recordings	Seizure detection, DBS signal optimization	Federated EEG/MEG model training across distributed centers	Enhances model robustness and cross-cohort adaptability
Digital biomarkers and remote monitoring	Smartphone, wearable sensors, voice, motion data	Early detection of neurodegenerative or motor disorders	Edge-device FL for behavioral and speech data	Enables decentralized and real-time monitoring
Cognitive and behavioral neuroscience	Behavioral task data, cognitive metrics	Modeling cognition, learning and emotion	Collaborative multi-site model training	Improves reproducibility and cross-cultural generalization
Neurodegenerative and psychiatric disorders	Multimodal (MRI, genetics, clinical data)	Early detection, prognosis, treatment response	Collaborative AI integrating multimodal datasets	Facilitates precision diagnosis and equitable inclusion
Brain–computer interfaces (BCI)	Invasive/non-invasive neural signals	Adaptive decoding, real-time rehabilitation	Federated BCI model learning across users	Protects privacy while improving device performance

Table 16.1. *Applications of federated learning and collaborative AI in neuroscience research*

The neural computing population patterns of multiple users and collaborative frameworks from different users have neural decoding accuracy improvements for real-time applications. This is groundbreaking for clinical rehabilitation. More communication devices for patients with motor limitations, and adaptive neuroprosthetic systems, have better integrated and rehabilitative systems (Soltan et al. 2024). In addition, collaborative AI neurotechnologies also respond to adaptive closed-loop systems with portable neural devices. This is more responsive to the rapid neural plasticity and variability of individuals. Table 16.1 shows applications of FL and collaborative AI in neuroscience research.

16.5. Challenges and limitations of FL and collaborative AI in neuroscience

16.5.1. *Technical challenges*

The chief technical problem in FL is the lack of data homogeneity between institutions. Neuroscience data is almost never independent and similarly distributed (non-IID) due to variations in hardware, acquisition conditions and subject (demographic) variables. Indicatively, fMRI evidence using a 1.5-Tesla incidence may be significantly distinct from information taken on a 3-Tesla apparatus. Learning FL models on these heterogeneous data may slow down the learning process and destabilize the gradients and result in biased global models (Kairouz et al. 2021).

The other issue is that FL is subject to communication restrictions. The repeated interactions between the clients and the central server of the model parameters/gradients need a robust bandwidth and a stable connection. Electrophysiology and large-scale neuroimaging projects may involve terabyte-scale data, so regular updates to the model can be computationally expensive. Communication bottlenecks are a feasible issue, although compression methods and asynchronous updates are currently under investigation.

Moreover, privacy protection is not enough to reduce the security risks of FL, as it is privacy-preserving. The threat of gradient inversion attacks, in which the attackers incorporate shared gradients to reconstruct original data, does exist. There are privacy calculation trade-offs between privacy, model accuracy and the cost of computation mitigated through techniques such as differential privacy or homomorphic encryption (Yin et al. 2018).

Finally, the problem of model interpretability is still present. Applications in neuroscience require outputs that are easy to read and understand and that we can have confidence in, without concerns of verification. The federated deep neural networks are often regarded as black boxes, which makes their application in clinical decision-making unproductive unless deciphered through explainable AI methods.

16.5.2. *Regulatory and ethical impediments*

Ethically, FL and collaborative AI have to deal with the multi-layered problems of consent, responsibility and equity. Guidance on informed consent is especially difficult to establish in longitudinal research within neuroscience because they may not have checked in advance that their data could be used in decentralized AI systems. Institutions should make sure that the procedures of consent consider disseminated information utilization and possible model provision.

The propagation of prejudice is another ethical issue. In the event that the datasets of underrepresented groups are scarce or excluded, collaborative models might restore systemic inequities. Neurodegenerative disease predictive models that are primarily trained using wealthier countries might not extrapolate to low-resource environments (Singh et al. 2025). This aids in making sure that diversity in the provision of data is observed to prevent a further intensification of health disparities.

Privacy-protective practices have been promoted by regulatory frameworks (including the GDPR, the HIPAA and others); however, these laws also create constraints, which may impede cooperation. As an example, GDPR mandates a clear explanation of cross-border data handling, which complicates teamwork between institutions in a federated setup. Striking a balance between regulation and scientific advancement is a sensitive matter.

16.5.3. *Challenges in the infrastructures*

Institutes of neuroscience differ considerably in their processing power, technical knowhow and secure information systems. High-performance computing clusters can be used in large research hospitals to support FL workloads, but smaller clinics or academic laboratory facilities do not have the means to train models locally. This unequal arrangement gives a weak balance in the cooperative projects where certain participants are more effective than the rest.

It has been suggested to use cloud-based FL systems and distributed computing infrastructure, which create a dependency on commercial institutions and can lead to issues of expense, data ownership and sustainability in the long term. The fair accessibility of computational infrastructure is therefore one of the main issues in scaling collaborative neuroscience.

Standardization is another infrastructural issue. A harmonization of the data format, the preprocessing pipelines and the annotation protocols between institutions are needed in collaborative AI. Loss of standardization brings in noise and variability which may compromise the performance of the model. Although data harmonization, such as the Brain Imaging Data Structure (BIDS), has been developed, its use is still inconsistent.

16.5.4. *Cultural and collaborative barriers*

In addition to technical and ethical factors, cultural issues affect the effectiveness of computer-assisted AI in neuroscience. Universities and hospitals tend to work in highly competitive settings in which information is regarded as intellectual property and not a common source of scientific literature. This spirit of competition may deter them from taking part in joint projects, even where technical protection schemes such as FL are involved.

Authorship issues, intellectual property and recognition are other problems that make collaborations more complex. The institutions might be unwilling to allocate resources to a project in which the contribution to the project cannot easily be quantified or noticed. Government structures should come up with clear rules in regard to credit allocation, authorship and ownership of jointly trained models.

The concept of trust is especially important in the collaborations between multiple institutions. Despite the technical protection, the fact that institutions are probably unwilling to trust the confidentiality of their data contributions is likely to occur. To establish trust, there must be transparency, proper communication and, more importantly, illustrations of proposed security measures.

16.5.5. *Striking a balance between innovation and responsibility*

The final problem of FL and cooperating AI in neuroscience is the issue of balancing innovation and responsibility. On the one hand, such methods introduce groundbreaking achievements in accuracy diagnostics, on-the-fly monitoring and massive thinking modeling. However, when challenges are left unaddressed, it may result in loss of privacy, biased results and unfair access.

The future solutions will most likely address hybrid solutions such as a method that incorporates technical innovation with effective government, moral guidelines and cultural change toward cooperation. Federated algorithms that consider the heterogeneity of data, combined with explainable AI and secure aggregation methods, are one of the directions to be taken. Policies with an international element that promote data inclusivity, equal access to infrastructure and rewarding of different contributions are also important.

16.6. Future directions

As a relatively new discipline, FL and collaborative AI have some way to go, yet the literature indicates potential areas of growth that can accelerate their expansion and increase their impact.

A key direction is to come up with adaptive federated algorithms that can better manage non-IID and multimodal data. Neuroscience tends to integrate neuroimaging, electrophysiology and genomic information, each of which possesses its own statistical pattern. More robustness and generalizability could be achieved with new FL optimization techniques that consider such heterogeneity, for example, personalized FL or meta-learning (Woo 2025).

The other significant direction is edge computing integration. This takes FL back to wearables, BCIs and mobile devices to allow the real-time performance of decentralized monitoring of brain activity in natural environments. As an example, neural-BCI with FL-enablement would enable patients with neural disorders to be provided with adaptive therapies without central servers having access to the raw neural information.

One more barrier is explainability and transparency. Neuroscience needs models that are interpretable because clinicians and patients can trust the predictions. The further development of the work will yield explainable federated structures of AI, which will show how distributed models draw conclusions without violating privacy.

International partnerships will also make a noticeable difference. International consortia and open-science efforts are seen as advantageous to neuroscience, and in this context, FL can offer a medium that does not interfere with the existing laws of data sovereignty. It will be necessary to build infrastructure to support standardized pipelines, federated governance and interoperability across borders that is secure (Stripelis et al. 2024).

16.7. Conclusion

Neuroscience research is changing the nature of FL and collaborative AI models. They are decentralized and privacy-safe and unique to long-term data sharing, security and scale issues. Institutions can participate in high-performance models without relinquishing sensitive data, thereby enabling accurate diagnosis, cognitive assessment, and targeted treatment. However, there are still numerous challenges. Technical challenges include data heterogeneity, slow communication and opaque models, which are examples of why it is difficult to apply FL to neuroscience. The effort is also complicated by ethical, infrastructural and cultural problems. To overcome these challenges, innovative algorithm designs, solid governance systems and a change of perspective toward improved communication and teamwork are needed. FL, collaborative AI and neuroscience might be integrated in the future to transform our understanding of the brain and offer a better clinical care process. When constructed in a responsible way, the decentralized structures will make it possible to promote fair, scaling and moral innovations that will eventually make the diagnostics, therapy and management of neurological diseases more effective.

16.8. References

Baghersalimi, S., Teijeiro, T., Atienza, D., Aminifar, A. (2021). Personalized real-time federated learning for epileptic seizure detection. *IEEE Journal of Biomedical and Health Informatics*, 26(2), 898–909.

Basnin, N., Mahmud, T., Islam, R.U., Andersson, K. (2025). An evolutionary federated learning approach to diagnose Alzheimer's disease under uncertainty. *Diagnostics*, 15(1), 80.

Cheplygina, V., De Bruijne, M., Pluim, J.P. (2019). Not-so-supervised: A survey of semi-supervised, multi-instance, and transfer learning in medical image analysis. *Medical Image Analysis*, 54, 280–296.

Dayan, I., Roth, H.R., Zhong, A., Harouni, A., Gentili, A., Abidin, A.Z., Liu, A., Costa, A.B., Wood, B.J., Tsai, C.S. et al. (2021). Federated learning for predicting clinical outcomes in patients with COVID-19. *Nature Medicine*, 27(10), 1735–1743.

Dentamaro, V., Impedovo, D., Musti, L., Pirlo, G., Taurisano, P. (2024). Enhancing early Parkinson's disease detection through multimodal deep learning and explainable AI: Insights from the PPMI database. *Scientific Reports*, 14(1), 20941.

Dou, Q., So, T.Y., Jiang, M., Liu, Q., Vardhanabhuti, V., Kaissis, G., Li, Z., Si, W., Lee, H.H., Yu, K. et al. (2021). Federated deep learning for detecting COVID-19 lung abnormalities in CT: A privacy-preserving multinational validation study. *NPJ Digital Medicine*, 4(1), 60.

Dubey, P., Dubey, P., Bokoro, P.N. (2025). Federated learning for privacy-enhanced mental health prediction with multimodal data integration. *Computer Methods in Biomechanics and Biomedical Engineering: Imaging & Visualization*, 13(1), 2509672.

Ghader, M., Farahani, B., Rezvani, Z., Shahsavari, M., Fazlali, M. (2023). Exploiting federated learning for EEG-based brain-computer interface system. In *2023 IEEE International Conference on Omni-layer Intelligent Systems (COINS)*, Berlin, 1–6.

Huang, J., Chen, H., Deng, J., Liu, X., Shu, T., Yin, C., Duan, M., Fu, L., Wang, K., Zeng, S. (2023). Interpretable machine learning for predicting 28-day all-cause in-hospital mortality for hypertensive ischemic or hemorrhagic stroke patients in the ICU: A multi-center retrospective cohort study with internal and external cross-validation. *Frontiers in Neurology*, 14, 1185447.

Jiang, W., Zhang, Y., Han, H., Liu, X., Gwak, J., Gu, W., Shankar, A., Maple, C. (2025). Fuzzy ensemble-based federated learning for EEG-based emotion recognition in Internet of Medical Things. *Journal of Industrial Information Integration*, 44, 100789.

Kairouz, P., McMahan, H.B., Avent, B., Bellet, A., Bennis, M., Bhagoji, A.N., Bonawitz, K., Charles, Z., Cormode, G., Cummings, R. et al. (2021). Advances and open problems in federated learning. *Foundations and Trends® in Machine Learning*, 14(1–2), 1–210.

Kaissis, G.A., Makowski, M.R., Rückert, D., Braren, R.F. (2020). Secure, privacy-preserving and federated machine learning in medical imaging. *Nature Machine Intelligence*, 2(6), 305–311.

Li, X., Gu, Y., Dvornek, N., Staib, L.H., Ventola, P., Duncan, J.S. (2020). Multi-site fMRI analysis using privacy-preserving federated learning and domain adaptation: ABIDE results. *Medical Image Analysis*, 65, 101765.

Munaweera, I. and Yapa, P. (2024). *Principles and Applications of Nanotherapeutics*. CRC Press, Boca Raton.

Perera, G., Broadbent, M., Callard, F., Chang, C.K., Downs, J., Dutta, R., Fernandes, A., Hayes, R.D., Henderson, M., Jackson, R. et al. (2016). Cohort profile of the South London and Maudsley NHS Foundation Trust Biomedical Research Centre (SLaM BRC) case register: Current status and recent enhancement of an electronic mental health record-derived data resource. *BMJ Open*, 6(3), e008721.

Rai, M. and Avila-Quezada, G. (eds) (2024). *Nanotechnology in Plant Health*. CRC Press, Boca Raton.

Sheller, M.J., Edwards, B., Reina, G.A., Martin, J., Pati, S., Kotrotsou, A., Milchenko, M., Xu, W., Marcus, D., Colen, R.R. et al. (2020). Federated learning in medicine: Facilitating multi-institutional collaborations without sharing patient data. *Scientific Reports*, 10(1), 12598.

Singh, T.M., Reddy, C.K., Puttanapura, J., Doss, S. (2025) Optimizing neural disorder treatment through federated learning and multi-institutional data collaboration. In *Federated Learning for Neural Disorders in Healthcare 6.0*, Reddy C., K.K. and Nag, A. (eds). CRC Press, Boca Raton.

Soltan, A.A., Thakur, A., Yang, J., Chauhan, A., D'Cruz, L.G., Dickson, P., Soltan, M.A., Thickett, D.R., Eyre, D.W., Zhu, T. et al. (2024). A scalable federated learning solution for secondary care using low-cost microcomputing: Privacy-preserving development and evaluation of a COVID-19 screening test in UK hospitals. *The Lancet Digital Health*, 6(2), e93–e104.

Stripelis, D., Ambite, J.L., Lam, P., Thompson, P. (2021). Scaling neuroscience research using federated learning. In *2021 IEEE 18th International Symposium on Biomedical Imaging (ISBI)*, 1191–1195.

Stripelis, D., Gupta, U., Saleem, H., Dhinagar, N., Ghai, T., Anastasiou, C., Sánchez, R., Ver Steeg, G., Ravi, S., Naveed, M. et al. (2024). A federated learning architecture for secure and private neuroimaging analysis. *Patterns*, 5(8), 101031.

Torre, D., Chennamaneni, A., Rodriguez, A. (2023). Privacy-preservation techniques for IoT devices: A systematic mapping study. *IEEE Access*, 11, 16323–16345.

Wang, X., Hu, J., Lin, H., Liu, W., Moon, H., Piran, M.J. (2022). Federated learning-empowered disease diagnosis mechanism in the internet of medical things: From the privacy-preservation perspective. *IEEE Transactions on Industrial Informatics*, 19(7), 7905–7913.

Warnat-Herresthal, S., Schultze, H., Shastry, K.L., Manamohan, S., Mukherjee, S., Garg, V., Sarveswara, R., Händler, K., Pickkers, P., Aziz, N.A. et al. (2021). Swarm learning for decentralized and confidential clinical machine learning. *Nature*, 594(7862), 265–270.

Wen, J., Zhang, Z., Lan, Y., Cui, Z., Cai, J., Zhang, W. (2023). A survey on federated learning: Challenges and applications. *International Journal of Machine Learning and Cybernetics*, 14(2), 513–535.

Woo, S.K. (2025). The role of artificial intelligence in advancing theranostics dosimetry for cancer therapy: A review. *Nuclear Medicine and Molecular Imaging*, 59(5), 329–341.

Xu, J., Glicksberg, B.S., Su, C., Walker, P., Bian, J., Wang, F. (2021). Federated learning for healthcare informatics. *Journal of Healthcare Informatics Research*, 5(1), 1–9.

Yang, D., Xu, Z., Li, W., Myronenko, A., Roth, H.R., Harmon, S., Xu, S., Turkbey, B., Turkbey, E., Wang, X. et al. (2021). Federated semi-supervised learning for COVID region segmentation in chest CT using multi-national data from China, Italy, Japan. *Medical Image Analysis*, 70, 101992.

Yin, D., Pananjady, A., Lam, M., Papailiopoulos, D., Ramchandran, K., Bartlett, P. (2018). Gradient diversity: A key ingredient for scalable distributed learning. In *International Conference on Artificial Intelligence and Statistics*. PMLR, Lanzarote, 1998–2007.

Zhang, Y., Wang, L., Su, K.J., Zhang, A., Zhu, H., Liu, X., Shen, H., Calhoun, V.D., Wang, Y., Deng, H. (2025). A privacy-preserving domain adversarial federated learning for multi-site brain functional connectivity analysis. *arXiv preprint*. doi: 10.48550/arXiv.2502.01885.

17

AI-enabled Approaches for Pain Prediction, Assessment and Management

Pain is an ambiguous, subjective experience, which is difficult to measure, forecast rapidly and treat efficiently in a clinical practice. The conventional methods, in the form of patient self-reports, numeric rating scales and clinician observations, tend to lack the dynamic, individualized and multidimensional experience of pain. The recent development of artificial intelligence (AI) has revolutionized the field of healthcare and provided novel means of comprehending, preventing and treating pain in diverse groups of individuals and circumstances. Physiological, behavioral and clinical signals are associated with pain and analyzed by AI-driven models, based on machine learning (ML) and deep learning (DL) models, natural language processing (NLP) and multimodal integration of data. Such tools enhance the objectivity of pain measurement and permit making personal predictions, tracking and real-time monitoring, as well as adapting their actions. Examples include wearable sensors to predict postoperative pain, implant-based automatic assessment of facial expression in children and optimization of analgesic dosing using reinforcement learners. Another partnership area of AI technology is with telemedicine apps and digital therapeutics to radically transform chronic pain management, in which real-time and constant monitoring are possible. In spite of such encouraging developments, there are still challenges. The fear of data privacy, the bias of algorithms, the enterprise of ethical issues, as well as the necessity of large-scale, clinically valid research remain. This chapter summarizes the latest AI scenarios in predicting, assessing and managing pain; it critically analyzes how it would enhance clinical decisions and patient outcomes; and explains how future studies and regulatory responses are required to use AI responsibly in pain management.

17.1. Introduction

Pain is also one of the most universal and complex phenomena in all of modern medicine. It is the leading cause of medical visits among individuals and a primary cause of disability and socioeconomic costs throughout the world

Chapter written by Mario ANTONY and Salim Allauddin CHAVAN.

(Adams et al. 2025). Acute pain (post-surgery and post-injury) may extend the healing process and increase hospitalization, and chronic pain impacts nearly one-third of the world's population by lowering quality of life and productivity (Abd-Elsayed et al. 2024). Since pain is sensory, emotional and cognitive, it is in a peculiar state of being difficult to measure, predict and manage. Traditional pain assessment tools, such as the Visual Analogue Scale (VAS) and the Numeric Rating Scale (NRS), remain the clinical standard, even though they are subjective and may not provide accurate assessments for young children, critically ill patients, or individuals with cognitive impairments (Srinivasan et al. 2024).

In recent years, pain care has gained new opportunities due to the rapid development of artificial intelligence (AI). Machine learning (ML), deep learning (DL) and natural language processing (NLP) are all elements of AI, which can also be defined as computational systems that replicate human intelligence. These methods are effective in the analysis of large and contemplated datasets, and the discovery of nonlinear trends that are not identified by the usual statistical models. Most importantly, AI is able to combine the multimodal data, including physiological data, imaging data, behavioral data and patient stories to provide a more objective perspective on pain (Meier et al. 2024).

Pain medicine AI can be divided into three general areas: prediction, assessment and management. Prediction tries to predict when pain will begin, how severe it will be or the progress of the process by examining clinical, physiological or environmental responses. Postoperative pain, i.e. the forecasting of the exacerbated stage of the chronic pain, allows early prevention, rather than remedy. Evaluation aims at the development of objective measures of pain with the help of such data as facial expression, voice, movement or brain activity, which are particularly effective with patients who cannot depend on self-reporting. Finally, there is AI-enabling management. This is carried out a through decision support system with customized analgesics doses, reinforcement learning (RL) to assist adaptive therapy and the collaboration with digital health platforms to ensure ongoing and remote care (Casarin et al. 2024).

There are still challenges with such promises. The only limitation on AI systems is the data they are trained on. Pain datasets are frequently large but unrepresentative and overly mislabeled. There are ethical concerns such as the privacy of data, the bias embedded in algorithms and patient consent, which only complicate the matter. Clinicians can also have reluctance to embrace AI insights in cases whereby they are not interpretable and have strong real-world validation.

This chapter provides an in-depth perspective of AI-based solutions for pain prediction, evaluation and treatment. We begin with existing methods of prediction in the areas of postoperative, chronic, and neuropathic pain management and assessment. Secondly, there are methods of AI assessment that focus on physiological, behavioral and neuroimaging data. After that, we consider AI-based inventions that assist in managing pain, including personalized treatment algorithms and digital therapeutics. Finally, we refer to outstanding issues, ethical concerns and future perspectives that will determine the responsible AI usage in pain medicine.

17.2. AI for pain prediction

Pain is always subjective; hence, it is not easy to predict pain in any field of medicine since it is caused by numerous factors. All pain is influenced by biological factors, psychology factors and even social factors, and none of the biomarkers is a reliable indicator of when pain begins and when pain will appear and become severe. The currently used clinical tools often assess pain once a patient complains of discomfort, thereby making it unaware of a future patient experiencing severe pain or when a flare-up is likely to take place. AI alters this and provides proactive treatments for pain. The scope of the data AI algorithms can analyze is massive, with the examples of the physiological signals that have been recorded in operation and daily activity logs all showing subtle patterns that precede pain. These trends allow AI models to forecast acute pain events: How will chronic pain evolve over the long-term and what is the probability of acute pain developing into chronic pain (Zhang et al. 2021)?

17.2.1. *Foundations of AI-based prediction*

ML and DL are largely used as AI prediction. Learning algorithms used to classify patients (such as support vector machines and random forests) are typically trained on supervised data (e.g. to answer the question of whether an individual will get high or low postoperative pain). Recurrent models and others are well adapted to work with time-series data such as physiological measurements or journal entries. Multimodal learning has been recently developed (as a result of integrating various types of data), which ensures improved accuracy of prediction because it contains imaging, sensor readings and clinical histories (Akhtar 2025).

17.2.2. *Postoperative pain prediction*

Among the first and most commonly researched fields in AI-based prediction of pain is postoperative pain. Postoperative pain management is crucial since management of acuteness failure to control pain may eventually induce healing retardation, increase the use of opioid and sometimes may result in chronic pain.

The common traditional predictors, such as the nature of surgery or age of a patient, seldom give reliable information.

Models that make use of AI to analyze perioperative data, such as anesthesia logs, vital signs, surgical information or other data, can detect those patients who are at risk of developing severe pain during the first 24 hours after surgery (Chustecki 2024). Through this, clinicians will have the opportunity to initiate preventive analgesic measures at the earliest stage rather than responding toward pain that has already developed.

Other studies have also included information of wearable devices, including heart-rate monitors and activity trackers, to the predictive model. Constant observing of these signs can assist physicians in managing the administered pain specifically, especially limiting patient time in the hospital and enhancing patient satisfaction.

17.2.3. *Chronic pain forecasting*

Chronic pains include arthritis, fibromyalgia and low back pain, which may fluctuate in intensity on a daily basis and flare impulsively. Major unmet needs are to understand when these flare-ups would take place. AI models, with the help of patient-reported outcomes, wearable sensor data and other lifestyle data, can reasonably predict the level of pain on a daily basis (Cascella et al. 2024b).

17.2.4. *Nociceptive and neuropathic pain*

The pain that is caused by the harm or malfunctioning of the nervous system is known as neuropathic pain and is notoriously difficult to predict. AI assists in studying complicated data collections, including the outcomes of quantitative sensory testing, electrophysiology and brain scanning. The initial results indicate that the models are able to identify these higher-risk patients who may develop neuropathic pain after the injury or surgery (Nagireddi et al. 2022).

17.2.5. *Multimodal data integration*

The greatest benefit of AI is its ability to combine a large number of various sources of data into individual models. As an example, electroencephalography (EEG) recording in conjunction with the analysis of facial expressions has been reported to enhance the prediction of procedural pain among children (Salama et al. 2024). Similarly, integrated genetic models, medication history and free-text clinical note models perform better as compared to single-variable models in predicting postoperative opioid requirements.

17.2.6. *Barriers to implementation*

Despite progress, AI-based pain prediction faces notable challenges. First, datasets are often small, heterogeneous and specific to single institutions, raising concerns about generalizability. Second, individual variability in pain perception – shaped by genetics, culture and psychosocial context – remains difficult to capture in models. Third, the "black box" nature of many DL algorithms limits interpretability, making clinicians hesitant to rely on predictions for high-stakes decisions such as opioid prescribing. Ethical issues, including privacy of continuously monitored data and the risk of biased predictions in underrepresented populations, further complicate clinical adoption (Nunes et al. 2024).

17.3. AI for pain assessment

17.3.1. *Deficiencies of traditional pain assessment*

The traditional pain scoring methods are mainly affected by culture, psychology and circumstances resulting in biased reporting. Indicatively, patients with chronic pain tend to under-report due to fears of stigma, whereas others may over-report so as to be offered better medication (Amirian et al. 2023). The greatest subjectivity is also observed in the clinical interpreters of pain behaviors such as grimacing or guarding. Also, these tools provide a limited number of snapshots instead of constant monitoring and, therefore, cannot provide the best results in a dynamic setting such as surgery or intensive care (Xing et al. 2024). These deficiencies would indicate the pressing necessity of AI-capable systems that would offer coherent and situation-free pain evaluation.

17.3.2. *Measuring using physiological signals*

Physiological indicators can be used as useful biomarkers that are indicative of nociception and stress. Heart rate variability (HRV), electrodermal activity (EDA), skin conductance, electromyography (EMG) and EEG have been investigated as parameters with which the intensity of pain is correlated. The complex nonlinear relationships between these signals and pain states are detected by AI models, in particular, ML and DL.

Supervised algorithms categorize the physiological patterns as no pain, mild pain or severe pain. Deep neural networks (DNNs) embrace the dynamics over time, which improves the real-time observational processes in the course of anesthesia or in postoperative recovery (Cascella et al. 2024a).

17.3.3. *Face recognition*

Facial expressions signal pain, and they are universal and, in most cases, can be in the form of micro-expressions such as the lowering of the brows, orbital tightening or a wrinkling of the nose. Computer-vision systems that are enhanced with AI are very effective at detecting these nuances. Convolutional neural networks (CNNs) recognize and label facial expressions of pain displayed in videos, which cannot be detected by the human since they are so fast. Such systems are used in pediatric and neonatal care, where verbal reporting is not possible to measure pain (Lu et al. 2023). It enhances their clinical capability by being integrated with portable devices and bedside monitors.

17.3.4. *Voice and speech analysis*

Pain changes the acoustic characteristics of speech: its pitch, intensity, rhythm and spectral characteristics. The speech recognition systems with AI pick these changes up and present an assessment tool of pain that is not invasive. NLP classifies patient stories, which involves deriving patterns in words, feel and linguistic signals that are tied to pain. Such methods prove particularly useful in telemedicine, where physically examining the patient is minor and the clinician gets another layer of insight into patient experiences (Nunes et al. 2024).

17.3.5. *Neuroimaging-based evaluation*

The advances in neuroimaging suggest neural pain involvement. The brain's activities are repeatedly activated while in pain through the use of functional magnetic resonance imaging (fMRI), near-infrared spectrosopy (NIRS) and EEG focused on the anterior cingulate cortex, insula and somatosensory cortex. Such activities are categorized into distinct pain radars through AI classifiers such as support vector machines (SVMs) and DL models. This neural signature approach has provided objective pain biomarkers, but the remaining challenges involve the cost, accessibility and scalability (Cascella et al. 2024a).

17.3.6. *Multimodal fusion approaches*

Pain occurs in various modalities, which include physiological expression, facial expressions, speech and the brain. Multimodal fusion techniques are used more and more often by the researchers who combine heterogeneous streams of data into a single model. This combines negativity and extrapolation and enhances pain evaluation. For example, combining facial recognition with physiological monitoring can reduce false positives caused by unrelated emotional expressions. Ensemble learning techniques and hybrid DL architectures have demonstrated superior performance compared to unimodal models. Such systems are particularly well suited for complex clinical environments such as intensive care units (ICUs), where continuous and accurate pain monitoring is critical (Cascella et al. 2024b).

17.4. AI in pain management

However, even though precise prediction and evaluation of pain are crucial, the final aim of the clinical practice is to have the pain under control. Management of pain is very personal and is based on the etiology, intensity, duration, comorbidities and psychosocial circumstances. Conventional interventions are comprised of opioid, non-steroidal anti-inflammatory drugs (NSAIDs), adjuvant medications, physical interventions, psychological strategies and interventional procedures. Limitations of these strategies include variability in patient response, risks of side effects and the inability to continue the monitoring on a long-term basis. New directions are provided by AI and are able to individualize treatment, make corrective decisions, continually check patients and fill the void created by traditional approaches (Sajdeya and Narouze 2024).

17.4.1. *Personalized analgesic dosing*

One of the issues that has posed a significant problem in the treatment of drugs is the difference in the patient response to medication. Safety and effectiveness are affected by genetics, age, sex, comorbid conditions and other drugs. AI models are supervised learning and RL, which optimize pain medication doses. These models forecast the patients who actually respond to a certain painkiller and those who are more vulnerable to issues linked to the use of opioid painkillers by studying massive amounts of pharmacogenomic and electronic health records (EHRs) (Antel et al. 2025). The systems facilitate the customization of opioid prescriptions, minimizing under-treatment and abuse.

17.4.2. *Prediction of risk and leadership in opioid stewardship*

Opioid misuse and addiction are now classed as global health emergencies. Opioids are potent and dangerous outside of close observation. The use of AI to predict misuse is based on prescription history, behavioral health records and socioeconomic factors. Quantitatively predictive models enable clinicians to prescribe alternatives, provide more monitoring or refer patients to addiction specialists at the earliest opportunity, upon detecting high-risk patients. Subtle warnings that are not observed in the structured records are also identified in the process of NLP of clinical notes. Through opioid stewardship, AI contributes to the increased patient safety and addresses one of the key public health issues (Borges 2024).

17.4.3. *Non-pharmacological interventions for pain*

AI promotes non-pharmacological ways of treatment such as physiotherapy, psychological interventions and neuromodulation. AI-powered wearable sensors are used in physiotherapy to monitor the movement, activity and compliance with rehab. Feedback makes the recovery optimal. ML optimizes exercise programs, establishing appropriate intensity and development. AI chatbots and virtual reality (VR) offer cognitive behavioral therapy (CBT) and mindfulness in chronic pain management in psychological care (Cascella and Naveed Shariff 2024). These tools are particularly helpful in underserved locations, making them more accessible and upholding evidence-based standards. AI is also beneficial to neuromodulation, where the spinal cord and deep brain stimulation are fine-tuned in real time to achieve optimal benefits and reduce side effects.

17.4.4. *Digital therapeutics and remote monitoring*

Digital health technologies make AI-enhanced pain treatment venture out of clinics. Mobile applications, wearables and telehealth solutions gather continuous patient-reported results, sensor and behavioral indicators. AI can be used to analyze such streams and identify patterns of pain flare-ups and implement the necessary interventions in time (Antel et al. 2025). Predictive alerts have the ability to inform patients and clinicians about an impending exacerbation and adjust their therapy in advance. Long-term follow-ups can be supported with the help of remote monitoring and help in providing proactive care instead of reactive care. These techniques are associated with the trend toward patient-centered, value-based healthcare.

17.4.5. *Integrative decision-support systems*

The treatment of pain is a complicated matter, as it involves the application of numerous treatment methods, side effects and the personal preference of the patient. The clinical decision support systems (CDSSs) provided by AI will include EHRs, imaging, genomics and data from wearables. They come up with individualized treatment prescriptions. CDSS assists clinicians in selecting the most appropriate therapies, perceiving the response and modifying plans in a dynamic manner. They provide doable information at the point of care, lowering the cognitive burden of the provider and enhancing evidence-based practice (Zhang et al. 2023). Pilot experiments demonstrate beneficial results when AI CDSS tools are added to pain processes.

17.4.6. *RL and adaptive learning models*

RL is a sub-discipline of AI, which learns by trial and error. RL is good at changing pain management. Closed-loop reinforcement learning (CRL) algorithms can adapt medication dosages, optimize neuromodulator settings, and dynamically design behavioral interventions, rather than relying on rigid, rule-based approaches. The adaptive systems continually update the recommendations according to the response of patients and formulate a feedback loop through which they do updates whenever the clinical requirements change.

The use of RS in chronic pain is promising because the symptoms become uneven and need an individualized approach (Meier et al. 2024).

17.4.7. *AI-based pain management dilemmas*

Even though it has been advanced, there are obstacles to its extensive implementation. Key factors that act as a barrier include regulatory approval, data privacy and integration in existing health systems. The absence of the clarification of the logic behind the decision can lead clinicians to distrust AI. Addressing these concerns requires serious clinical testing, user design and constant interaction between designers and clinicians. Equal access should also be achieved in a way that AI innovations do not exacerbate the existing disparity.

Table 17.1 lists AI techniques, data sources and applications in pain prediction, assessment and management.

17.5. Challenges and limitations of AI in pain medicine

The concept of integrating AI into the process of anticipating, evaluating and treating pain has huge potential, yet it cannot be implemented without encountering severe challenges. These issues touch upon technical, clinical and social aspects, and unless they are addressed together, they may restrict the practical implications of AI innovations.

Domain	AI technique/model	Data source/modality	Objective/function	Clinical outcome/benefit
Pain prediction	ML (SVM, random forests)	EHRs, perioperative data, vitals	Predict postoperative or chronic pain severity	Enables proactive analgesia and early intervention
Pain prediction	Deep neural networks (RNN, LSTM)	Wearable sensors, HRV, EDA	Forecast acute/chronic pain flare-ups	Supports preventive care and home monitoring
Pain assessment	CNN-based facial recognition	Video, facial micro-expressions	Objective pain scoring in non-verbal patients	Improves assessment accuracy in children and ICUs
Pain assessment	NLP and speech analysis	Voice recordings, clinical narratives	Detects pain intensity from acoustic and linguistic cues	Enables remote and telehealth-based evaluation
Pain assessment	Physiological signal modeling (DNN, transformers)	EEG, EMG, ECG, skin conductance	Classifies nociceptive responses into pain levels	Facilitates real-time intraoperative monitoring
Pain management	RL	Pharmacogenomic data, EHR	Adaptive optimization of analgesic dosing	Reduces opioid misuse, supports personalized therapy
Pain management	AI-powered decision support systems (CDSS)	Integrated EHR, imaging, sensor data	Tailor treatment plans dynamically	Enhances clinician confidence and treatment precision
Pain management	Digital therapeutics and federated learning	Mobile apps, wearables, patient feedback	Continuous remote care and personalized adjustment	Enables decentralized, privacy-preserving pain management
Multimodal integration	Ensemble/hybrid DL	Neuroimaging, physiological and behavioral data	Combines heterogeneous data streams for robust prediction	Improves diagnostic accuracy and real-time assessment

Table 17.1. *AI techniques, data sources and applications in pain prediction, assessment and management*

17.5.1. *Data scarcity and data quality concerns*

Effective AI models are based on high-quality and large-scale data. Standardized datasets are, however, not common in medicine of pain. The pain information is usually inconsistent because of the fluctuating self-report scales, small number of clinical trials and cross-population heterogeneity. As an example, a model that is trained on postoperative pain in adults may not be generalized properly to the children or the elderly (Chustecki 2024). Physiological measurements of wearables or patient outcomes may also be noisy and incomplete, making it difficult to effectively train a model.

17.5.2. *Applicability to some populations*

AI tools in pain medicine are often trained on controlled research in settings with insufficient populace diversities. Model accuracy can be influenced by ethnicity, age, comorbid and cultural perception of pain. Algorithms used to perform facial recognition can inaccurately decode expressions belonging to different ethnic groupings and models based on speech may overlook language and accent differences (De Sario et al. 2023). These raise some doubts regarding the possible biases and unequal treatment in case the models are deployed without validation.

17.5.3. *Embedding in clinical workflow*

Hospitals are complicated settings, and the introduction of AI systems requires a thorough consideration of the process of incorporating them into the current routine. Clinicians already have large workloads of EHRs, and AI should not introduce additional administrative responsibility. Besides, the lack of interoperability between health–IT systems may also hinder the implementation of AI. Even well-adjusted models can still be left to go to waste when they are not integrated in a way that is smooth enough to apply in practice (Chustecki 2024).

17.5.4. *Interpretability and trust*

Most AI models, particularly DL models, are black boxes that provide predictions but not explanations. Interpretability is necessary in pain medicine because decisions directly influence the safety of a patient. To make informed choices in high-stakes settings, such as when prescribing opioids or more or less neuromodulation, clinicians must understand the rationale behind a particular intervention given by a model. This limits the adoption of AI systems because clinicians do not trust them (El-Tallawy et al. 2024).

17.5.5. *Cost and resource constraints*

The development, implementation and maintenance of AI-based systems are expensive. Most medical institutions, particularly those that are resource constrained, do not have the required financial and technical resources to support advanced AI applications. Another significant issue is fair access to the AI-enhanced pain solutions since the presence of digital-health disparities has the potential to increase the divide between the high- and low-resource healthcare systems (Taha et al. 2025).

17.6. Ethical, legal and future directions

17.6.1. *Data privacy and security*

AI systems employ various data on patients including physiological indicators and medical records as well as behavioral data. This data is essential, and its protection is very important, as its breach may lead to loss of the patient's confidence and even lawsuits. Although the laws, such as General Data Protection Regulation (GDPR) and Health Insurance Portability and Accountability Act (HIPAA) provide guidelines, it is difficult to translate them into a daily routine. In order to maintain privacy without reducing data utility, techniques such as deidentification, federation learning and strong encryption are under testing (Chustecki 2024).

17.6.2. *Unbiased and fair work environments*

The greatest danger in pain medicine is bias in AI. Models may strengthen current inequalities when they are trained on inadequate sets of data that do not represent some groups. As an example, when learning facial-recognition models that are trained primarily with light-skinned faces, they make false estimations about the amount of pain in dark-skinned patients (De Sario et al. 2023). Remedy of bias refers to the attempt to explicitly incorporate varied information, bias audits and ML structures that facilitate fairness.

17.6.3. *Legal liability and accountability*

The legal landscape surrounding AI in healthcare is still evolving. A critical question is: Who is responsible when an AI system makes an incorrect recommendation that leads to harm? Current frameworks place responsibility on clinicians, but as AI becomes more autonomous, shared liability between developers, healthcare institutions and practitioners may become necessary. Clear guidelines and regulatory pathways are essential to establish accountability and ensure safe deployment (El-Tallawy et al. 2024).

17.6.4. *Patient autonomy and consent*

AI-enabled pain management must respect patient autonomy. Patients should have the right to understand how their data is used, what role AI plays in their care and the ability to opt out if desired. Transparent communication and informed consent are therefore critical. Moreover, involving patients in the design and evaluation of AI systems may enhance usability, trust and acceptance (Taha et al. 2025).

17.6.5. *Future directions*

Looking forward, AI in pain medicine is expected to evolve in several key directions:

– *Multimodal integration*: combining signals from wearable sensors, imaging, genomics and patient-reported data to provide holistic, personalized pain management solutions.

– *Edge AI and real-time monitoring*: deploying algorithms directly on wearable devices to enable continuous, low-latency monitoring of pain in real-world environments.

– *Explainable AI (XAI)*: developing interpretable models that allow clinicians to understand the rationale behind predictions, fostering greater trust.

– *Collaborative AI systems*: moving toward human-in-the-loop frameworks, where AI supports but does not replace clinician decision-making, ensuring safety and accountability.

17.7. Conclusion

The introduction of AI technology is revolutionizing the practice of pain medicine by proposing innovative ways of predicting, assessing and treating pain. AI attempts to produce a more objective and continuous assessment of pain by integrating multiple data sources, including physiological data, facial analysis, neuroimaging and self-reported data. The use of predictive models and adaptive decision-support systems along with RL and digital therapeutics enables proactive pain management. The integration of these systems and technologies will assist pain management in surpassing the subjective standards that have characterized pain management for decades. AI's widespread use is impeded by inadequate data, biased algorithms, challenges in workflow integration and the ubiquitous use of opaque models. Ethical and legal concerns such as privacy, accountability and equity remain inadequately addressed. Addressing these issues requires the collaborative efforts of several disciplines in the field, along with the practical application of governance that balances patient safety with innovative disruption.

17.8. References

Abd-Elsayed, A., Robinson, C.L., Marshall, Z., Diwan, S., Peters, T. (2024). Applications of artificial intelligence in pain medicine. *Current Pain and Headache Reports*, 28(4), 229–238.

Adams, M.C., Bowness, J.S., Nelson, A.M., Hurley, R.W., Narouze, S. (2025). A roadmap for artificial intelligence in pain medicine: Current status, opportunities, and requirements. *Current Opinion in Anesthesiology*, 38(5), 680–688.

Akhtar, Z.B. (2025). Exploring AI for pain research management: A deep dive investigative exploration. *Journal of Pain Research and Management*, 1(1), 28–42.

Amirian, S., Carlson, L.A., Gong, M.F., Lohse, I., Weiss, K.R., Plate, J.F., Tafti, A.P. (2023). Explainable AI in orthopedics: Challenges, opportunities, and prospects. In *2023 Congress in Computer Science, Computer Engineering, & Applied Computing (CSCE)*. IEEE, Las Vegas, 1374–1380.

Antel, R., Whitelaw, S., Gore, G., Ingelmo, P. (2025). Moving towards the use of artificial intelligence in pain management. *European Journal of Pain*, 29(3), e4748.

Borges, M.D. (2024). Artificial intelligence in pain management: Advancing translational science in digital health research from bench to bedside review article. *Advances in Machine Learning & Artificial Intelligence*. doi: 10.2139/ssrn.4983858.

Casarin, S., Haelterman, N.A., Machol, K. (2024). Transforming personalized chronic pain management with artificial intelligence: A commentary on the current landscape and future directions. *Experimental Neurology*, 382, 114980.

Cascella, M. and Naveed Shariff, M. (2024). Why is applying artificial intelligence to pain so challenging? *Current Medical Research and Opinion*, 40(12), 2021–2024.

Cascella, M., Leoni, M.L., Shariff, M.N., Varrassi, G. (2024a). Artificial intelligence-driven diagnostic processes and comprehensive multimodal models in pain medicine. *Journal of Personalized Medicine*, 14(9), 983.

Cascella, M., Monaco, F., Piazza, O. (2024b). Artificial intelligence and pain medicine: An introduction. *Journal of Pain Research*, 17, 509–518.

Chustecki, M. (2024). Benefits and risks of AI in health care: Narrative review. *Interactive Journal of Medical Research*, 13(1), e53616.

De Sario, G.D., Haider, C.R., Maita, K.C., Torres-Guzman, R.A., Emam, O.S., Avila, F.R., Garcia, J.P., Borna, S., McLeod, C.J., Bruce, C.J. et al. (2023). Using AI to detect pain through facial expressions: A review. *Bioengineering*, 10(5), 548.

El-Tallawy, S.N., Pergolizzi, J.V., Vasiliu-Feltes, I., Ahmed, R.S., LeQuang, J.K., El-Tallawy, H.N., Varrassi, G., Nagiub, M.S. (2024). Incorporation of "artificial intelligence" for objective pain assessment: A comprehensive review. *Pain and Therapy*, 13(3), 293–317.

Lu, Z., Ozek, B., Kamarthi, S. (2023). Transformer encoder with multiscale deep learning for pain classification using physiological signals. *Frontiers in Physiology*, 14, 1294577.

Meier, T.A., Refahi, M.S., Hearne, G., Restifo, D.S., Munoz-Acuna, R., Rosen, G.L., Woloszynek, S. (2024). The role and applications of artificial intelligence in the treatment of chronic pain. *Current Pain and Headache Reports*, 28(8), 769–784.

Nagireddi, J.N., Vyas, A.K., Sanapati, M.R., Soin, A., Manchikanti, L. (2022). The analysis of pain research through the lens of artificial intelligence and machine learning. *Pain Physician*, 25(2), E211.

Nunes, D.A., Ferreira-Gomes, J., Neto, F., de Matos, D.M. (2024). Computational analysis of the language of pain: A systematic review. *arXiv preprint*. doi: 10.48550/arXiv.2404.16226.

Sajdeya, R. and Narouze, S. (2024). Harnessing artificial intelligence for predicting and managing postoperative pain: A narrative literature review. *Current Opinion in Anesthesiology*, 37(5), 604–615.

Salama, V., Godinich, B., Geng, Y., Humbert-Vidan, L., Maule, L., Wahid, K.A., Naser, M.A., He, R., Mohamed, A.S., Fuller, C.D. et al. (2024). Artificial intelligence and machine learning in cancer pain: A systematic review. *Journal of Pain and Symptom Management*, 68(6), e462–e490.

Srinivasan, B., Venkataraman, A., Raja, S.N. (2024). Artificial intelligence and pain management: Cautiously optimistic. *Pain Management*, 14(7), 331–333.

Taha, H.A., Zeilani, R.S., Haddad, R.H., Abdalrahim, M.S. (2025). Artificial intelligence and machine learning techniques for predicting neuropathic pain in patients with cancer: A systematic review. *Digital Health*, 11, 20552076251358315.

Xing, Y., Yang, K., Lu, A., Mackie, K., Guo, F. (2024). Sensors and devices guided by artificial intelligence for personalized pain medicine. *Cyborg and Bionic Systems*, 5, 0160.

Zhang, M., Zhu, L., Lin, S.Y., Herr, K., Chi, N.C. (2021). Using artificial intelligence to improve pain assessment and pain management: A scoping review. *Innovation in Aging*, 5(Suppl 1), 633.

Zhang, M., Zhu, L., Lin, S.Y., Herr, K., Chi, C.L., Demir, I., Dunn Lopez, K., Chi, N.C. (2023). Using artificial intelligence to improve pain assessment and pain management: A scoping review. *Journal of the American Medical Informatics Association*, 30(3), 570–587.

18

Conversational AI and Virtual Assistants for Neurological Patient Support

Diseases of the nervous system such as Parkinson's disease, Alzheimer's disease, multiple sclerosis and epilepsy, as well as post-stroke disorders, have devastating effects on the cognitive, motor and emotional function of patients. Such chronic conditions need continuous assistance, regular observations and adaptive rehabilitation that extend beyond the regular clinical attendance. Virtual assistants and conversational artificial intelligence (AI) are now seen as potential solutions to these gaps. They are able to deliver real-time advice, medication reminders, emotional companionship, cognitive stimulation and connections with healthcare providers by offering interactive, convenient and patient-centered assistance. With patient history, behavioral data and preferences, these assistants are capable of creating scalable solutions to supplement clinical treatment. The introduction of wearable devices and electronic health records, as well as Internet of Things (IoT) ecosystems, will allow them to provide continuous monitoring solutions and interactive care. However, there are still issues such as privacy of data, bias in algorithms, lack of use in various populations and the inability to recognize insidious neurological symptoms. To be safe in the deployment of health settings, ethical and regulatory frameworks, as well as clinical validation, are necessary. With the evolution of AI, conversational AI, affective computing and multimodal interaction, not to mention growing independence, more pleasant lives and better clinical outcomes, it is possible to revolutionize the support for neurological patients. This chapter provides an analysis of the status quo, future trends, clinical use and opportunities of conversational AI and virtual assistants in neurological care.

18.1. Introduction

Among the various neurological diseases, such as Alzheimer's disease, Parkinson's disease, multiple sclerosis, epilepsy and post-stroke disabilities, are growing causes of disability and diminished quality of life globally. They place

---

Chapter written by Nikhilchandra MAHAJAN and Piyush Ashokrao DALKE.

increasing challenges on the patients, those who provide care and those that promote healthcare systems; and they are usually difficult to handle in the long term and through multidisciplinary means (Tran et al. 2025). Traditional methods of treating the nervous system, including periodic visits to hospitals, prescribed medication and face-to-face rehabilitation, are often not enough to satisfy the ongoing needs of patients. Poor accessibility to experts, compliance challenges and social isolation also make chronic condition management more complicated (Cai et al. 2025).

Digital health technologies have become a potential solution that can address gaps in neurological care in recent years. Conversational artificial intelligence (AI) and virtual assistants have shown their potential. Based on natural language and speech recognition and learning adaptation algorithms, such systems are used to mimic human-like interactions so that patients can interact with healthcare devices in a natural and personalized way (Rizzo 2025). Conversational AI is also able to modify responses as needed in accordance with patient preferences, monitor behaviors and give reminders or coach readers that promote autonomy and compliance with treatment, unlike other forms of digital resources (static).

The rising adoption of conversational AI in healthcare is related to the general trends in telemedicine, remote monitoring and personalized medicine. Virtual assistants provide a chance for cognitive stimulation in their everyday lives, emotional support, as well as physical exercises and medication assistance to neurological patients, in particular. This chapter is a broad overview of the role of conversational AI and virtual assistants in support of neurological patients, focusing on the basis of technology, clinical uses, issues and prospects.

18.2. Technological foundations of conversational AI in healthcare

Conversational AI systems are systems of artificially intelligent computational linguistics and human–computer interaction that allow machines to comprehend and respond to natural human speech. In the healthcare industry, these systems should be more dependable, situational and individualized compared to the general chatbots (Rizzo and Dawson 2025). They are effective because of three areas that are connected to each other: natural language processing (NLP), dialogue management and collaboration with healthcare infrastructure.

18.2.1. *NLP and understanding*

This generally enables the user to understand and communicate with a speech-dependent yet speech-independent computer program that is based on a natural language.

NLP allows virtual assistants to convert patient speech or written data into a format of action. Speech recognition and meaning extraction processes have become more precise due to the implementation of deep learning and transformer models, in particular (Liu et al. 2025a). This is crucial for neurological patients whose speech may be impaired due to dysarthria, aphasia or mental challenges. Healthcare systems with good use of NLP will incorporate specialized training data and adaptive models that deal with such unusual patterns of language.

In addition to word recognition, natural language understanding (NLU) goes beyond words to comprehend the intent of a patient who has input it. For example, in the case where a patient with Parkinson's explains that they are feeling stiff this morning, the AI must conclude that there is a medication problem and not that the patient is talking casually. Disagreement over patient language is prevented through proper disambiguation and appropriate patient response, which develops trust and clinical utility.

18.2.2. *Discussion management and individualization*

Dialogue management refers to the way a system organizes the conversation, maintains the context and selects the response. To support their neurological purposes, it will have to sustain coherent, empathetic and goal-oriented interactions, rather than provide generic responses. It should be personalized: a virtual assistant achieves maximum efficiency when it adjusts to a personal status, a history and habits (Feng et al. 2025). One system may be simplified and repeat-key-point based on dementia patients, and another on exercises that correspond with the recovery objectives in stroke survivors.

New developments in reinforcement learning and adaptive dialogue approaches enable assistants to learn during continuous interactions. They are able to determine the best prompts, reminders and incentives to use with each user, enhancing long-term involvement and therapeutic recovery.

18.2.3. *Multimedia interfaces and accessibility*

Speech, motor control or cognitive neurological disorders may also be involved, and therefore, a single-mode interface is not always sufficient. Multimodal systems are a mix of voice, text and touch and visual systems, making the communication between patients with different impairments comfortable. A patient with motor impairment could use voice commands, and a patient with speech impairment may use text or pictorial information. This redundancy eliminates misunderstanding and increases availability (Aljanahi 2025).

New technologies introduce wearable gadgets, brain–computer interfaces (BCIs) and virtual reality, building more engaging communication methods. Such tools allow conversational AI to progress beyond a chat with the virtual assistant that can provide exercises in real-time, track physiological conditions and modify interventions in real time.

18.2.4. *Data integration and healthcare ecosystems*

Next-generation conversational AI has links to electronic health records, IoTs and telehealth devices. This type of integration allows virtual assistants to access patient histories, medication compliance and notifications of worrying patterns (Gupta and Malhotra 2025). As an example, an AI may be able to see that a patient has switched the date in a couple of drug notifications and alerts a caregiver or provider.

Data that are self-reported together with objective health indicators such as gait, sleeping patterns or wearable biometric results make the process of personalization more effective. This, however, demands high standards of interoperability and the presence of good data-security provisions to abide by healthcare regulations.

18.3. Clinical applications of conversational AI in neurological care

The transfer of conversational AI technologies that were originally based on general-purpose tools to the clinical context has provided possibilities of working with neurological patients. Virtual assistance may offer a range of complementing interventions that assist in traditional care through integrating real-time communication with adaptive feedback. The use of cognitive rehabilitation, emotional support and better communication between patients and healthcare providers is not limited to their daily use in managing various symptoms. This section contains a description of the most important spheres where conversational AI has proven to be productive in neurological practice.

18.3.1. *Medication adherence and symptom tracking*

Patients with long-term neurological conditions have a chronic adherence dilemma with medication. Losing dosages, mismanagement of complicated drug regimes or lack of communication of side effects may aggravate symptoms and increase hospital readmission. Assistants based on AI conversation can be useful because they provide individuals with personalized reminders, determine whether drugs have been taken and invite users to report symptoms (Yeung et al. 2023).

As an example, a patient with Parkinson's can be reminded every day that they should be taking levodopa at certain times. In case the patient complains of continued tremors despite compliance, the system will prompt the patient to record the details to be reviewed later by their clinician.

On top of the alerts, AI assistants can be used more proactively to monitor the presence of symptoms, posing patients with focused questions related to moods, mobility, pain or cognitive alterations. These data points can help clinicians over time to make valuable insights and switch to proactive care rather than reactive care, including adjusting the treatment plans.

18.3.2. *Cognitive rehabilitation and training*

Loss of thinking ability is a characteristic of numerous diseases such as Alzheimer's disease, dementia and muscle lesion from a stroke. The interactive exercises promoted by conversational AI systems can maintain memory, attention and problem-solving abilities.

A virtual assistant can suggest memory games, word games or orientation exercises for patients, which can keep their minds active. Contrary to the case with static programs, conversational systems adjust the difficulty and frequency with regard to personal progress (Sandrone 2024).

These interventions are also applied to speech therapy amongst stroke victims. Conversational agents may offer repetitive language training, word-remembering tasks and pronunciation aids and make the patient practice between their sessions with a specialist. This motivation enhances compliance with therapy and accelerates the results of recovery.

18.3.3. *Emotional support and companionship*

As a result of brain diseases, people tend to become socially isolated, anxious and depressed. Conversational AI provides an option of delivering companionship in terms of responsive and understanding interactions. Although virtual assistants cannot substitute human bonds, they may alleviate loneliness through daily conversations with the patients, inspirational support and relaxation or mindfulness meditation (Liu et al. 2025b). Frequent, minor contact may result in positive psychological effects in the case of patients who have limited access to care.

Affective computing applications enable virtual assistants to identify and respond to emotional messages in spoken or written language with adequate empathy. As an example, in the case when a patient is upset about the need to move, the assistant may provide encouraging messages and propose relaxation methods. This helping relationship creates a feeling of trust and motivates the patients to continue participating in care routines.

18.3.4. *Improvement of communication with speech-impaired patients*

Conversational AI can be applied as an assistive communication method by patients with speech or language disabilities who have amyotrophic lateral sclerosis (ALS) or have suffered a severe stroke. Voice synthesis, speech-to-text and predictive typing provide virtual assistants with the ability to assist people in formulating their requests (Todericiu 2025). A patient with poor speech may be able to type or use words that are voiced by the assistant when the patient interacts with clinicians or other people who attend to them.

They may be integrated with multimodal systems, as such assistants are capable of employing gestures, text and voice simultaneously, which leads to easier everyday communication and makes the process of communication less frustrating in terms of the emotional state it evokes.

18.3.5. *Remote monitoring and telehealth integration*

Conversational AI has been emphasized as a valuable way of interacting between healthcare providers and patients through telemedicine. Virtual assistants can serve as a gateway to patient data, symptom triaging and report creation to provide clinicians with the required data.

For example, a patient communicating with the assistant about new neurological symptoms arranges the information and passes it to the rest of the care team to follow up (Rahsepar Meadi et al. 2025).

Combined with wearable tools, conversational AI systems make it possible to monitor gait, heart rate or sleep habits without interruption remotely. The insights can enable clinicians to identify the fluctuations of early worsening and take effective action.

The clinical decision-making process is improved through the use of conversational interfaces in combination with remote monitoring, as well as making patients active participants in their own care. Table 18.1 lists the clinical applications of conversational AI in neurological patient support.

Clinical area	Purpose of an AI assistant	Example functionality	Neurological conditions benefited	Expected outcomes
Medication adherence	Improve compliance with prescribed drugs	Daily reminders, symptom check-ins, alerts for missed doses	Parkinson's, epilepsy, multiple sclerosis	Fewer relapses, reduced hospital readmissions
Cognitive rehabilitation	Enhance memory, speech and attention	Interactive games, word recall, speech repetition training	Alzheimer's, strokes, dementia	Improved cognitive performance and engagement
Emotional support	Reduce loneliness and anxiety	Conversational companionship, mindfulness guidance	All chronic neurological patients	Better mental health, emotional stability
Communication aid	Assist speech-impaired patients	Speech-to-text, voice synthesis, predictive typing	ALS, post-stroke aphasia	Enhanced communication and independence
Remote monitoring	Enable continuous observation	Integration with wearables, symptom tracking, clinician alerts	Parkinson's, stroke survivors	Early detection of symptom progression, timely intervention

Table 18.1. *Clinical applications of conversational AI in neurological patient support*

18.4. Benefits and opportunities of conversational AI for neurological support

The application of conversational AI and virtual assistants has numerous advantages for patients with neurological disorders, their caregivers and healthcare systems. The outcomes of these advantages extend past clinical care and influence psychological health, patient autonomy and the efficiency of the system. With the acceleration of digital health adoption, chances to implement the tools in common neurological practice are increasing swiftly.

18.4.1. *Improving patient engagement and empowerment*

Among the most effective applications of conversational AI is that it can also be actively used to engage patients in the process of their care. Neurological conditions can be used to teach practices on a daily routine, yet with time, compliance tends to lapse as weariness, aggravation or forgetfulness sets in. Virtual assistants can be beneficial because they provide reminders and motivational prompts, along with engagement in dialogues that assist in accountability (Alshami et al. 2025). An assistant may inquire about how a patient feels, monitor their reactions and change reminders according to the adherence to the plan, instead of merely reminding a patient to take medication.

Along with adherence, conversational AI provides patients with greater health management authority. This sense of agency particularly applies to individuals who have progressive conditions such as Parkinson's disease or dementia, in which the psychological factor of being able to stay autonomous is paramount.

18.4.2. *Accessibility and scalability*

Neurology would be resource-intensive, as it requires the expertise of specialists, rehabilitation centers and further monitoring. Numerous patients, especially in the low-resource environments, have a problem accessing regular care. Conversational AI is a commonly scalable approach, as it is able to provide support anywhere without geographic or other logistical constraints (Calderone et al. 2024). Smartphones, tablets or smart speakers may be used to access a virtual assistant, which would serve a wide range of potential customers.

Scalability is also useful to healthcare, which is regularly short of neurologists and rehab practitioners. Automated daily operations such as medication reminders or check-ups give virtual assistants the freedom to allow clinicians to attend to the more complicated cases, and thus, there is a fairer allocation of care resources.

18.4.3. *Customized and modifiable interventions*

The capability of personalization of conversational AI is one of its strengths. Vital cues by studying interaction and previous data and understanding the context can help the virtual assistants to adapt their answers to the needs of the individual patient. As an example, a stroke survivor undergoing speech therapy would get progressively more complicated exercises as their language abilities develop, whereas a dementia patient would respond well to repetition and simplified prompting (Schiza et al. 2019).

Adaptive interventions enhance the effectiveness of therapeutic processes by matching the content of the therapy with the progress, preference and ability of a patient. In the long run, this will create more interactions and improved results, making conversational AI more of a living companion and less of a machine.

18.4.4. *Minimization of social isolation and emotional support*

Neurological conditions may pose social loneliness, as well as emotional suffering to both the patient and the caregiver. Conversational AI may serve to overcome loneliness with trustful and sympathetic communication (Stasolla et al. 2021). Although a virtual assistant is unable to substitute human companionship, it can be used as a source of daily conversations, encouragement and light entertainment, which can enhance emotional well-being.

This will be particularly handy to elderly patients who lead independent lives and have mobility difficulties. This can be alleviated through the use of simple check-ins, facilitated relaxation exercises and conducive dialogue that can reduce feelings of abandonment and enable patients to feel integrated into their care system. To caregivers, it is reassuring to understand that an AI assistant is in action and eliminates emotional exhaustion.

18.4.5. *Interoperability with other broader digital health ecosystems*

The biggest opportunity is in the execution of conversational AI together with broader healthcare and digital health systems. Related to electronic health records, wearable technologies and telehealth software, virtual assistants are smart intermediaries between patients and clinicians. As an example, an assistant may track the activity by means of a smartwatch, compare it with medicine records and send a condensed version of the report to the neurologist prior to the next appointment (Keserwani et al. 2024).

This type of integration improves continuity of care and facilitates data-based decision-making. In the long run, such systems may become all-inclusive digital companions, oversee several health factors and integrate seamlessly between the domestic and clinical environments.

18.5. Challenges and limitations

18.5.1. *Accuracy and reliability of interactions*

A significant problem is to ensure that conversational AI provides correct answers. Dysarthria, aphasia or intellectual disabilities characterize the speech of a neurological patient. There is a likelihood that most of the natural language models are trained on healthy speech and thus cause misinterpretation of such patterns (Tu et al. 2025). Mistakes may result in frustration, lack of trust and even harmful misunderstanding related to treatment or symptoms. Despite the advancement in deep learning in speech recognition, we require more patient-specific data sets and algorithms, which should be able to consider the specifics of various groups of patients.

18.5.2. *Data privacy and security issues*

Healthcare applications should be of high quality to avoid sensitive information. The deep personal data of conversational AI, including physician records of habits and feelings, are gleaned. One of the most important concerns is the protection of such data against any breach or misuse (Kummer and Busis 2024). The interconnection of these systems with electronic health records and IoT devices increases the vulnerability even more.

It is also possible that the patients would not be willing to provide any personal information because they are not certain what their information will be used for. To build trust, serious consideration should be paid to laws such as HIPAA and GDPR that allow it to be used in a broader way.

18.5.3. *Ethical and social implications*

Another complex factor is ethics. Autonomy, consent and possible exploitation among neurological patients are a dicey realm, to be approached with caution. Assistants designed to be unwelcoming may intentionally enforce prejudices, not notice cultural peculiarities or provide unsuitable responses (Kalani and Anjankar 2024). These results also cast doubts on substituting human empathy with AI interactions due to the over-reliance on AI as a companion.

There is a danger that AI can further increase healthcare inequality, should it be oriented more toward high-resource locations. Individuals whose devices have little or no digital literacy may not be reached, which will compromise the aim of providing equitable care.

18.5.4. *Barriers to usability and accessibility*

Even the most developed AI should be available to patients with different capacities. Neurology has the ability to influence the vision, action, hearing and thinking of the user by affecting the interaction with the system. Multifaceted interfaces and unreliable reactions may disillusion patients, decrease participation and damage compliance (Ruscu et al. 2023). Inclusive design demands more than one mode of interaction, plain interfaces and continuous user feedback during the development.

Caregivers also are central to it. A large number of caregivers assist in the care of a patient; hence, assistants that do not pay attention to the needs of a caregiver are unlikely to offer real utility.

18.5.5. *Integration and clinical validation problems*

Although the use of conversational AI in neurological care is becoming increasingly popular, its efficacy is poorly defined. Most applications remain small in scale, with short follow-ups. Strict clinical testing is also needed to confirm the improvements in patient outcomes, adherence and quality of life (Das et al. 2022). In the absence of such assistance, healthcare providers can remain cynical.

There have been challenges in integrating AI into the existing health systems. Conformability with electronic health records, medical device interoperability and congruence with clinical workflows are complicated. The resources of most healthcare bodies are limited, and hence, it becomes even more challenging to implement and maintain these technologies.

18.6. Future directions and research opportunities

Stable development of conversational AI and virtual assistants will introduce a sunny side of working with neurological patients. Accountable instruments that enhance conformity, restoration and emotional health are currently present. The next generation of patient-centered digital health can be developed based on the findings in the future to produce more sophisticated and personalized systems.

18.6.1. *Multisensory interfaces and multimodal interfaces*

Making use of many senses is the next major advancement of conversational AI. Voice or text is primarily used by the present assistants, although a large portion of neurological patients require more than simple communication. It is possible that future systems will combine speech, gesture detection, expression analysis and haptic feedback to provide more lifelike interactions (Salem and Shaalan 2023). A stroke patient that cannot talk much may use their hands to communicate, so the assistant would decipher the movements and combine them with whatever they say in order to give the right response.

Rehabilitation can also take place on these multimodal systems. With a combination of graphics, physical activities and sound stimuli, virtual assistants are able to provide therapy experiences that are virtually close to an actual clinical session.

18.6.2. *Integrates BCIs*

BCI technology is used to supplement conversational AI when it allows brain-to-computer communication. This is avoided by motor or speech defects. BCI could be used to activate an AI agent by patients with ALS or locked-in syndrome to read their words and thus enable them to speak with a degree of independence never seen before (Cross et al. 2024).

The combination of BCIs, wearable sensors and AI dialogue management, in the form of hybrid systems, can make assistive tools a full-fledged neurological care platform.

18.6.3. *Preventive and predictive healthcare paradigms*

Another important direction is to change reactive care to predictive care. Chatbots combined with machine learning will be able to examine long-term patient records to predict situations, including medication non-adherence, symptom exacerbation or cognitive impairment (McDermott et al. 2024). For example, when the answers of a dementia patient grow more chaotic, the system may alert caregivers about the first signs of its worsening, in order to provide medical care in time.

Predictive models are supportive of preventive plans, which involve shorter hospital stays, better living and lowering expenditure. Their data and validation of quality are based on good quality and proper validation to guarantee accuracy and reliability.

18.6.4. *Federated learning and privacy-preserving AI*

The way AI should be used in the future should be more privacy-regulated, yet personalized. Federated learning allows the models to be trained at distributed devices without centralizing the sensitive data at a single point (Patel et al. 2021). This makes personalization localized, maintains privacy and allows patients to enjoy the advantages of aggregated knowledge across populations.

Ranging across neurological care, federated models have the ability to learn using multiple classes of patients while maintaining patient privacy and can lessen AI biases by covering the difference in linguistic and cultural backgrounds.

18.6.5. *Emotional intelligence, affective computing*

Emotion recognition and response will also be one of the central aspects of next-generation AI. Affective computing includes additions of emotional sensitivity that include recognition of tone of voice, facial expression and even the tone of language (Ceradini et al. 2024). Emotionally intelligent assistants would be able to deliver context-sensitive care, especially to patients who are likely to be depressed, anxious or frustrated with their conditions.

Such systems can also become early mental-health detection aids, and they will trigger a clinical referral. Emotional tact and moral protection are paramount in order to not pursue manipulation and reliance (Bernini et al. 2021).

18.6.6. *Broadening clinical evidence and policy frameworks*

Clinical validation and favorable policies are needed to facilitate widespread adoption. The efficacy, safety and cost-efficacy have to be demonstrated using large-scale randomized controlled trials. The policymakers need to formulate control policies that are sensitive to the patients yet encourage innovation. These systems should encompass liability, certification and ethical issues such that the AI is on par with other medicine technologies (Zeka and Mikroelektrot 2025).

18.7. Conclusion

There are hardships in neurological disorders that extend well beyond the normal clinical environment. Chronic disease poses an emotional burden on patients, who tend to have complicated medication regiments, sluggish mental or physical abilities and extra complications. The resources and access issues of traditional health systems are hampered. They are not always able to give out the in-depth, individualized care patients require. Conversational AI and virtual assistants can be regarded, in this context, as powerful tools that introduce care in the daily lives of patients. These systems have the potential to make a conversation with the patient natural, fast and flexible by integrating NLP, dialogue management and multimodal interaction. Clinical data already demonstrates positive outcomes across most sectors and will help clients to adhere to their medication, enhance cognition, enhance emotional well-being, support speech-impaired individuals and connect to telehealth services. In addition to clinical measures, the technologies make patients more independent, reduce social isolation and foster a sense of ownership of their health process. There are still numerous challenges, though. Issues connected to accurately decoding non-standard speech, safeguarding privacy, ethics and inclusivity may reveal the necessity of designing very carefully. Moreover, pilots should be followed by easy scaling, and it is necessary to support them with solid clinical validation and the functionality of new health systems. In the absence of such steps, the conversational AI may remain under-utilized despite its massive potential.

18.8. References

Aljanahi, M.H. (2025). Leading with data: AI-driven decision making. In *AI in Learning, Educational Leadership, and Special Education: Innovations and Ethical Dilemmas: Innovations and Ethical Dilemmas*, Efstratopoulou, , M., Argyriadi, A., Argyriadis, A. (eds). IGI Global Scientific Publishing, Hershey, PA.

Alshami, A., Nashwan, A., AlDardour, A., Qusini, A. (2025). Artificial intelligence in rehabilitation: A narrative review on advancing patient care. *Rehabilitación*, 59(2), 100911.

Bernini, S., Stasolla, F., Panzarasa, S., Quaglini, S., Sinforiani, E., Sandrini, G., Vecchi, T., Tassorelli, C., Bottiroli, S. (2021). Cognitive telerehabilitation for older adults with neurodegenerative diseases in the COVID-19 era: A perspective study. *Frontiers in Neurology*, 11, 623933.

Cai, T., Ma, S., Zhong, R. (2025). Can intelligent virtual assistants improve cognitive function in older adults? A two-wave mediation study. *Digital Health*, 11, 20552076251317355.

Calderone, A., Latella, D., Bonanno, M., Quartarone, A., Mojdehdehbaher, S., Celesti, A., Calabrò, R.S. (2024). Towards transforming neurorehabilitation: The impact of artificial intelligence on diagnosis and treatment of neurological disorders. *Biomedicines*, 12(10), 2415.

Ceradini, M., Losanno, E., Micera, S., Bandini, A., Orlandi, S. (2024). Immersive VR for upper-extremity rehabilitation in patients with neurological disorders: A scoping review. *Journal of NeuroEngineering and Rehabilitation*, 21(1), 75.

Cross, S., Bell, I., Nicholas, J., Valentine, L., Mangelsdorf, S., Baker, S., Titov, N., Alvarez-Jimenez, M. (2024). Use of AI in mental health care: Community and mental health professionals survey. *JMIR Mental Health*, 11(1), e60589.

Das, A., Sen, V., Rose, A.C. (2022). Developing a chatbot/intelligent system for neurological diagnosis and management. In *Augmenting Neurological Disorder Prediction and Rehabilitation Using Artificial Intelligence,* Pillai, A.S. and Menon, B. (eds). Academic Press, New York, 273–291.

Feng, Y., Hang, Y., Wu, W., Song, X., Xiao, X., Dong, F., Qiao, Z. (2025). Effectiveness of AI-driven conversational agents in improving mental health among young people: Systematic review and meta-analysis. *Journal of Medical Internet Research*, 27, e69639.

Gupta, A. and Malhotra, D. (2025). Advancing rare neurological disorder diagnosis: Addressing challenges with systematic reviews and AI-driven MRI meta-trans learning framework for neurodegenerative disorders. *Ageing Research Reviews*, 111, 102831.

Kalani, M. and Anjankar, A. (2024). Revolutionizing neurology: The role of artificial intelligence in advancing diagnosis and treatment. *Cureus*, 16(6), e61706.

Keserwani, P.K., Das, S., Sarkar, N. (2024). A comparative study: Prediction of Parkinson's disease using machine learning, deep learning and nature inspired algorithm. *Multimedia Tools and Applications*, 83(27), 69393–69441.

Kummer, B.R. and Busis, N.A. (2024). Beyond audio-video Telehealth: Perspective on the current state and future directions of digital neurological care in the United States. *JMIR Neurotechnology*, 3(1), e46736.

Liu, J., Cao, W., Yuan, B., Xie, W., Wang, C., Liu, S. (2025a). ChatGPT vs DeepSeek: A comparative study of diagnostic accuracy and clinical reasoning in rare and complex diseases. *medRxiv*. doi: 10.1101/2025.08.28.25331796.

Liu, C., Ran, Y., Hu, C., Wang, M., Li, N., Yang, Z., Ding, Z., Qiao, C., Xi, J., Su, W. et al. (2025b). Nanomedicines and stroke: Advantages in chronic inflammation treatment and neural regeneration. *Neural Regeneration Research*. doi: 10.4103/NRR.NRR-D-25-00120.

McDermott, E.R., DeFoor, M.T., Dekker, T.J., DePhillipo, N.N. (2024). Artificial intelligence in rehabilitation. In *Artificial Intelligence in Orthopaedic Surgery Made Easy,* Familiari, F., Galasso, O., Gasparini, G. (eds). Springer, Cham, 197–204.

Patel, U.K., Anwar, A., Saleem, S., Malik, P., Rasul, B., Patel, K., Yao, R., Seshadri, A., Yousufuddin, M., Arumaithurai, K. (2021). Artificial intelligence as an emerging technology in the current care of neurological disorders. *Journal of Neurology*, 268(5), 1623–1642.

Rahsepar Meadi, M., Sillekens, T., Metselaar, S., van Balkom, A., Bernstein, J., Batelaan, N. (2025). Exploring the ethical challenges of conversational AI in mental health care: Scoping review. *JMIR Mental Health*, 12, e60432.

Rizzo, M. (2025). AI in neurology: Everything, everywhere, all at once Part 3: Surveillance, synthesis, simulation, and systems. *Annals of Neurology*, 98(4), 651–667.

Rizzo, M. and Dawson, J.D. (2025). AI in neurology: Everything, everywhere, all at once Part 1: Principles and practice. *Annals of Neurology*, 98(2), 211–230.

Ruscu, M., Cercel, A., Kilic, E., Catalin, B., Gresita, A., Hermann, D.M., Albu, C.V., Popa-Wagner, A. (2023). Nanodrugs for the treatment of ischemic stroke: A systematic review. *International Journal of Molecular Sciences*, 24(13), 10802.

Salem, M. and Shaalan, K. (2023). ChatGPT: Advancing education with virtual assistants. In *International Conference on Business Intelligence and Information Technology*. Springer, Singapore, 283–293.

Sandrone, S. (2024). Chatbots in neurology and neuroscience: Interactions with students, patients and neurologists. *Brain Disorders*, 15, 100145.

Schiza, E., Matsangidou, M., Neokleous, K., Pattichis, C.S. (2019). Virtual reality applications for neurological disease: A review. *Frontiers in Robotics and AI*, 6, 100.

Stasolla, F., Matamala-Gomez, M., Bernini, S., Caffò, A.O., Bottiroli, S. (2021). Virtual reality as a technological-aided solution to support communication in persons with neurodegenerative diseases and acquired brain injury during COVID-19 pandemic. *Frontiers in Public Health*, 8, 635426.

Todericiu, I.A. (2025). Virtual assistants: A review of the next frontier in AI interaction. *Acta Universitatis Sapientiae, Informatica*, 17(1), 1.

Tran, H.H., Thu, A., Twayana, A.R., Fuertes, A., Gonzalez, M., Basta, M., James, M., Frishman, W.H., Aronow, W.S. (2025). The role of generative artificial intelligence and large language models in atrial fibrillation: Clinical research and decision support. *Cardiology in Review*, 10–97.

Tu, T., Schaekermann, M., Palepu, A., Saab, K., Freyberg, J., Tanno, R., Wang, A., Li, B., Amin, M., Cheng, Y. et al. (2025). Towards conversational diagnostic artificial intelligence. *Nature*, 642, 442–450.

Yeung, J.A., Wang, Y.Y., Kraljevic, Z., Teo, J.T. (2023). Artificial intelligence (AI) for neurologists: Do digital neurones dream of electric sheep? *Practical Neurology*, 23(6), 476–488.

Zeka, S.A. and Mikroelektrot, M.A. (2025). Investigation of an open AI model in the analysis of STN microelectrode recordings: Consistency with clinicians and potential for DBS targeting. *Medical Journal of Bakirköy*, 21(3), 288–295.

19

Brain–Computer Interfaces Enhanced by Artificial Intelligence

A brain–computer interface (BCI) facilitates direct interaction between brain activity and external equipment, by passing through normal neuromuscular and synaptic interfaces. The technology is swiftly changing the interaction with machines. Recent years have witnessed a significant enhancement of the performance of BCIs through their combination with artificial intelligence (AI) and adoption of more adaptable and relevant applications in practice. Machine learning and deep neural AI models focus on recurrent neural signals and increase the accuracy of decoding neural signals in complex cases and also maximize noise removal. They are also capable of real-time interpretation of brain activity, which immediately permits the interaction with external devices. These innovations have expanded the application of BCI from medical rehabilitation and assistive communication for people with motor impairments up to immersive virtual reality, computer gaming and military technologies. The collaboration of AI and BCIs addresses the old problems of signal acquisition, feature extraction and accuracy of classification. Adaptive algorithms are now being used to tailor the system response based on single neural patterns, enhancing better usability and reducing time training for users. Intelligent predictive models are also AI-based, and they are used to control prosthetics, exoskeletons and neurofeedback to enhance the quality of life for patients with neurodegenerative or spinal cord disorders. However, scalability, ethical issues and data privacy continue to be significant challenges, as neural data is sensitive. This chapter recapitulates the recent studies in AI-enhanced BCI, addressing the technical approaches, fields of application of the tools and the emerging issues and the necessity to use the tools safely and ethically within an interdisciplinary context.

19.1. Introduction

BCIs connect neuronal processing to external machines by connecting the brain and computer together without the involvement of skeletal muscles (Craik et al. 2019). They hold a lot of potential for those who are motor impaired or those with

Chapter written by Rahul S.S. and Mrudula NIMBARTE.

motor deficiencies, in that they are able to operate computers, prosthetics and assistive devices simply through thoughts. Beyond therapeutic applications, researchers also explore BCIs for cognitive enhancement, gaming, military use, and immersive human–machine interaction. In spite of the accelerated progress of both computational neuroscience and signal-acquisition technologies over the last 20 years, BCIs still have serious issues with accuracy, adaptability and practical application.

Artificial intelligence (AI) is an effective solution to these issues when incorporated into BCIs. Conventional BCIs are based on manual feature extraction and classical machine learning (ML) methods and typically do not represent the nonlinear and dynamic nature of neural signals. The latest AI, and especially deep learning (DL), acquires hierarchic features in large datasets, automatically enhancing neural-signal decoding (Escorcia-Gutierrez et al. 2022). It is also possible to use these AI models to deliver real-time adaptability and make BCIs more accurate and user-friendly.

Signal acquisition is one of the pillars of the development of BCI. Electroencephalography (EEG), functional near-infrared spectroscopy (fNIRS) and magnetoencephalography (MEG) provide a safe and relatively affordable method of monitoring brain activity, although they all tend to have low signal-to-noise ratios and artifacts. More invasive methods such as the electrocorticography (ECoG) and intracortical microelectrodes have better resolution but are more unsafe and not as stable (Roy et al. 2019). A process boosted by AI, such as deep denoising networks, is also being used to remove obtrusions and identify pertinent neural properties in a more efficient manner than its conventional counterparts.

Another important step is to decode the signals captured. Classical algorithms such as linear discriminant analysis (LDA), support vector machines (SVMs) and hidden Markov models have proved prevalent, but they find it difficult to be user adaptive or make non-stationary predictions. Convolutional and recurrent deep neural networks have been demonstrated to have a higher capacity of modeling – both temporal and spatial interaction in neural data (Asgher et al. 2023). These developments enable the use of BCIs in real-world dynamic environments, as opposed to the controlled laboratory settings only.

AI-BICs are not just a technical novelties. Applied in healthcare, they make intuitive use of neuroprosthetics, exoskeleton and communication assistance, and they enable individuals with ALS, spinal cord injuries or paralysis due to a stroke to use them. They are also increasingly used in cognitive monitoring, neurorehabilitation and monitoring neuro-disorders at an early stage. Beyond the medical industry, the integration of AI and BCIs is still expanding the possibilities of entertainment, immersion gaming and virtual reality (VR), and defense and security, where making decisions quickly and having a thorough situational awareness greatly matters (Hossain et al. 2023).

AI-BCIs involve great challenges despite the level of excitement they are stirring. Ethical issues concerning neural-data privacy, autonomy and abuse are the primary issues of research and policy discussion. The few big and uniform datasets of the brain are obstacles to neural network training and extrapolation. Furthermore, DL systems require a lot of computation, which restricts real-time BCI applications, which leads to hardware acceleration and edge AI.

This chapter represents an excellent summary of AI-enhanced BCIs, including their technical basis, usage and issues. Section 19.2 describes the process of acquiring and preprocessing neural signals. Section 19.3 outlines AI-based decoding and feature-extraction techniques. Section 19.4 also describes real-life applications in the medical profession and the rehabilitation process, among others. Section 19.5 will overview the current barriers and future trends with reference to the ethical, computational and scalability issues. With the help of this synthesis, we will be able to showcase the changing nature of the world of AI-enhanced BCIs and their transformational capabilities in various areas.

19.2. Neural signal acquisition and preprocessing

19.2.1. *Neural signal acquisition modalities*

There are both invasive and non-invasive ways of neural acquisition in BCI systems. Some methodologies involve invasive procedures, for example, ECoG and intracortical microelectrodes, where activity is being recorded directly off the cortex. They provide great time and spatial resolution as well as perform well in decoding both motor and sensory signals. Nevertheless, they have the potential of causing surgical complications and infections, as well as prolonged biocompatibility issues (Nicolas-Alonso and Gomez-Gil 2012). Other, safer methods include non-invasive (EEG, fNIRS, MEG and functional magnetic resonance imaging (fMRI)). However, they typically have a poor signal-to-noise ratio and a low spatial resolution (Jiang et al. 2019).

The most popular non-invasive method is EEG. It is cheap, free-sized and provides millisecond time dissemination. It is also susceptible to muscle movement artifacts, eye movements and noise, as well as environmental noise. On the contrary, fNIRS measures the hemodynamic responses via brain activity. It is also not easily affected by electrical interference but is poorer in its temporal resolution. MEG and fMRI are excellent in providing high-packet spatial mapping, but they are prohibited due to their high price, and being stationary and inconvenient to use in real-time. A combination of multiple modalities of hybrid BCIs is hence being designed to overcome complementary strengths (Abiri et al. 2019).

19.2.2. *Challenges in raw signal quality*

Raw neural signals are vulnerable to various distortions, including biological artifacts (e.g. electromyographic or ocular activity) and external noise sources (e.g. power line interference). These distortions complicate signal interpretation and reduce system performance. Traditional preprocessing pipelines rely on filtering techniques such as bandpass filters, independent component analysis (ICA) and common average referencing. While effective to some extent, these approaches often fail in dynamic real-world environments where noise characteristics vary.

Using AI-geared techniques to boost primary signal quality continues to rise. As an example, DL signal CNNs can be trained to eliminate noise while preserving task-relevant features of the signal (Jaipriya and Sriharipriya 2024). In contrast to traditional noise filters, such DL models have the ability to adjust to different artifact situations and can generalize to different sessions and people, thus providing an even greater scalable solution.

19.2.3. *Feature extraction and dimensionality reduction*

During preprocessing, one of the first steps is the extraction of meaningful features from the high-dimensional neural data. In BCI literature, Fourier transforms, wavelet decompositions and common spatial patterns (CSPs) are conventional approaches. However, due to the reliance on handcrafted heuristics, such approaches are prone to intersubject variability.

Conversely, AI-based approaches to feature extraction handle the task considerably better, as they learn to represent the data on their own from raw or lightly processed data. For instance, deep CNNs learn the spatial and temporal patterns of EEG and do the work of recurrent neural networks (RNNs) and long short-term memory (LSTM) for temporal modeling. Furthermore, to enhance efficiency, we can apply dimensionality reduction approaches such as autoencoders and variational autoencoders. These techniques reduce the high-dimensional input data to lower-dimensional latent spaces that are more suited for the classifiers (Merlin Praveena et al. 2022).

19.2.4. *Adaptive preprocessing and personalization*

One of the most persistent challenges in BCIs is inter- and intra-subject variability. Neural patterns differ not only across individuals but also within the same person over time due to fatigue, mood or physiological changes. Static preprocessing pipelines are often inadequate in such contexts. AI-driven adaptive preprocessing frameworks enable dynamic recalibration of filters and feature extractors to accommodate variability.

19.3. AI-driven neural decoding and feature extraction

The systems based on brain–computer interface (BCI) have their foundation in decoding neural activity into meaningful commands. The effectiveness, flexibility and precision of such a decoding process define the success of BCIs in general life. The old pipelines were handcrafted with superficial classifiers, which could be linear disciplined examination (LDA) or help vehicles (SVM). These methods worked well in controlled laboratories and were unable to generalize across individuals, recording sessions and tasks. The implementation of AI, more notably, ML and DL, transformed neural decoding. AI techniques are automatic to learn features, temporal–spatial correlations and personalize themselves to individual users, which significantly enhances performance (Song et al. 2024).

19.3.1. *Classical versus AI-based decoding approaches*

Classical decoding is based on statistical assumptions with regard to neural data. LDA or SVM-based CSPs have been popular in motor-imagery BCIs. They, however, are sensitive to noise, electrode placement and variation of signal as time progresses. Their artificial features (normally made by hand) frequently lack the nonlinear dynamics of the brain. Procedures that make use of AI avoid these problems, where the features are learned directly on raw or minimally processed data (Anumanchipalli et al. 2019).

Convolutional neural networks (CNNs) are used to identify the spatial patterns of EEG or ECoG channel records, whereas RNNs and LSTM networks are used to predict signal development. Newer architectures (attention-based and graph neural networks (GNNs)) are superior to older ones because they incorporate the important feature of modeling connectivity and relationships across electrodes.

19.3.2. *Feature extraction using DL*

The next generation is DL, which has been adopted as the best decoding tool of BCIs. CNNs are fine at identifying spatially local patterns of EEG data. CNN decoders invariably outperform conventional approaches in motor-imaging experiments, i.e. in situations where frequency-specific and electrode-specific cues are involved. RNNs and LSTMs are well suited to the representation of time-varying signals, and hence continuous-control BCIs, such as robotic arm control or speech synthesis, are well represented (Pandarinath et al. 2017). The hybrid CNN-RNN pipelines are the pipelines that pair spatial and temporal extraction, which results in enhanced speed and accuracy. Autoencoders – particularly variational autoencoders (VAEs) – are unsupervised models that learn meaningful features, reduce dimensionality, and preserve task-relevant information.

19.3.3. *Transfer learning and domain adaptation*

The biggest obstacle is inter-subject variability. The reactions of the brain in various individuals vary due to anatomy, physiology and psychology. The model requires time and resources to be trained separately on a case-by-case basis. The solution to this is through transfer learning, which uses a large pretrained dataset and fine-tunes it to a new user. The labeled data required is reduced through this approach (Willett et al. 2021). The methods of domain adaptation, including adversarial neural networks, also enhance the generalization process by matching the distribution of the features in one subject or session with those of the other ones. These techniques accelerate penetration and increase stability of performance over time with regard to BCI.

19.3.4. *Attention-based GNNs and mechanisms*

New developments incorporate the attention and graph-based learning in decoding. Attention allows a model to take note of the most informative time windows, or channels, of electrodes, maximizing interpretability and accuracy. As an illustration, the attention-based RNNs deliver state-of-the-art performance in EEG emotion recognition and motor-imaging classification. GNNs view the brain as interconnected nodes (Mitchell et al. 2023). Functional connectivity establishes edges between electrodes or brain regions. The fact that GNNs can model both spatial and temporal dependence in a graph gives them a biologically reasonable structure, being particularly useful when higher-order cognition is needed, such as decision-making or speech synthesis.

AI technique	Key characteristics	Applications in BCI	Advantages	Limitations
CNN (convolutional neural networks)	Captures spatial features from EEG/ECoG signals	Motor imagery classification, prosthetic control	High spatial accuracy; automatic feature extraction	Sensitive to electrode placement; requires large datasets
RNN/LSTM (recurrent neural networks)	Models' temporal dependencies in signals	Continuous control, speech decoding	Handles time-varying signals effectively	Computationally expensive; slower training
Autoencoders/VAEs	Learns compressed latent representations	Dimensionality reduction, noise removal	Enhances signal clarity; unsupervised learning	Limited interpretability
Graph neural networks (GNNs)	Models brain connectivity as graphs	Emotion recognition, decision-making	Biologically interpretable; captures spatial–temporal relations	Complex architecture; requires connectivity data
Attention-based models	Focus on the most relevant time windows/channels	EEG emotion recognition, adaptive decoding	Improved interpretability; high performance	High computational cost
Reinforcement learning (RL)	Learns adaptively via feedback loops	Motor rehabilitation, prosthetic adaptation	Real-time adaptability; user personalization	Training instability; high data need
Transfer learning	Adapts pre-trained models across subjects	Cross-user generalization, fast calibration	Reduces data requirement; faster deployment	Risk of overfitting to base domain

Table 19.1. *Comparative summary of AI-Based neural decoding techniques in brain–computer interfaces*

19.3.5. *Adaptive and online learning*

BCI usually works in conditions whereby neural signals vary due to fatigue, mood or noises. Under such circumstances, the accuracy of the static AI models is lost. The use of adaptive learning, such as reinforcement learning and online transfer learning, enables models to keep on updating as new information comes in. In motor imagery BCIs, reinforcement learning has maximized feedback loops to help the user engage in the device and learn. The frameworks of online learning optimize models on-the-fly to the changing neural signature of each user. This flexibility is very important in long-term application, particularly in clinical groups where neural activity varies with time as a result of rehabilitation or disease course.

19.3.6. *On the way to real-time neural decoding*

BI research eventually aims at real-time, closed-loop communication. This is achievable using AI-powered decoders that minimize latency and improve robustness. Architectures composed of lightweight components, supported by efficient GPU and neuromorphic chip acceleration, enable real-time decoding for practical applications such as speech synthesis, robotic control, and immersive virtual reality. Neural networks that are obtained through edge computing, i.e. by lightweight neural networks, can minimize the use of cloud servers not only in terms of latency but also in terms of privacy.

19.4. Applications of AI-enhanced BCIs

The opportunities of the BCI application have been magnified by the use of AI, which has enhanced the way we decode signals in the brain, accommodate various users and address noise. BCIs, which were once restricted to the laboratory environment, have been invading real-world environments, particularly in healthcare, rehabilitation, communication, entertainment and defense. The AI and BCI collaboration accelerates the transformation of research concepts and practice-oriented tools, which can enhance human capabilities and recover the functions that have been lost (Moses et al. 2021).

19.4.1. *Medical and neurorehabilitation applications*

19.4.1.1. *Motor rehabilitation*

AI-enhanced BCIs are particularly applicable in motor rehabilitation in stroke affected, spinal cord injured or neurodegenerative disease patients. Traditional approaches rely on repetitive physical exercises, which can sometimes be excessive. Teaching robotic exoskeletons or functional electrical stimulation (FES) through motor intentions, BCIs can be used to detect motor intentions directly and in turn control them (Collinger et al. 2018). The convolutional and recurrent neurons enhance decoding of the motor imagery and the correlated brain signals and thus increasing the performance in rehabilitation.

Recent research indicates that neuroplasticity can be enhanced through AI-driven BCIs because they maintain feedback through a closed loop, which accelerates the recovery process and can sustain long-term benefits. Adaptive algorithms also help customize interventions to the individual neural patterns of a patient; this reduces the amount of training required.

19.4.1.2. *Communication for locked-in patients*

The barrier to effective communication between nurses and locked-in patients is highly noteworthy. Numerous patients face significant risks due to the existing communication challenges enforced by patients as determinants.

BCIs are crucial in the restoration of communication in individuals who have either locked-in syndrome (LIS) or amyotrophic lateral sclerosis (ALS). Classical P300 spellers also create text by means of visual information, although they are not only inaccurate but also have high mental loads (Ajiboye et al. 2017).

The concept of AI-enhanced decoding uses DL to enhance event-related potential (ERP) recognition to provide faster and more effective communication. BI systems that incorporate natural language processing (NLP) forecast words or phrases, reducing the cognitive burden required to construct sentences. The innovations are important in enhancing the quality of life of patients with profound communication challenges.

19.4.1.3. *Cognitive and emotional monitoring*

The applications of AI-BCIs in the context of cognitive monitoring in clinical and non-clinical environments continue to increase. EEG-based BCIs linked to AI classifiers have a high accuracy in determining fatigue, stress and emotional conditions. Application areas encompass psychiatric health and custom therapy, as well as the adaptive learning environment (Flesher et al. 2021). The AI-based neurofeedback BCIs offer insights into brain activity in real-time and are beneficial in the process of treating a patient with depression or anxiety, as they support specific interventions.

19.4.2. *Assistive technologies and neuroprosthetics*

19.4.2.1. *Prosthetic limb control*

One of the central objectives of BCI research has been controlling prosthetic limbs. Motor intentions can be decoded using AI and provide more natural and precise control. CNNs and RNNs will decode delicate neural events related to fine motions, which will allow the control of robotic limbs in the multi-degree-of-freedom (Benabid et al. 2019). The learning in reinforcement also hones down prosthetic techniques, allowing the systems to constantly evolve based on the preferences of the users.

19.4.2.2. *Intelligent wheelchairs and mobility aids*

AI-BCIs are not only limited to the field of prosthetic but also include mobility aids such as smart wheelchairs. The user is able to control wheelchairs without using a manual or voice control, instead the wheelchair deciphers neural signals to navigate. AI enhances better results in classifications, particularly in noisy conditions, which makes navigation safe. Blended systems comprising the integration of computer vision and AI obstacle detectors with BCIs allow individuals with severe motor disabilities to move.

19.4.3. *Human–computer interaction and entertainment*

19.4.3.1. *Immersive virtual and augmented reality*

BCIs with AI improvements are becoming more often embedded into VR and augmented reality (AR). These BCIs can currently alter VR/AR content in real-time, based on the decoded neural signals of attention, engagement or emotional valence to make the content more engaging. Indicatively, AI models can detect when a user is tired or distracted and reduce or increase the level of difficulty in the task (Lebedev and Nicolelis 2017).

Such applications do not only cover gaming. The AI-driven neuroadaptive systems in education, military and healthcare can be used to tailor virtual training to enhance learning. They provide personalized experiences, which react to the mental state of a user in real-time.

19.4.3.2. *Gaming and entertainment interfaces*

In the gaming industry, BCIs represent the next frontier of user interaction. AI decoding of neural signals allows players to control in-game actions through thought, creating novel gameplay experiences. Emotion recognition BCIs also enable adaptive storytelling and interactive narratives where the plot responds to the player's emotional state (Polo-Hortigüela et al. 2025).

The combination of BCIs with AI-based content generation models further enhances engagement by enabling personalized entertainment tailored to the user's mental and emotional profile.

19.4.4. *Defense and security applications*

19.4.4.1. *Cognitive augmentation for soldiers*

Defense organizations are exploring AI-enhanced BCIs for augmenting soldier performance in high-stress environments. BCIs can monitor cognitive load, situational awareness and fatigue, providing real-time feedback to optimize decision-making. AI-driven models ensure accurate detection of neural states in complex environments, where noise and stress would otherwise compromise reliability (Machado et al. 2013).

19.4.4.2. *Drone and robotic control*

AI-integrated BCIs are being piloted for the control of drones and other robotic systems for military and security purposes. BCI systems, unlike manual and voice-command systems, facilitate rapid and intuitive command execution. Under difficult circumstances, AI systems can confidently determine intent, which could provide significant advantages in military and emergency response situations.

19.4.5. *Education and workplace applications*

19.4.5.1. *Neuroadaptive learning systems*

In education, the use of AI-enhanced BCIs is fostering the creation of neuroadaptive learning systems. These systems monitor brain activity to evaluate classroom attention, engagement and understanding in real-time. Based on this information, AI adjusts the customer learning materials and personalizes instruction to optimize learning efficiency (Tonin et al. 2025).

These systems are particularly beneficial for individuals with learning disabilities, offering adaptive and flexible support for cognitive development.

19.4.5.2. *Brain-to-brain communication*

Recent studies indicate that the direct brain-to-brain communication can be achieved using AI-enhanced BCIs. These systems transmit deciphered neuronal signals between individuals, although they are still experimental and deciphered, which enables individuals to collaborate to solve problems or gain control of the devices. To complete the efficient transmission and decoding of signals among users, the assistance of AI is required (Khan et al. 2021).

19.5. Challenges, ethical considerations and future directions

Even though the gains made by AI-driven BCIs have been quite impressive, it is important to note that there are several hurdles hindering their wide usage. These barriers cut across technical, ethical, legal and social levels. The introduction of AI to BCIs presents unique issues regarding the privacy of data, bias and interpretability and long-term safety. Introduction of laboratory prototypes into the real world also requires cost, infrastructure and regulatory control solutions. We identify these challenges in this section, mention ethical concerns and encourage future directions.

19.5.1. *Technical challenges*

19.5.1.1. *Data scarcity and variability*

AI models typically require large amounts of labeled data to achieve high performance. However, the collection of large-scale neural datasets is constrained by practical, ethical and financial limitations. Neural signals exhibit high inter-subject and intra-subject variability, which complicates the generalization of models. The scarcity of standardized, open-access datasets further hampers the training and benchmarking of AI models across different laboratories and applications (Roy et al. 2019).

19.5.1.2. *Signal quality and robustness*

Neural activity always contains noise and may be corrupted by muscle and movement activity or outside factors. To some extent, AI-based methods have improved the quality of the signals. From a practical standpoint, however, the outdoor and prolonged use of such systems poses unpredictable challenges to the system's robustness. This continues to provide obstacles for reliable decoding.

19.5.1.3. *Computational and energy constraints*

In the case of real-time BCIs, the systems have to be designed for the requisite quick and efficient decoding. This is a challenge, not only because DL systems are inherently more computationally intensive but also because their use in wearables and implantable devices triggers questions surrounding latency, resource use and the feasibility of the necessary hardware. Although edge AI and neuromorphic computing are offered as possible answers, their practical use in BCI systems is still in the very preliminary stage of development (Khan et al. 2019).

19.5.2. *Ethical and societal considerations*

19.5.2.1. *Privateness and safety of neural data*

Neural signals are one of the highly vulnerable types of personal data. They express motives, feelings and subconscious activity. Privacy invasion in this area caused by unauthorized access may be unparalleled. Thus, it is essential to keep the storage, transmission and processing safe. AI models are not any simpler; they may incorporate sensitive data due to their model inversion or an adversarial attack, as mentioned in (Ligthart et al.).

19.5.2.2. *Autonomy and agency*

This has the potential of influencing user autonomy through AI-based BCIs. Algorithms that make predictions about intentions may lead to the consideration of intentions, which are not particularly focused between choices. There must be a balance where both the system and the user control the unit so that agency and trust are maintained.

19.5.2.3. *Bias and fairness*

The models of AI that are trained on biased datasets can stabilize inequalities. There can be the underrepresentation of cultural, gender or neurological diversity with the result of disproportionate performance. To overcome the prejudices, it is necessary to include data and provide equal algorithms that should be generalized and cover users.

19.5.2.4. *Psychological and social effects*

BCIs are able to change the self of the users. The blurring of the boundary between the biological and the technological agency poses psychological challenges to adaptation in cases of patients who resort to the use of BCIs to manage their prosthetics or even their communication devices. Neural technology overused in non-medical settings (gaming or workplace surveillance) may have an impact on social life.

19.5.3. *Regulatory and legal challenges*

Regulation of AI-enabled BCI remains in its infancy. Accurate risk assessment models such as the ones that have been implemented by the European Medicines

Agency (EMA) and the US Food and Drug Administration (FDA) provide some guidelines but fail to cover the specific risks linked to the neural technologies. The questions regarding the safety of the long-term implants, continuous software updates and liability in the case of the system malfunctioning have not yet been answered (Yuste et al. 2017).

Intellectual property rights over neural data and AI models also present complex legal questions. For example, if an AI-decoded neural signal generates creative content, questions of authorship and ownership arise. Similarly, in defense applications, accountability for AI-driven BCI actions must be clearly defined to avoid ethical gray zones.

19.5.4. *Future directions*

19.5.4.1. *Advances in neural interfaces*

Future research is likely to focus on developing less invasive yet high-resolution neural interfaces. Emerging technologies such as flexible bioelectronics, optogenetic interfaces and ultrasound-based neural recording promise to improve signal fidelity while reducing risks associated with traditional implants (Li et al. 2020). AI models tailored for these new modalities will be critical for unlocking their full potential.

19.5.4.2. *Multimodal and hybrid systems*

Combining multiple biosignals (e.g. EEG, fNIRS, electromyography (EMG), eye tracking) can compensate for the limitations of individual modalities. AI is particularly well suited for fusing multimodal data, extracting synergistic features and improving robustness. Hybrid systems could enable richer and more reliable interactions in real-world settings, from healthcare to entertainment.

19.5.4.3. *Explainable and trustworthy AI*

One of the barriers to clinical adoption is the "black-box" nature of DL models. Explainable AI (XAI) techniques can provide insights into why specific neural patterns are associated with certain outputs, enhancing trust among clinicians and users. Transparent models will also facilitate regulatory approval and reduce resistance to adoption.

19.6. Conclusion

The combination of AI and BCIs will be a revolutionary leap in the human–machine interaction. Through highly sophisticated ML and DL algorithms, AI enhances the neural-signal decoding process by lowering the noise enhancing real-time flexibility. The advances increase the usability and reliability of BCIs. Such advances have put BCIs out of the laboratory and into the field in healthcare, rehabilitation, communication, game and defense. BCIs that are being enhanced by AI are likely to not only provide motor performance, allow assistive communication and create immersive experiences but also better understand the brain. Nevertheless, the discipline continues to experience immense problems. The scale and confidence of BCIs require the solution of technical issues such as data insufficiency, subject variability and insufficient computing capacity. There are also ethical, legal and social issues, which may be related to gathering, analyzing and using sensitive neural data. Innovation must focus on privacy, fairness and autonomy of the users. The future is projected to have additional enhancements of BCI capped with emerging hardware, integration of multimodal signal reading and XAI.

19.7. References

Abiri, R., Borhani, S., Sellers, E.W., Jiang, Y., Zhao, X. (2019). A comprehensive review of EEG-based brain–computer interface paradigms. *Journal of Neural Engineering*, 16(1), 011001.

Ajiboye, A.B., Willett, F.R., Young, D.R., Memberg, W.D., Murphy, B.A., Miller, J.P., Walter, B.L., Sweet, J.A., Hoyen, H.A., Keith, M.W. et al. (2017). Restoration of reaching and grasping movements through brain-controlled muscle stimulation in a person with tetraplegia: A proof-of-concept demonstration. *The Lancet*, 389(10081), 1821–1830.

Anumanchipalli, G.K., Chartier, J., Chang, E.F. (2019). Speech synthesis from neural decoding of spoken sentences. *Nature*, 568(7753), 493–498.

Asgher, U., Ayaz, Y., Taiar, R. (2023). Advances in artificial intelligence (AI) in brain computer interface (BCI) and Industry 4.0 for human machine interaction (HMI). *Frontiers in Human Neuroscience*, 17, 1320536.

Benabid, A.L., Costecalde, T., Eliseyev, A., Charvet, G., Verney, A., Karakas, S., Foerster, M., Lambert, A., Morinière, B., Abroug, N. et al. (2019). An exoskeleton controlled by an epidural wireless brain–machine interface in a tetraplegic patient: A proof-of-concept demonstration. *The Lancet Neurology*, 18(12), 1112–1122.

Collinger, J.L., Gaunt, R.A., Schwartz, A.B. (2018). Progress towards restoring upper limb movement and sensation through intracortical brain-computer interfaces. *Current Opinion in Biomedical Engineering*, 8, 84–92.

Craik, A., He, Y., Contreras-Vidal, J.L. (2019). Deep learning for electroencephalogram (EEG) classification tasks: A review. *Journal of Neural Engineering*, 16(3), 031001.

Escorcia-Gutierrez, J., Beleno, K., Jimenez-Cabas, J., Elhoseny, M., Alshehri, M.D., Selim, M.M. (2022). An automated deep learning enabled brain signal classification for epileptic seizure detection on complex measurement systems. *Measurement*, 196, 111226.

Flesher, S.N., Downey, J.E., Weiss, J.M., Hughes, C.L., Herrera, A.J., Tyler-Kabara, E.C., Boninger, M.L., Collinger, J.L., Gaunt, R.A. (2021). A brain-computer interface that evokes tactile sensations improves robotic arm control. *Science*, 372(6544), 831–836.

Hossain, K.M., Islam, M.A., Hossain, S., Nijholt, A., Ahad, M.A. (2023). Status of deep learning for EEG-based brain–computer interface applications. *Frontiers in Computational Neuroscience*, 16, 1006763.

Jaipriya, D. and Sriharipriya, K.C. (2024). Brain computer interface-based signal processing techniques for feature extraction and classification of motor imagery using EEG: A literature review. *Biomedical Materials & Devices*, 2(2), 601–613.

Jiang, X., Bian, G.B., Tian, Z. (2019). Removal of artifacts from EEG signals: A review. *Sensors*, 19(5), 987.

Khan, W.Z., Ahmed, E., Hakak, S., Yaqoob, I., Ahmed, A. (2019). Edge computing: A survey. *Future Generation Computer Systems*, 97, 219–235.

Khan, H., Naseer, N., Yazidi, A., Eide, P.K., Hassan, H.W., Mirtaheri, P. (2021). Analysis of human gait using hybrid EEG-fNIRS-based BCI system: A review. *Frontiers in Human Neuroscience*, 14, 613254.

Lebedev, M.A. and Nicolelis, M.A. (2017). Brain-machine interfaces: From basic science to neuroprostheses and neurorehabilitation. *Physiological Reviews*, 97(2), 767–837.

Li, H., Wang, J., Fang, Y. (2020). Bioinspired flexible electronics for seamless neural interfacing and chronic recording. *Nanoscale Advances*, 2(8), 3095–3102.

Ligthart, S., Ienca, M., Meynen, G., Molnar-Gabor, F., Andorno, R., Bublitz, C., Catley, P., Rainey, S., Kellmeyer, P. et al. (2023). Minding rights: Mapping ethical and legal foundations of 'neurorights'. *Camb. Q Healthc. Ethics*, 15, 1–21. doi: 10.1017/S0963180123000245..

Machado, S., Almada, L.F., Annavarapu, R.N. (2013). Progress and prospects in EEG-based brain–computer interface: Clinical applications in neurorehabilitation. *Journal of Rehabilitation*, 1(1), 29.

Merlin Praveena, D., Angelin Sarah, D., Thomas George, S. (2022). Deep learning techniques for EEG signal applications – a review. *IETE Journal of Research*, 68(4), 3030–3037.

Mitchell, P., Lee, S.C., Yoo, P.E., Morokoff, A., Sharma, R.P., Williams, D.L., MacIsaac, C., Howard, M.E., Irving, L., Vrljic, I. et al. (2023). Assessment of safety of a fully implanted endovascular brain–computer interface for severe paralysis in 4 patients: The stentrode with thought-controlled digital switch (SWITCH) study. *JAMA Neurology*, 80(3), 270–278.

Moses, D.A., Metzger, S.L., Liu, J.R., Anumanchipalli, G.K., Makin, J.G., Sun, P.F., Chartier, J., Dougherty, M.E., Liu, P.M., Abrams, G.M. et al. (2021). Neuroprosthesis for decoding speech in a paralyzed person with anarthria. *New England Journal of Medicine*, 385(3), 217–227.

Nicolas-Alonso, L.F. and Gomez-Gil, J. (2012). Brain computer interfaces, a review. *Sensors*, 12(2), 1211–1279.

Pandarinath, C., Nuyujukian, P., Blabe, C.H., Sorice, B.L., Saab, J., Willett, F.R., Hochberg, L.R., Shenoy, K.V., Henderson, J.M. (2017). High performance communication by people with paralysis using an intracortical brain-computer interface. *eLife*, 6, e18554.

Polo-Hortigüela, C., Ortiz, M., Soriano-Segura, P., Iáñez, E., Azorín, J.M. (2025). Time-frequency analysis of motor imagery during plantar and dorsal flexion movements using a low-cost ankle exoskeleton. *Sensors*, 25(10), 2987.

Roy, Y., Banville, H., Albuquerque, I., Gramfort, A., Falk, T.H., Faubert, J. (2019). Deep learning-based electroencephalography analysis: A systematic review. *Journal of Neural Engineering*, 16(5), 051001.

Song, J., Zhai, Q., Wang, C., Liu, J. (2024). EEGGAN-Net: Enhancing EEG signal classification through data augmentation. *Frontiers in Human Neuroscience*, 18, 1430086.

Tonin, A., Semprini, M., Kiper, P., Mantini, D. (2025). Brain–computer interfaces for stroke motor rehabilitation. *Bioengineering*, 12(8), 820.

Willett, F.R., Avansino, D.T., Hochberg, L.R., Henderson, J.M., Shenoy, K.V. (2021). High-performance brain-to-text communication via handwriting. *Nature*, 593(7858), 249–254.

Yuste, R., Goering, S., Arcas, B.A., Bi, G., Carmena, J.M., Carter, A., Fins, J.J., Friesen, P., Gallant, J., Huggins, J.E. et al. (2017). Four ethical priorities for neurotechnologies and AI. *Nature*, 551(7679), 159–163.

20

The Future of AI in Neurology: Innovations, Challenges and Strategic Directions

Artificial intelligence (AI) is an increasingly popular technology that is transforming contemporary medicine, particularly the area of neurology. Neurological diseases present a great burden to the population. They have complicated causes, courses and limited treatment opportunities. AI brings the benefits of diagnosing, predicting, personalizing and the long-term management of patients. With machine learning, deep learning and the combination of multiple types of data, AI can find hidden imaging facts, predict disease outcomes and assist clinicians in making more rational decisions in less time. Digital health technologies based on AI, including wearability devices and mobile apps, transform how patients are watched and rehabilitated to enable them to play a more active role. However, there are actual obstacles in AI in the field of neurology. The challenges that need to be tackled are the standardization of data, transparency, as well as the fairness of algorithms, interpretability, bias and safeguarding privacy and clarifying clinician responsibility. Validation and regulation procedures also should keep abreast of the rapid changes in technologies. Success in the future will rely on collaboration across various spheres, a stable infrastructure and equitable access to the technology all over the world. This chapter is a review of the most recent advances, obstacles and future plans in AI in neurology, with the emphasis placed on imaging, predictive analytics, digital therapies and ethics. The findings demonstrate that it is critical to adopt AI in a balanced way, considering the benefits of patients, as well as the technical, ethical and systemic barriers.

20.1. Introduction

Neurological complications form one of the biggest global health burdens. They are the cause of disability-adjusted life years (DALYs) and affect hundreds of millions of people across the world. Diseases such as Alzheimer's, dysfunction,

Chapter written by Sunil Ramrao YADAV and Mrudula NIMBARTE.

stroke, epilepsy and traumatic brain injury are difficult to manage by healthcare systems due to their complexity, diversity and unpredictability (Feigin et al. 2020). Traditional diagnosis and treatment rely upon clinical knowledge, neuroimaging and invasive studies. These methods are not time-efficient, and they are not sensitive or even specific. The incidence of neurological diseases is increasing with an increasing aging population, so there is an acute need to seek new ways of diagnosis, prognosis and treatment.

Machine learning (ML), deep learning (DL), natural language processing (NLP) and artificial intelligence (AI) are changing the field of medicine. They can be applied to epidemiology and neurology, auto-neuroimaging interpretation and disease progression prediction and individualized therapy prescription. Contrary to traditional statistical applications, AI is capable of working with large, non-homogeneous datasets of medical images, electrophysiological data, genomic data, patient feedback, etc. at a scale and speed that is entirely beyond human capabilities (Topol 2019). This could make AI a keystone for exploiting neurology, where healthcare routes are built based on intricate data aggregation.

One of the possible promising fields of AI application is neuroimaging. High-level DL methods are able to identify hidden radiographical biomarkers, which could be overlooked by human specialists. As an illustration, when trained on massive datasets, convolutional neural networks (CNNs) have a high accuracy in distinguishing between a normal and a pathological brain structure. Electroencephalogram (EEG) and magnetoencephalography (MEG) data are being exposed to AI models, which could be used to advance epilepsy monitoring and seizure prediction.

Another up-and-coming field is digital health. Mobile apps and wearable devices that are powered by AI and constantly monitor neurological operations are now part of our day-to-day lives. These systems are able to monitor movement, speech and thought and identify when a disease is progressing and aid in adaptive treatments. Even further, the integration of AI into electronic health records (EHRs) assists clinicians by merging the history of the patient and the tests and outcomes into useful information (Roy et al. 2019).

Despite the availability of these opportunities, the application of AI in neurology is characterized by a variety of challenges. Health equity, algorithm transparency, clinical validation and data confidentiality are not established. There are numerous AI models that are black box, which can lead to issues of trust, responsibility and regulatory acceptance. Since neurology has life-altering effects, there must be an adherence to safety, reliability and ethics (Yin et al. 2021).

This chapter reviews the future of AI in the field of neurology by exploring the existing advances, the most significant challenges and requirements in striving to achieve strategic needs in responsible clinical use. It explains the use of AI in diagnostics, prognosis, therapies and rehabilitation and also highlights the ethical and systemic issues that are required to make the use of AI sustainable. This chapter will help clinical professionals, scientists and policymakers navigate the fluctuating relationship between AI and neurology and provide an overview of the recent advancements and actionable points.

20.2. AI in neurological diagnostics

Proper and timely diagnosis is one of the most significant problems in neurology. Numerous neurological illnesses are similar to one another, with an insidious onset, or a differing course of progression in patients. Conventional methods such as magnetic resonance imaging (MRI), computed tomography (CT), positron emission tomography (PET), electroencephalogram (EEG) and neuropsychological testing are essential, although generally not sensitive and specific, particularly at the onset of the disease process. The AI system, due to its sophisticated pattern-recognition tools, has become an effective addition to support the accuracy needed in the diagnosis of many of the neurological diagnoses.

20.2.1. *AI in neuroimaging*

One of the earliest and most successful places in which AI has had a presence in the field of neurology is neuroimaging. DL, and in particular CNNs, are effective in the segmentation of brain structures, detection of abnormalities and disease classification. When applied in a stroke care setting, CNN models are capable of detecting ischemic lesions in CT scans with an accuracy that can match custom radiologists, reducing the time to initiate treatment. Similarly, automated analysis of MRI can identify all lesions of multiple sclerosis (MS) and thus give accurate measurements and reduce inter-observer variability (Amirian et al. 2025).

In the case of neurodegenerative disease such as Alzheimer's, multi-imaging AI models (such as structural MRI, functional Magnetic Resonance Imaging (fMRI) and PET) can identify the early signs of brain injury well before patients show any symptoms. This assists in grouping the patients in clinical research and scheduling preventive care. It is also useful in Parkinson's disease (PD): DL models can identify when a specific part of the brain, which contains a lot of dopamine, is altered, as shown by PET and single-photon emission computed tomography (SPECT) images.

20.2.2. *Electrophysiological diagnostics through AI*

AI is also effective in imaging-based power assays, particularly in electrophysiological analyses. EEG and MEG record brain activity in real-time but generates huge, multimodal data, which is difficult to analyze manually. ML models are excellent at discovering latent patterns. When used in epilepsy they are able to identify interictal spikes, locate the seizure focus and even predict the seizures minutes in advance (Truong et al. 2018). These benefits enhance treatment and assist in planning surgery on patients whose seizures are unresponsive to medication.

In addition, AI-based EEG may be used to distinguish between psychiatric and neurological conditions, for example, minor depression versus initial dementia. The application of AI with evoked potentials is also used to diagnose MS since they identify small evidence of demyelination.

20.2.3. *Cognitive and behavioral diagnostics AI*

Conventional neuropsychology relies on subjective scoring, which may have inconsistencies among examiners. AI provides objective and standard measures through the analysis of speech, movement and the performance of a task. Examples of biomarkers of Alzheimer's identified by NLP models include word-finding problems and simplified syntax. AI studies of handwriting, gait and fine-motor tasks in those with PD compared to normal aging also make the difference (Fraser et al. 2015). This can be extended to mobile applications and wearables, which can notify of an early loss of neurological functioning by continuously monitoring voice, sleep or movement. Indicatively, accelerometers have been used with ML to pick up subtle motor changes in the pre-symptomatic phase of Parkinson's to treat the disease earlier.

20.2.4. *AI in uncommon and complex neurological diseases*

Symptoms in neurological conditions are often variable, and there is a lack of awareness about them, resulting in a slow diagnosis of rare neurological disorders. Imaging and genetic data have been combined with clinical information to create AI systems capable of diagnosing patients faster because patient data is compared to vast database collections. Indicatively, machine-trained models, which analyze MRI, can successfully categorize leukodystrophies and other infrequent neurodevelopmental disorders (Voigtlaender et al. 2024). Genomic AI systems can be used to detect disease-causing variants, which can be particularly helpful with inherited disorders.

20.2.5. *Multimodal and integrated diagnostics*

Multimodal and integrated diagnostics is another area that is experiencing intense development within HRI circles.

The multimodal integration of AI into neurology is the next step to be taken. Rather than performing a single analysis on the data type alone, sophisticated AI systems combine neuroimaging, electrophysiology, genomics, biomarkers and electronic health data to create a multi-faceted diagnosis. As an example, when structural MRI and cerebral fluid biomarkers are integrated using AI, they enhance the diagnosis of Alzheimer's compared to both individually. Similarly, by combining gait data collected by wearable technology with clinical data, the sensitivity of wearables to Parkinsonian syndromes is also enhanced (Goudarzi et al. 2025). Precision medicine is also supported with these integrated models, where they detect patient-specific phenotypes. Due to the ongoing development of AI, the capacity to produce various inputs will probably alter the criteria of neurological diagnosis.

20.2.6. *Clinical translation and current limitations*

While AI has demonstrated significant promise in diagnostic applications, clinical translation remains restricted. Most models are developed on retrospective datasets with limited generalizability across populations. Biases in training data can reduce performance in underrepresented groups, potentially exacerbating healthcare disparities (Meskó and Görög 2020).

20.3. AI in prognosis and disease progression modeling

One of the most demanding and, at the same time, the most important aspects of neurology is prognostication. Most neurological diseases have an unpredictable course of evolution, a fluctuating speed of the process, relapse or recovery. Predictions at the population level using statistics and personal experience are standard by clinicians, yet the tools might fail to capture individual variations. Longitudinal data and multimodal data can be analyzed by AI.

20.3.1. *Predicting cognitive decline in Alzheimer's disease*

Alzheimer's disease (AD) and associated dementias are conditions in which determining the next step is vital in the treatment of the patients. Predictors such as the common biomarkers, like amyloid-2 and tau imaging, are only partially predictive and ignore all the variations in the disease progression (Luppi et al. 2023).

AI models incorporating imaging, fluid biomarkers and genetic information have a greater ability to predict the time when a person with mild cognitive impairment (MCI) is going to get AD. DL techniques applied over long-term periods are capable of detecting subtle changes in the brain long before overt cognitive deterioration occurs, providing opportunities to intervene earlier and select clinical-trial populations.

NLP is also useful to predict disease based on the speech and writing styles of people. Minor language changes can inform on future cognitive impairment, to which imaging predictors can be added. These AI applications are more frequently being applied in remote follow-up of at-risk individuals.

20.3.2. *Progression modeling in PD*

The progression of PD varies significantly across individuals, with some patients experiencing rapid decline while others maintain relative stability for years. ML algorithms have been used to predict motor and non-motor symptom trajectories based on wearable sensor data, neuroimaging and genetic profiles (Ferrante et al. 2025). For example, recurrent neural networks (RNNs) trained on longitudinal gait data can forecast motor deterioration, guiding therapeutic adjustments such as deep brain stimulation (DBS) settings.

20.3.3. *Stroke recovery prediction*

Stroke is among the leading causes of disability in the world. The information about how a patient is going to be treated is imperative in the planning of their rehabilitation. The use of such tools as the National Institutes of Health Stroke Scale provides the approximate estimates but fails to focus on personal differences. AI models that evaluate acute images, demographic and clinical variables have demonstrated improved validity to differentiate a patient who will be functionally independent three to six months following a stroke (Heo et al. 2019).

DL algorithms learning with CT perfusions and MRI scans have the potential to approximate the growth of an infarct and the amount of penumbra that can be preserved. This is information that facilitates individualized acute treatment programs. Furthermore, AI models can be trained using rehabilitation data that can confidently predict patient response to physical, occupational or speech therapy, which can be used to personalize patient rehabilitation suggestions.

20.3.4. *MS prognosis*

MS is a progressive disease that arises following several stages of advancement of myelin sheath infiltration and inflammation of the central nervous system.

MS demonstrates a very diverse range of disease courses, both mild and in the form of rapid progression and disabilities. The frequency of relapse and alteration of lesion loads through time and long-term disability accumulation have been predicted using ML methods. Indicatively, MRI lesion feature models paired with immunological biomarkers are more effective in predicting relapse than the traditional feature prediction models (Eitel et al. 2019).

Prognostic models of MS can also be used to make a choice of treatment. Disease-modifying treatment is more effective in some patients than in others. Predicting the course of every patient, AI will help clinicians to choose the most appropriate approach that will be beneficial and risk-free.

20.3.5. *Prognostic models and their applications to clinical practice*

The true advantage of AI prognosis is with implementation into daily care. Clinical decision-providers based on AI have the potential to provide real-time prognostic feedback at the bedside. As an example, AI dashboards integrating the history of a patient, imaging and biomarkers can show the risk score of disability or relapse in the future, enabling clinicians to tailor interventions (Esteva et al. 2019).

However, there are a number of barriers to extensive use. Various models are trained using homogeneous populations, which limits their use in different populations. Besides that, some AI models are too intricate, which makes them difficult to interpret, and clinicians must have confidence in the predictions to act. Explainable artificial intelligence (XAI) methods focus on making the reasoning transparent, which improves the confidence of clinicians.

20.4. AI in therapeutics and rehabilitation

20.4.1. *AI in pharmacological and therapeutic development*

The process of drug discovery and optimization of therapy is becoming extremely popular with AI. The reason as to why neurological diseases are difficult to treat is due to the complexity of the central nervous system and slow drug penetration through the blood–brain barrier as well as the different reactions among patients. Conventional drug development is costly and time-consuming since it can take over a decade before a compound is brought to market. AI is able to increase the speed of these procedures by predicting drug-to-target interactions, repurposing current compounds and modeling clinical outcomes (Vamathevan et al. 2019).

In one example, DL predictors are used to filter large libraries of chemicals as treatments to help treat AD by targeting amyloid-2 protein and tau. In the case of PD, AI applications process the genomic and proteomic data to propose neuroprotective and symptom-reducing drugs. Drug repurposing based on ML finds new uses for drugs, reducing the cost and time of development.

AI is also useful in personalized medicine. AI systems use a combination of genetic, biomarker and clinical data to make predictions of individual reactions. Predictive models are used in epilepsy so that the drug can be predictive of the patient's response to antiseizure drugs, thus decreasing the trial-and-error-treatment of the disease (Yao et al. 2019). Among other things, dosing regimens are also optimized, resulting in increased efficacy and reduced side effects.

AI is beneficial in invasive therapies. In the DBS of PD and dystonia, AI models are used to optimize the position of electrodes, as well as electrode stimulation parameters. In adaptive DBS systems, neural feedback is used to change the stimulation with real-time AI algorithms, which may result in better symptom control and a reduction in side effects.

20.4.2. *Neurorehabilitation with AI*

Neurology rehabilitation is one of the foundations of neurology, particularly in patients who have suffered a stroke, traumatic brain injury or progressive neurological conditions such as MS. Standard rehab is based on the manual use of therapists, where it does not have the capacity to be personalized or to undergo constant observation. AI-powered technologies, including robotics, virtual reality (VR) and wearables are redesigning this picture.

20.4.2.1. *Robotics-assisted rehabilitation*

Assistive devices, robot exoskeletons and other gadgets are increasingly being paired with AI algorithms to improve motor recovery. These systems can customize the intensity of training and patterns of movement to the progress of the patient, providing individualized rehabilitation programs (Kumthornthip et al. 2024). For stroke victims, AI-controlled robot arms and gait trainers provide highly intensive repetitive training that is difficult to obtain with traditional treatment. Biomechanical data can be analyzed with embedded ML models that could refine assistance and facilitate independence progressively.

20.4.2.2. *Virtual and augmented reality*

AI has been developed into VR and auxiliary reality (AR) settings, which are becoming popular for neurological rehabilitation. Gamified experiences and immersion increase patient adherence, as well as patient engagement in therapy programs. AI models control performance, task adaptation to cognitive or motor capacity and real-time feedback. In the case of PD, VR-based gait training is beneficial in terms of balance and mobility (Arntz et al. 2023). Cognitive VR exercises help stroke patients to activate their memory, recall and executive functioning.

20.4.2.3. *Remote rehabilitation and wearables*

Continuous monitoring of motor and physiological parameters is made possible by wearable sensors, i.e. accelerators, gyroscopes, electromyography (EMG) devices, which allow patients to be monitored outside of the clinic. Together with AI analytics, they allow the real-time evaluation of a patient's status and rehabilitation plans can be changed remotely (Vanmechelen et al. 2023). To set an example, AI programs that analyze gait behaviors can also identify slight improvements or degradations in stroke victims to intervene in time. Remote rehabilitation is also made easier through remote monitoring, particularly where there are underserved areas with limited access to specialists.

20.4.3. *Therapeutic AI implementation issues*

Although they have potential, AI-based therapeutics and rehabilitation devices have barriers to their adoption. The limited high-quality CNS-specific data, the biological complexity of neurological disorders and the difficulty in clinically validating AI-specific targets are all barriers to pharmacological applications. In rehabilitation, high prices, the technological literacy of patients and inconsistent access to cutting-edge equipment limit the usage of AI.

The unregulated environment where there is no standardization is also an issue facing AI. Real-time DBS or robotic platforms are adaptive AI systems that must be carefully validated with regard to safety. The inclusion of digital therapeutics into healthcare systems requires interoperability with EHRs and reimbursement models that consider digital therapeutics.

20.4.4. *The new paradigm of individualized neurotherapeutics*

As a prospective solution, AI in therapeutics and rehabilitation is expected to have a converging point of holistic care and an individualized model. Through the incorporation of pharmacological optimization and adaptive rehabilitation, AI may be used to prescribe holistic treatment plans where each patient is treated according to the profile of the patient. As an example, a stroke patient may be targeted with an AI-predicted thrombolytic treatment, AI-controlled gait training performed by robots, monitored using wearables and constantly controlled by forecasting algorithms.

This paradigm has improved results, and neurology has moved to a precision rehabilitation model wherein the therapy is adapted according to the increasing patient requirements. Table 20.1 shows the applications of AI in neurology: domains, approaches and clinical impact.

Neurological domain	AI techniques used	Key applications	Clinical benefits	Challenges/ limitations
Neuroimaging diagnostics	CNNs, 3D U-Nets, transfer learning	MRI/CT lesion detection in stroke, tumor, MS; Alzheimer's biomarker detection via PET/fMRI	Rapid, automated image interpretation; early diagnosis; reduced observer bias	Dataset heterogeneity; model generalizability
Electrophysiology (EEG/MEG)	RNNs, CNNs, ensemble ML, SVM	Epileptic seizure prediction; focus localization; differentiation of psychiatric vs. neurological disorders	Real-time analysis; pre-seizure alerts; improved surgical planning	Noise, inter-subject variability
Cognitive and behavioral analysis	NLP, computer vision, random forests	Speech and handwriting analysis for Alzheimer's, Parkinson's	Objective cognitive assessment; early biomarkers	Requires large labeled datasets; language bias
Prognosis and disease progression	Deep learning, LSTM, Bayesian ML	Predicting cognitive decline (AD), relapse (MS), stroke recovery	Personalized risk prediction; better rehabilitation planning	Interpretability; limited longitudinal data

Therapeutic optimization	Deep learning, reinforcement learning	Drug repurposing; treatment response prediction (epilepsy, PD)	Shorter drug development cycles; personalized dosing	Biological complexity; validation required
Neurorehabilitation	Robotics + ML, VR/AR + AI, wearables + DL	Robotic-assisted motor recovery; cognitive VR training; telerehabilitation	Personalized therapy; remote monitoring; enhanced engagement	Cost; accessibility; regulatory validation
Ethical and systemic AI	XAI, federated learning, fairness-aware ML	Explainable models; privacy-preserving training; bias mitigation	Improved clinician trust; equitable AI use	Technical complexity; limited global adoption

Table 20.1. *Applications of artificial intelligence in neurology: domains, approaches and clinical impact*

20.5. Challenges and ethical considerations

20.5.1. *Technical challenges*

20.5.1.1. *Data quality and standardization*

The models created by AI require large amounts and high-quality training and validation data. Such datasets in the field of neurology are commonly shared across facilities, use varying imaging regimes and are not commonly annotated. As an example, brain MRI results at different hospitals can differ in terms of their resolution or acquisition parameters, decreasing the generalizability of a model. The data also lacks representation of rare neurological disorders, thereby crippling the performance of algorithms among such patients. The inconsistency in the accuracy of AI tools across the different clinical settings depends on the absence of standardized data pipelines.

20.5.1.2. *Algorithm bias and generalizability*

AI prejudice is a grave issue. In situations where the data used in training is biased towards certain groups such as individuals in affluent nations, or even a certain ethnicity, the AI can provide misrepresentations when applied to other individuals (Char et al. 2018). This exacerbates health disparities, particularly in the field of neurology, wherein disparities in African and American regions and populations vary according to disease patterns. Models fail miserably in practical life where real-world data is less ideal than laboratory data.

20.5.1.3. *Interpretability and explainability*

Deep learning (DL) models are not only highly powerful but are also often described as "black boxes." They make precise predictions but fail to demonstrate how they come to their conclusions. In neurology, where diagnostic and prognostic forecasts can alter life-saving judgments, physicians must view the construction of predictions. In order to explain these processes, XAI is emerging with tools to visualize these processes, such as heatmaps with images or feature attribution with prognostic models (Holzinger et al. 2019). Nevertheless, it is still difficult to have a high level of complexity and complete transparency.

20.5.2. *Ethical challenges*

20.5.2.1. *Privacy and data security*

Neurology data, which can be imaging, genomic profiles and electrophysiological records, is very sensitive. Special harm might be inflicted on patients if this information were to be disclosed. Large volumes of data are required to train AI models, and this raises concerns on the treatment of health records in terms of data storage, sharing and anonymization (Sheller et al. 2020). A potential solution is federated learning, in which the institution models are trained on the data of each institution without transferring any sensitive information to the central server. The practice of federated learning has not yet been established, despite its potential.

20.5.2.2. *Equity and access*

AI innovations in neurology are often developed in technologically advanced healthcare systems, raising questions about global equity. Low- and middle-income countries (LMICs), where neurological care is often limited, risk being excluded from the benefits of AI due to cost barriers, infrastructure deficits and a lack of digital health integration (Wahl et al. 2018). Without deliberate strategies to ensure equitable access, AI could widen the neurological care gap rather than narrow it.

20.5.2.3. *Accountability and liability*

Accountability issues are caused when AI systems affect or make clinical decisions. A diagnostic tool that implements AI can cause mismanagement by misinterpreting the information, and the responsibility may be disputed between the developers, clinicians and healthcare institutions. Legal systems will need to change to define liability in care mediation with AI. AI is supposed to be more of an aid rather than a replacement for clinicians, who should be the decision-makers.

20.5.2.4. *Trust and human–AI interaction*

The adoption of AI in neurology requires the trust of the patient and the clinician. It is likely that patients will be reluctant to accept algorithm-informed care when they perceive decisions as being impersonal or opaque. Clinicians will be opposed to AI when they perceive it as threatening their work or putting more supervision onto them. The dynamics of trust are established through open modeling, strict clinical testing and the involvement of a broad spectrum of stakeholders.

20.6. Strategic directions for the future

20.6.1. *Clinical translation and regulatory frameworks*

AI tools require rigorous evaluation in clinics to move beyond the preliminary laboratory research stages. Although the existing AI solutions excel in controlled research environments, they will have to deal with real-life clinical variety. As such, multi-hospital, premeditated, clinical trials should demonstrate that these tools are safe, effective and functional in a wide population of patients (Liu et al. 2019). The regulators, such as the FDA in the US and the European Medicines Agency (EMA) in the EU, are beginning to develop guidelines on AI that are able to learn by new data, although there is not a worldwide set of consistent standards. Achieving the development of trust between clinicians and patients requires transparent and open testing procedures, entailing explainability and requiring constant monitoring post-launch.

20.6.2. *Integration into healthcare systems*

To be of real value, AI has to be assimilated into existing clinical processes. The most common enablers are interoperation with EHRs, user-friendly interfaces for clinicians and real-time decision support systems (Jiang et al. 2017). Moreover, the reimbursement systems should be restructured to consider AI-based diagnostics and digital therapeutics as billing services. To have smooth AI implementation in neurology, hospitals and health systems will have to invest in digital infrastructure, employee training and an approach focused on multidisciplinary collaboration.

20.6.3. *Research priorities*

There are many more data types (imaging, genomics, electrophysiology, wearables, etc.) that need to be integrated into one set of the patient profile in the future (Yasmin et al. 2025). The advancements in neuroinformatics and federated learning will enable researchers to work together without sacrificing privacy. Moreover, any emphasis must be placed on the uncommon neurological conditions where the training data of AI have traditionally been lacking. Through the creation of global, inclusive data repositories, we are able to increase the accuracy of diagnosis and create equity.

20.6.4. *Global equity and access*

Neurology AI must not be yet another asset of high-resource health systems. These technologies need to be incorporated into LMICs through strategic initiatives, which have high neurologic disease burdens (Yousef and Schmollgruber 2024). Advanced diagnostic and therapeutic tools can be made accessible to additional individuals with the assistance of cloud-based AI systems, inexpensive wearable gadgets and open-source software. The way to bridge the digital gap is through international collaborations and the partnership of governments and businesses (McKinney et al. 2020).

20.7. Conclusion

Neurology will gain from AI to enhance diagnostic accuracy, augment prognosticism models and allow new interventions and rehabilitation. AI is capable of identifying trends beyond the conventional approach, customizing patient services and accelerating the decision-making process in neuroimaging, electrophysiology, digital health and drug discovery. AI leads to robotics, VR and wearables as methods of administering specific neurotherapeutics in the rehabilitation process. Treatment regimens can be altered in response to the progress of a patient. Yet challenges remain. Technical barriers such as disaggregated information, algorithm bias and uninterpretability slow down the adoption of technology in clinics. There are also the ethical concerns of privacy, responsibility, and equality, which should be addressed attentively. Neurology issues seriously affect identity and autonomy; consequently, the priority is safety, transparency and faithfulness to patients. To solve such issues, it is necessary to work with clinicians, data scientists, ethicists, regulators and patients. The next step is to focus on intensive clinical validation and the harmonization of regulatory requirements and the creation of a universal and complete data infrastructure. It is important to make AI tools available to the global community, in particular, in low- and middle-income nations where neurological pathology is prevalent and limited specialists are available.

20.8. References

Amirian, S., Gao, F., Littlefield, N., Hill, J.H., Yates, A.J., Plate, J.F., Pantanowitz, L., Rashidi, H.H., Tafti, A.P. (2025). State-of-the-art in responsible, explainable, and fair AI for medical image analysis. *IEEE Access*, 13, 58229–58263.

Arntz, A., Weber, F., Handgraaf, M., Lällä, K., Korniloff, K., Murtonen, K.P., Chichaeva, J., Kidritsch, A., Heller, M., Sakellari, E. et al. (2023). Technologies in home-based digital rehabilitation: Scoping review. *JMIR Rehabilitation and Assistive Technologies*, 10(1), e43615.

Char, D.S., Shah, N.H., Magnus, D. (2018). Implementing machine learning in health care – Addressing ethical challenges. *The New England Journal of Medicine*, 378(11), 981.

Cho, J., Lee, K., Shin, E., Choy, G., Do, S. (2015). How much data is needed to train a medical image deep learning system to achieve necessary high accuracy? arXiv preprint, arXiv:1511.06348.

Eitel, F., Soehler, E., Bellmann-Strobl, J., Brandt, A.U., Ruprecht, K., Giess, R.M., Kuchling, J., Asseyer, S., Weygandt, M., Haynes, J.D. et al. (2019). Uncovering convolutional neural network decisions for diagnosing multiple sclerosis on conventional MRI using layer-wise relevance propagation. *NeuroImage: Clinical*, 24, 102003.

Esteva, A., Robicquet, A., Ramsundar, B., Kuleshov, V., DePristo, M., Chou, K., Cui, C., Corrado, G., Thrun, S., Dean, J. (2019). A guide to deep learning in healthcare. *Nature Medicine*, 25(1), 24–29.

Feigin, V.L., Vos, T., Nichols, E., Owolabi, M.O., Carroll, W.M., Dichgans, M., Deuschl, G., Parmar, P., Brainin, M., Murray, C. (2020). The global burden of neurological disorders: Translating evidence into policy. *The Lancet Neurology*, 19(3), 255–265.

Ferrante, F.J., Escobar Grisales, D., López, M.F., Lopes da Cunha, P., Sterpin, L.F., Vonk, J.M., Chaná Cuevas, P., Estienne, C., Hesse, E., Amoruso, L. et al. (2025). Cognitive phenotyping of Parkinson's disease patients via digital analysis of spoken word properties. *Movement Disorders*, 40(11), 2354–2366.

Fraser, K.C., Meltzer, J.A., Rudzicz, F. (2015). Linguistic features identify Alzheimer's disease in narrative speech. *Journal of Alzheimer's Disease*, 49(2), 407–422.

Goudarzi, N., Taheri, Z., Nezhad Salari, A.M., Kazemzadeh, K., Tafakhori, A. (2025). Recognition and classification of facial expression using artificial intelligence as a key of early detection in neurological disorders. *Reviews in the Neurosciences*, 36(5), 479–495.

Heo, J., Yoon, J.G., Park, H., Kim, Y.D., Nam, H.S., Heo, J.H. (2019). Machine learning-based model for prediction of outcomes in acute stroke. *Stroke*, 50(5), 1263–1265.

Holzinger, A., Langs, G., Denk, H., Zatloukal, K., Müller, H. (2019). Causability and explainability of artificial intelligence in medicine. *Wiley Interdisciplinary Reviews: Data Mining and Knowledge Discovery*, 9(4), e1312.

Jiang, F., Jiang, Y., Zhi, H., Dong, Y., Li, H., Ma, S., Wang, Y., Dong, Q., Shen, H., Wang, Y. (2017). Artificial intelligence in healthcare: Past, present and future. *Stroke and Vascular Neurology*, 2(4). doi: 10.1136/svn-2017-000101.

Kumthornthip, W., Tassatarn, S., Chotiyarnwong, C. (2024). Does early rehabilitation admission improve functional outcomes of stroke patients after a short hospital stay? A Thai retrospective study on 596 patients. *Journal of the Medical Association of Thailand*, 107(12), 1013–1020.

Liu, X., Faes, L., Kale, A.U., Wagner, S.K., Fu, D.J., Bruynseels, A., Mahendiran, T., Moraes, G., Shamdas, M., Kern, C. et al. (2019). A comparison of deep learning performance against health-care professionals in detecting diseases from medical imaging: A systematic review and meta-analysis. *The Lancet Digital Health*, 1(6), e271–e297.

Luppi, A.I., Ching, S., Diringer, M.N. (2023). Please let us know how this document benefits you. *NeuroImage*, 275, 120162.

McKinney, S.M., Sieniek, M., Godbole, V., Godwin, J., Antropova, N., Ashrafian, H., Back, T., Chesus, M., Corrado, G.S., Darzi, A. et al. (2020). International evaluation of an AI system for breast cancer screening. *Nature*, 577(7788), 89–94.

Meskó, B. and Görög, M. (2020). A short guide for medical professionals in the era of artificial intelligence. *NPJ Digital Medicine*, 3(1), 126.

Roy, Y., Banville, H., Albuquerque, I., Gramfort, A., Falk, T.H., Faubert, J. (2019). Deep learning-based electroencephalography analysis: A systematic review. *Journal of Neural Engineering*, 16(5), 051001.

Sheller, M.J., Edwards, B., Reina, G.A., Martin, J., Pati, S., Kotrotsou, A., Milchenko, M., Xu, W., Marcus, D., Colen, R.R. et al. (2020). Federated learning in medicine: Facilitating multi-institutional collaborations without sharing patient data. *Scientific Reports*, 10(1), 12598.

Topol, E.J. (2019). High-performance medicine: The convergence of human and artificial intelligence. *Nature Medicine*, 25(1), 44–56.

Truong, N.D., Nguyen, A.D., Kuhlmann, L., Bonyadi, M.R., Yang, J., Ippolito, S., Kavehei, O. (2018). Convolutional neural networks for seizure prediction using intracranial and scalp electroencephalogram. *Neural Networks*, 105, 104–111.

Vamathevan, J., Clark, D., Czodrowski, P., Dunham, I., Ferran, E., Lee, G., Li, B., Madabhushi, A., Shah, P., Spitzer, M. et al. (2019). Applications of machine learning in drug discovery and development. *Nature Reviews Drug Discovery*, 18(6), 463–477.

Vanmechelen, I., Haberfehlner, H., De Vleeschhauwer, J., Van Wonterghem, E., Feys, H., Desloovere, K., Aerts, J.M., Monbaliu, E. (2023). Assessment of movement disorders using wearable sensors during upper limb tasks: A scoping review. *Frontiers in Robotics and AI*, 9, 1068413.

Voigtlaender, S., Pawelczyk, J., Geiger, M., Vaios, E.J., Karschnia, P., Cudkowicz, M., Dietrich, J., Haraldsen, I.R., Feigin, V., Owolabi, M. et al. (2024). Artificial intelligence in neurology: Opportunities, challenges, and policy implications. *Journal of Neurology*, 271(5), 2258–2273.

Wahl, B., Cossy-Gantner, A., Germann, S., Schwalbe, N.R. (2018). Artificial intelligence (AI) and global health: How can AI contribute to health in resource-poor settings? *BMJ Global Health*, 3(4), e000798.

Yao, L., Cai, M., Chen, Y., Shen, C., Shi, L., Guo, Y. (2019). Prediction of antiepileptic drug treatment outcomes of patients with newly diagnosed epilepsy by machine learning. *Epilepsy & Behavior*, 96, 92–97.

Yasmin, F., Hasan, M., Hassan, M.M., Yu, X. (2025). Neuroinformatics in the era of personalized neuroscience. In *Brain Networks in Neuroscience: Personalization Unveiled Via Artificial Intelligence*, Hassan, M.M., Yasmin, F., Islam, S.M.S., Bairagi, A.K., Aung, S.T. (eds). River Publishers, Gistrup, 285–309.

Yin, J., Ngiam, K.Y., Teo, H.H. (2021). Role of artificial intelligence applications in real-life clinical practice: Systematic review. *Journal of Medical Internet Research*, 23(4), e25759.

Yousef, K. and Schmollgruber, S. (2024). Artificial intelligence in low-and middle-income countries: Reducing the gaps in health care, research, and education. *International Journal of Critical Care*, 18(2), 1–3.

List of Authors

J.P. ANANTH
Dayananda Sagar University
Bengaluru
India

Mario ANTONY
Department of Emergency Medicine
Krishna Institute of Medical Sciences
Krishna Vishwa Vidyapeeth
"Deemed to be University"
Taluka-Karad
India

Sanjay L. BADJATE
S. B. Jain Institute of Technology
Management and Research
Nagpur
India

Shrikrishna N. BAMNE
Department of Physiology
Krishna Institute of Medical Sciences
Krishna Vishwa Vidyapeeth
"Deemed to be University"
Taluka-Karad
India

Priya BATTA
Amity School of Engineering
and Technology
Amity University Punjab
Mohali
India

Salim Allauddin CHAVAN
Govindrao Wanjari College of
Engineering and Technology
Nagpur
India

Piyush Ashokrao DALKE
Mechanical Engineering Department
Shri Sant Gajanan Maharaj College
of Engineering
Shegaon
India

Ashwini R. GARGATE
Department of Physiology
Krishna Institute of Medical Sciences
Krishna Vishwa Vidyapeeth
"Deemed to be University"
Taluka-Karad
India

K. GAVHALE
Department of Information Technology
Yeshwantrao Chavan College of Engineering
Nagpur
India

Chaitnya GODBOLE
Department of Neurosurgery
Krishna Institute of Medical Sciences
Krishna Vishwa Vidyapeeth
"Deemed to be University"
Taluka-Karad
India

Sharifnawaj Y. INAMDAR
Jaywant College of Engineering and Polytechnic
K. M. Gad
Julewadi
India

Swati JAGTAP
Department of Physiology
Krishna Institute of Medical Sciences
Krishna Vishwa Vidyapeeth
"Deemed to be University"
Taluka-Karad
India

Dipali JANKAR
Department of Physiology
Krishna Institute of Medical Sciences
Krishna Vishwa Vidyapeeth
"Deemed to be University"
Taluka-Karad
India

Komal M. JUJAR
Jaywant College of Engineering and Polytechnic
K. M. Gad
Julewadi
India

Shrikant Rangrao KADAM
Jaywant College of Engineering and Polytechnic
K. M. Gad
Julewadi
India

Amruta B. KALE
Jaywant College of Engineering and Polytechnic
K. M. Gad
Julewadi
India

Swapna KAMBLE
Department of Information Technology
Yeshwantrao Chavan College of Engineering
Nagpur
India

Sharad KSHIRSAGAR
Department of Psychiatry
Krishna Institute of Medical Sciences
Krishna Vishwa Vidyapeeth
"Deemed to be University"
Taluka-Karad
India

Omkar KULKARNI
Department of Physiology
Krishna Institute of Medical Sciences
Krishna Vishwa Vidyapeeth
"Deemed to be University"
Taluka-Karad
India

Abhishek KUMAR
Department of Computer Science and Engineering
Chandigarh University
Mohali
India

Nikhilchandra MAHAJAN
Department of Emergency Medicine
Krishna Institute of Medical Sciences
Krishna Vishwa Vidyapeeth
"Deemed to be University"
Taluka-Karad
India

Kalpana MALPE
Department of Computer Science
Suryodaya College of Engineering
and Technology
Nagpur
India

Shamla MANTRI
Department of Electronics and
Communication
MIT World Peace University
Pune
India

Mrudula NIMBARTE
CSE Department
S. B. Jain Institute of Technology,
Management and Research
Nagpur
India

Ashish N. PATIL
Jaywant College of Engineering
and Polytechnic
K. M. Gad
Julewadi
India

Rahul PATIL
Department of Medicine
Krishna Institute of Medical Sciences
Krishna Vishwa Vidyapeeth
"Deemed to be University"
Taluka-Karad
India

Shilpa C. PATIL
Department of General Medicine
Krishna Institute of Medical Sciences
Krishna Vishwa Vidyapeeth
"Deemed to be University"
Taluka-Karad
India

Atul Namdev PAWAR
Jaywant College of Engineering
and Polytechnic
K. M. Gad
Julewadi
India

G.V. RAMDAS
Department of Neurosurgery
Krishna Institute of Medical Sciences
Krishna Vishwa Vidyapeeth
"Deemed to be University"
Taluka-Karad
India

Debabrata SAHANA
Department of Neurosurgery
Krishna Institute of Medical Sciences
Krishna Vishwa Vidyapeeth
"Deemed to be University"
Taluka-Karad
India

Anil SAHU
Department of Mechanical
Engineering
G. H. Raisoni College of Engineering
and Management
Pune
India

Fazil SHEIKH
Department of Computer Science and Engineering
Yeshwantrao Chavan College of Engineering
Nagpur
India

Rahul S.S
Department of Emergency Medicine
Krishna Institute of Medical Sciences
Krishna Vishwa Vidyapeeth
"Deemed to be University"
Taluka-Karad
India

G.M. VAIDYA
Department of Computer Technology
Yeshwantrao Chavan College of Engineering
Nagpur
India

Sunil Ramrao YADAV
Department of Neurosurgery
Krishna Institute of Medical Sciences
Krishna Vishwa Vidyapeeth
"Deemed to be University"
Taluka-Karad
India

Index

A, B

C, D

E, F

G, H

I, L

M, N

P, R

S, T

V, W

Other titles from

iSTE

in

Computer Engineering

2026

BHAMBRI Pankaj, DUTTA Pushan Kumar, KHAN Mudassir, STAROSTKA-PATYK Marta
Next-Gen Supply Chains: AI, Automation, and Sustainability in a Disrupted World

DARCHE Philippe
Computer Memories 1: Core Concepts
Computer Memories 2: Static Random-Access Memory

MAHOUT Vincent, ROCACHER Thierry, AURIOL Guillaume
Programming of Embedded Systems: Applications to SM32F10x μControllers

2025

CHIKH Azeddine
Systemic Approach to Categorizing and Modeling Requirements

KUMAR Abhishek, BATTA Priya, AHUJA Sachin, RATHORE Pramod Singh
AI-driven Innovations in Physiotherapy and Oncology 1
AI-driven Innovations in Physiotherapy and Oncology 2

TANEJA Ashu, KUMAR Abhishek, LIMKAR Suresh Vishnudas, OUAISSA Mariya, OUAISSA Mariyam
Driving Innovation through AI and Digital Twin for 6G Powered Sustainable Ultra Smart Cities

TANEJA Ashu, KUMAR Abhishek, LIMKAR Suresh Vishnudas, OUAISSA Mariya, OUAISSA Mariyam
6G Urban Innovation: AI and Digital Twin for Next-Gen Sustainable Cities

2024

CHAKRABORTY Rajdeep, GHOSH Anupam, KUMAR MANDAL Jyotsna, CHOUDHURY Tanupriya, CHATTERJEE Prasenjit
Smart Edge Computing: An Operation Research Perspective
(International Perspectives in Decision Analytics and Operations Research Set – Volume 2)

HOMÈS Bernard
Fundamentals of Software Testing (2nd edition, revised and updated)

JERBI Abdessalem
Discrete-Event Simulation: Concepts and Production in Arena

PRADHAN Devasis, KUMAR SAHU Prasanna, MYO TUN Hla, CHATTERJEE Prasenjit
Artificial and Cognitive Computing for Sustainable Healthcare Systems in Smart Cities
(International Perspectives in Decision Analytics and Operations Research Set – Volume 3)

2023

CHOUDHURY Tanupriya, KHANNA Abhirup, CHATTERJEE Prasenjit, UM Jung-Sup, BHATTACHARYA Abhishek
Blockchain Applications in Healthcare: Innovations and Practices
(International Perspectives in Decision Analytics and Operations Research Set – Volume 1)

PAI G A Vijayalakshmi
A Textbook of Data Structures and Algorithms 1: Mastering Linear Data Structures
A Textbook of Data Structures and Algorithms 2: Mastering Nonlinear Data Structures
A Textbook of Data Structures and Algorithms 3: Mastering Advanced Data Structures and Algorithm Design Strategies

2022

HOMÈS Bernard
Advanced Testing of Systems-of-Systems 1: Theoretical Aspects
Advanced Testing of Systems-of-Systems 2: Practical Aspects

MEHTA Shikha, TIWARI Sanju, SIARRY Patrick, JABBAR M.A.
Tools, Languages, Methodologies for Representing Semantics on the Web of Things

SIDHOM Sahbi, KADDOUR Amira
Systems and Uses of Digital Sciences for Knowledge Organization (Digital Tools and Uses Set – Volume 9)

ZAIDOUN Ameur Salem
Computer Science Security: Concepts and Tools

2021

DARCHE Philippe
Microprocessor 4: Core Concepts – Software Aspects
Microprocessor 5: Software and Hardware Aspects of Development, Debugging and Testing – The Microcomputer

DELHAYE Jean-Loïc
Inside the World of Computing: Technologies, Uses, Challenges

HARDIN Thérèse, JAUME Mathieu, PESSAUX François,
VIGUIÉ DONZEAU-GOUGE Véronique
Concepts and Semantics of Programming Languages 1: A Semantical Approach with OCaml and Python
Concepts and Semantics of Programming Languages 2: Modular and Object-oriented Constructs with OCaml, Python, C++, Ada and Java

MKADMI Abderrazak
Archives in The Digital Age: Preservation and the Right to be Forgotten (Digital Tools and Uses Set – Volume 8)

TOKLU Yusuf Cengiz, BEKDAŞ Gebrail, NIGDELI Sinan Melih
Metaheuristics for Structural Design and Analysis
(Optimization Heuristics Set – Volume 3)

2020

DARCHE Philippe
Microprocessor 1: Prolegomenes – Calculation and Storage Functions – Models of Computation and Computer Architecture
Microprocessor 2: Core Concepts – Communication in a Digital System
Microprocessor 3: Core Concepts – Hardware Aspects

DUVAUT Patrick, DALLOZ Xavier, MENGA David, KOEHL François,
CHRIQUI Vidal, BRILL Joerg
Internet of Augmented Me, I.AM: Empowering Innovation for a New Sustainable Future

LAFFLY Dominique
TORUS 1 – Toward an Open Resource Using Services: Cloud Computing for Environmental Data
TORUS 2 – Toward an Open Resource Using Services: Cloud Computing for Environmental Data
TORUS 3 – Toward an Open Resource Using Services: Cloud Computing for Environmental Data

LAURENT Anne, LAURENT Dominique, MADERA Cédrine
Data Lakes
(Databases and Big Data Set – Volume 2)

OULHADJ Hamouche, DAACHI Boubaker, MENASRI Riad
Metaheuristics for Robotics
(Optimization Heuristics Set – Volume 2)

SADIQUI Ali
Computer Network Security

VENTRE Daniel
Artificial Intelligence, Cybersecurity and Cyber Defense

2019

BESBES Walid, DHOUIB Diala, WASSAN Niaz, MARREKCHI Emna
Solving Transport Problems: Towards Green Logistics

CLERC Maurice
Iterative Optimizers: Difficulty Measures and Benchmarks

GHLALA Riadh
Analytic SQL in SQL Server 2014/2016

TOUNSI Wiem
Cyber-Vigilance and Digital Trust: Cyber Security in the Era of Cloud Computing and IoT

2018

ANDRO Mathieu
Digital Libraries and Crowdsourcing
(Digital Tools and Uses Set – Volume 5)

ARNALDI Bruno, GUITTON Pascal, MOREAU Guillaume
Virtual Reality and Augmented Reality: Myths and Realities

CARDON Alain
Beyond Artificial Intelligence: From Human Consciousness to Artificial Consciousness

HOMAYOUNI S. Mahdi, FONTES Dalila B.M.M.
Metaheuristics for Maritime Operations
(Optimization Heuristics Set – Volume 1)

JEANSOULIN Robert
JavaScript and Open Data

PIVERT Olivier
NoSQL Data Models: Trends and Challenges
(Databases and Big Data Set – Volume 1)

SEDKAOUI Soraya
Data Analytics and Big Data

SALEH Imad, AMMI Mehdi, SZONIECKY Samuel
Challenges of the Internet of Things: Technology, Use, Ethics
(Digital Tools and Uses Set – Volume 7)

SZONIECKY Samuel
Ecosystems Knowledge: Modeling and Analysis Method for Information and Communication
(Digital Tools and Uses Set – Volume 6)

2017

BENMAMMAR Badr
Concurrent, Real-Time and Distributed Programming in Java: Threads, RTSJ and RMI

BOUHAÏ Nasreddine, SALEH Imad
Internet of Things: Evolutions and Innovations
(Digital Tools and Uses Set – Volume 4)

HÉLIODORE Frédéric, NAKIB Amir, ISMAIL Boussaad, OUCHRAA Salma, SCHMITT Laurent
Metaheuristics for Intelligent Electrical Networks
(Metaheuristics Set – Volume 10)

MA Haiping, SIMON Dan
Evolutionary Computation with Biogeography-based Optimization
(Metaheuristics Set – Volume 8)

PÉTROWSKI Alain, BEN-HAMIDA Sana
Evolutionary Algorithms
(Metaheuristics Set – Volume 9)

PAI G A Vijayalakshmi
Metaheuristics for Portfolio Optimization: An Introduction using MATLAB®
(Metaheuristics Set – Volume 11)

REYES-GARCIA Everardo
The Image-Interface: Graphical Supports for Visual Information
(Digital Tools and Uses Set – Volume 3)

REYES-GARCIA Everardo, BOUHAÏ Nasreddine
Designing Interactive Hypermedia Systems
(Digital Tools and Uses Set – Volume 2)

SZONIECKY Samuel, BOUHAÏ Nasreddine
Collective Intelligence and Digital Archives: Towards Knowledge Ecosystems
(Digital Tools and Uses Set – Volume 1)

2016

BLUM Christian, FESTA Paola
Metaheuristics for String Problems in Bio-informatics
(Metaheuristics Set – Volume 6)

DEROUSSI Laurent
Metaheuristics for Logistics
(Metaheuristics Set – Volume 4)

DHAENENS Clarisse, JOURDAN Laetitia
Metaheuristics for Big Data
(Metaheuristics Set – Volume 5)

LABADIE Nacima, PRINS Christian, PRODHON Caroline
Metaheuristics for Vehicle Routing Problems
(Metaheuristics Set – Volume 3)

LEROY Laure
Eyestrain Reduction in Stereoscopy

LUTTON Evelyne, PERROT Nathalie, TONDA Alberto
Evolutionary Algorithms for Food Science and Technology
(Metaheuristics Set – Volume 7)

MAGOULÈS Frédéric, ZHAO Hai-Xiang
Data Mining and Machine Learning in Building Energy Analysis

RIGO Michel
Advanced Graph Theory and Combinatorics

ZELM Martin, DOUMEINGTS Guy, MENDONÇA Joao Pedro
Enterprise Interoperability: in the Digitized and Networked Factory of the Future

2015

BARBIER Franck, RECOUSSINE Jean-Luc
COBOL Software Modernization: From Principles to Implementation with the BLU AGE® Method

CHEN Ken
Performance Evaluation by Simulation and Analysis with Applications to Computer Networks

CLERC Maurice
Guided Randomness in Optimization
(Metaheuristics Set – Volume 1)

DURAND Nicolas, GIANAZZA David, GOTTELAND Jean-Baptiste, ALLIOT Jean-Marc
Metaheuristics for Air Traffic Management
(Metaheuristics Set – Volume 2)

MAGOULÈS Frédéric, ROUX François-Xavier, HOUZEAUX Guillaume
Parallel Scientific Computing

MUNEESAWANG Paisarn, YAMMEN Suchart
Visual Inspection Technology in the Hard Disk Drive Industry

2014

BOULANGER Jean-Louis
Formal Methods Applied to Industrial Complex Systems
Formal Methods Applied to Complex Systems: Implementation of the B Method

EXPOSITO Ernesto, DIOP Codé
Smart SOA Platforms in Cloud Computing Architectures

GARDI Frédéric, BENOIST Thierry, DARLAY Julien, ESTELLON Bertrand, MEGEL Romain
Mathematical Programming Solver based on Local Search

KRICHEN Saoussen, CHAOUACHI Jouhaina
Graph-related Optimization and Decision Support Systems

LARRIEU Nicolas, VARET Antoine
Rapid Prototyping of Software for Avionics Systems: Model-oriented Approaches for Complex Systems Certification

LAURAS Matthieu, ZELM Martin, ARCHIMÈDE Bernard, BÉNABEN Frédérick, DOUMEINGTS Guy
Enterprise Interoperability: Interoperability for Agility, Resilience and Plasticity of Collaborations

OUSSALAH Mourad Chabane
Software Architecture 1
Software Architecture 2

QUESNEL Flavien
Scheduling of Large-scale Virtualized Infrastructures: Toward Cooperative Management

RIGO Michel
Formal Languages, Automata and Numeration Systems 1: Introduction to Combinatorics on Words
Formal Languages, Automata and Numeration Systems 2: Applications to Recognizability and Decidability

SAINT-DIZIER Patrick
Musical Rhetoric: Foundations and Annotation Schemes

TOUATI Sid, DUPONT DE DINECHIN Benoit
Advanced Backend Code Optimization

2013

ANDRÉ Étienne, SOULAT Romain
The Inverse Method: Parametric Verification of Real-time Embedded Systems

BOULANGER Jean-Louis
Safety Management for Software-based Equipment

DELAHAYE Daniel, PUECHMOREL Stéphane
Modeling and Optimization of Air Traffic

FRANCOPOULO Gil
LMF — Lexical Markup Framework

GHEDIRA Khaled
Constraint Satisfaction Problems: CSP Formalisms and Techniques

GOVAERT Gérard, NADIF Mohamed
Co-Clustering: Models, Algorithms and Applications

LANDRAGIN Frédérick
Man–Machine Dialogue: Design and Challenges

LUCAS Laurent, LOSCOS Céline, REMION Yannick
3D Video: Models, From Capture to Diffusion

ROCHANGE Christine, UHRIG Sascha, SAINRAT Pascal
Time-Predictable Architectures

WAHBI Mohamed
Algorithms and Ordering Heuristics for Distributed Constraint Satisfaction Problems

ZELM Martin, VAN SINDEREN Marten, FERRAIRA PIRES Luis, DOUMEINGTS Guy
Enterprise Interoperability: Research and Applications in the Service-oriented Ecosystem

2012

ARBOLEDA Hugo, ROYER Jean-Claude
Model-Driven and Software Product Line Engineering

BLANCHET Gérard, DUPOUY Bertrand
Computer Architecture

BOULANGER Jean-Louis
Industrial Use of Formal Methods: Formal Verification
Formal Methods: Industrial Use from Model to the Code

CALVARY Gaëlle, DELOT Thierry, SÈDES Florence, TIGLI Jean-Yves
Computer Science and Ambient Intelligence

MAHOUT Vincent
Assembly Language Programming: ARM Cortex-M3 2.0: Organization, Innovation and Territory

MARLET Renaud
Program Specialization

SOTO Maria, SEVAUX Marc, ROSSI André, LAURENT Johann
Memory Allocation Problems in Embedded Systems: Optimization Methods

2011

BICHOT Charles-Edmond, SIARRY Patrick
Graph Partitioning

BOULANGER Jean-Louis
Static Analysis of Software: The Abstract Interpretation

CAFERRA Ricardo
Logic for Computer Science and Artificial Intelligence

KORDON Fabrice, HADDAD Serge, PAUTET Laurent, PETRUCCI Laure
Distributed Systems: Design and Algorithms
Models and Analysis in Distributed Systems

LORCA Xavier
Tree-based Graph Partitioning Constraint

RIDHA MAHJOUB A.
Progress in Combinatorial Optimization: ISCO2010

TRUCHET Charlotte, ASSAYAG Gerard
Constraint Programming in Music

VICAT-BLANC Pascale, GOGLIN Brice, GUILLIER Romaric, SOUDAN Sébastien
Computing Networks: From Cluster to Cloud Computing

2010

AUBRUN Christophe, SIMON Daniel, SONG Ye-Qiong
Co-design Approaches for Dependable Networked Control Systems

AUDIBERT Pierre
Mathematics for Informatics and Computer Science

BABAU Jean-Philippe, BLAY-FORNARINO Mireille, CHAMPEAU Joël, ROBERT Sylvain, SABETTA Antonino
Model Driven Engineering for Distributed Real-Time Systems: MARTE Modeling, Model Transformations and their Usages

BOULANGER Jean-Louis
Safety of Computer Architectures

SIGAUD Olivier, BUFFET Olivier
Markov Decision Processes in Artificial Intelligence

MONMARCHÉ Nicolas, GUINAND Frédérick, SIARRY Patrick
Artificial Ants

SOLNON Christine
Ant Colony Optimization and Constraint Programming

2009

FOURNIER Jean-Claude
Graph Theory and Applications: with exercises and problems

GUÉDON Jeanpierre
The Mojette Transform: theory and applications

JARD Claude, ROUX Olivier H.
Communicating Embedded Systems: Software and Design

LECOUTRE Christophe
Constraint Networks: Techniques and Algorithms

2008

BANÂTRE Michel, MARRON Pedro Jose, OLLERO Anibal, WOLITZ Adam
Cooperating Embedded Systems and Wireless Sensor Networks

MERZ Stephan, NAVET Nicolas
Modeling and Verification of Real-time Systems: Formalisms and Software Tools

PASCHOS Vangelis Th.
Combinatorial Optimization and Theoretical Computer Science: Interfaces and Perspectives

WALDNER Jean-Baptiste
Nanocomputers and Swarm Intelligence

2007

BENHAMOU Frédéric, JUSSIEN Narendra, O'SULLIVAN Barry
Trends in Constraint Programming

JUSSIEN Narendra
A to Z of Sudoku

2006

BABAU Jean-Philippe, CHAMPEAU Joël, GÉRARD Sébastien
From MDD Concepts to Experiments and Illustrations – DRES 2006

HABRIAS Henri, FRAPPIER Marc
Software Specification Methods: An Overview Using a Case Study

MURAT Cécile, PASCHOS Vangelis Th.
Probabilistic Combinatorial Optimization on Graphs

PANETTO Hervé, BOUDJLIDA Nacer
Interoperability for Enterprise Software and Applications: Proceedings of the Workshops and the Doctorial Symposium of the Second IFAC/IFIP I-ESA International Conference: EI2N, WSI, IS-TSPQ 2006

2005

GÉRARD Sébastien, BABAU Jean-Philippe, CHAMPEAU Joël
Model Driven Engineering for Distributed Real Time Embedded Systems

PANETTO Hervé
Interoperability of Enterprise Software and Applications: Workshops of the INTEROP-ESA 2005 International Conference (EI2N, WSI, ISIDI and IEHENA 2005)